ANTIVIRALS AGAINST AIDS

ANTIVIRALS AGAINST AIDS

edited by

Ronald E. Unger

Johannes Gutenberg-Universität Mainz Medical Center
Mainz, Germany

Jörg Kreuter

Johann Wolfgang Goethe-Universität
Frankfurt am Main, Germany

Helga Rübsamen-Waigmann

Bayer AG
Wuppertal, Germany

MARCEL DEKKER, INC.   NEW YORK · BASEL

Library of Congress Cataloging-in-Publication Data

Antivirals against aids / Ronald E. Unger, Jörg Kreuter, Helga Rübsamen-Waigmann.
    p. cm.
    Includes index.
    ISBN 0-8427-0358-8 (alk. paper)
    1. AIDS (Disease)—Chemotherapy. 2. Antiviral agents. I. Unger, Ronald E. II.
Kreuter, Jörg III. Rübsamen-Waigmann, Helga

    RC607.A26 A547 2000
    616.97'92061—dc21   00-031590

This book is printed on acid-free paper.

Headquarters
Marcel Dekker, Inc.
270 Madison Avenue, New York, NY 10016
tel: 212-696-9000; fax: 212-685-4540

Eastern Hemisphere Distribution
Marcel Dekker AG
Hutgasse 4, Postfach 812, CH-4001 Basel, Switzerland
tel: 41-61-261-8482; fax: 41-61-261-8896

World Wide Web
http://www.dekker.com

The publisher offers discounts on this book when ordered in bulk quantities. For more information, write to Special Sales/Professional Marketing at the headquarters address above.

Current printing (last digit):
10 9 8 7 6 5 4 3 2 1

PRINTED IN THE UNITED STATES OF AMERICA

Preface

Acquired immunodeficiency syndrome (AIDS) is the first human retroviral disease with a worldwide epidemiological impact. A disease transmitted primarily by sexual contact, AIDS was first observed in 1980 in the United States but has since spread rapidly throughout the world. Acquired immunodeficiency syndrome is a result of infection by either of two types of related human immunodeficiency viruses—HIV-1 or HIV-2—and eventually leads to the death of the infected individual. After the discovery of these two viruses as the cause of AIDS, it was hoped and believed that a cure would soon be found. Because of its viral etiology, it was thought that AIDS could soon be prevented by the use of a vaccine. However, because of the high genetic variability of HIV and the ability of the retrovirus to integrate into the genome of cells belonging to the immune system and to either go dormant or destroy these cells, these early expectations were not met.

Although significant advances have been made in the battle against AIDS, a cure has not been found. An enormous research effort is in progress to find ways to prevent the spread of the virus, to efficiently treat the infection, to cure patients of the virus, and, ultimately, to defeat the disease.

The aim of this book is to provide the layman, the medical practitioner, and the medical researcher with an overview and summary of current therapies and their benefits and shortcomings. In addition, the book presents next-generation therapies as well as alternative approaches such as gene therapy and nanoparticle technology to combat HIV. This combined information in one volume should be a valuable asset to researchers in the field and will hopefully stimulate innovative ideas and foster new collaborations that will lead to successful antiviral therapies and to eventual victory over HIV.

Ronald E. Unger
Jörg Kreuter
Helga Rübsamen-Waigmann

Introduction

After major victories were won in controlling and nearly eradicating many of the classic infectious diseases such as syphilis, smallpox, diphtheria, and cholera in the 1960s and 1970s, the developed world became complacent with respect to these killers of the past. Onto this scene emerged AIDS, or the acquired immunodeficiency syndrome. The agent responsible for AIDS, the human immunodeficiency virus (HIV), is an old virus of African origin. First observed in the United States, it has since spread throughout the world. Although it is not highly communicable (the transmission of the virus is primarily limited to intimate sexual contact, blood exchange, or from mother to child), its rapid worldwide dissemination was brought about by modern mass tourism. Little may change in the infected individual for a number of years, but eventually infection leads to the destruction of the cellular immune response, to the development of AIDS, and ultimately to the death of the individual.

Campaigns to prevent the spread of HIV have reduced the exponential growth of new infections observed at the beginning of the epidemic to a current rate of a roughly 5% increase in new infections per year in the developed world. However, in many developing countries, infection rates are increasing exponentially, despite many efforts to educate and assist populations in adopting a safer lifestyle. Thus, we are witnessing only the beginning of a catastrophe that will take a great toll on families and social structures, that will place a tremendous financial burden on governments, especially those of Third World countries, and that will extend well into the future.

Like no other disease before it, AIDS has initiated an unprecedented scientific effort to find the agent causing the disease, to determine its mode of transmission, and to develop therapies and vaccines against it. After the pioneering work by Francoise Barré-Sinoussi, Jean-Claude Chermann, and Luc Montagnier, who first isolated the virus, the possibility of generating a vaccine seemed within reach. However, researchers, including ourselves, who isolated additional viruses from infected individuals soon discovered that HIV is not a single virus. Each new isolate has its own characteristics and, with time, a continuous evolution takes place in infected individuals, resulting in a pool of closely related yet genotypically slightly different viruses or quasispecies. Thus, the longer the virus resides in a particular area of the world, the broader its genetic diversity becomes. In addition, soon after the first type of HIV was isolated, a related virus was discovered in West Africa. Currently, two large families of this lentivirus are known—HIV-1 and HIV-2—and although these viruses share similar genome structures, cell tropisms, and pathogenic outcomes resulting in AIDS, they exhibit extensive genetic diversity.

The genetic variability of the HIV isolated from individuals in different parts of the world has led to the additional classification of HIV-1 and HIV-2 into different subgroups. In the past, the subgroup B of HIV-1 was the most prevalent virus subgroup observed in the developed world. In recent years, however, infections with an increasing number of other subgroups of HIV-1 have been identified. These subgroups were not recognized early on, because testing for HIV in other parts of the world was not as prevalent as in North America and Europe and because these other subgroups had their primary transmission outside of these two regions. Furthermore, as time progressed and the population exposed to HIV increased, so did the spread of different viral subgroups. For example, while HIV-2 at first did not spread considerably outside of Africa, it reached India together with HIV-1 at the beginning of the 1990s. An additional difficulty in the classification of HIV into subgroups is the increased occurrence of recombination between different subgroups of HIV-1 and HIV-2. All these factors add further to the genetic diversity of the AIDS viruses.

The primary goal of this book is to present the current state of antiviral therapy, an area in which significant progress has been made in recent years. Suppression of viral replication by drugs has resulted in a clear clinical benefit for patients. However, despite this success, antiviral drug therapy and vaccine development still wrestle with the ability of HIV to generate variants. Rapid generation of such resistant viruses requires the use of combinations of drugs and leads to cumbersome drug regimens that are difficult for patients to adhere to. Recent drug developments have aimed at combining more than one drug compound in a single pill and at finding drugs of the second or third generation with pharmacokinetic parameters allowing a once-daily application. While this accomplishment will make following pill-taking regimens easier for the patients, it will not solve the problem of viral resistance. Increasing resistance against the drugs of the present classes makes absolutely necessary the development of new drug classes with novel mechanisms of action, as well as the use of new therapeutic strategies and approaches such as gene therapy.

This book describes current approaches to anti-HIV therapy as well as the various targets of novel antiviral strategies against AIDS. Attempts at antiretroviral treatment in the HIV-infected individual are presented as are problems encountered with resistance. Discussions include second- and third-generation approaches to anti-HIV therapies targeting the HIV reverse-transcriptase and protease proteins. Furthermore, the book examines the potential for targeting HIV receptors for entry into cells as a means of inhibiting the spread of HIV and uses of unique delivery systems to facilitate the uptake of drugs into specific cells as alternative methods to inhibit viral replication. Finally, the use and suitability of animal model systems for studying and evaluating the performance of these drugs are discussed.

To date, all efforts to develop a vaccine to safely protect humans from HIV infection have failed. This is due primarily to the enormous evolutionary potential and immune-evasive mechanisms of the AIDS viruses. New technologies and approaches are being intensively studied, but the hope for developing a safe and effective vaccine in the near future is slim. Nonetheless, the only chance for controlling the continued spread of HIV and for preventing a worldwide epidemic lies in the development of an inexpensive vaccine. One important chapter of this book is, therefore, devoted to vaccines against HIV.

Much has been achieved in the years since the virus was first discovered but much still needs to be done. Apart from coping with the constant evolution of virus variants that are resistant to current therapies, a major challenge is to develop therapeutic strategies and vaccines that arc financially affordable in those countries where they are needed most.

In this volume, we bring together the current approaches to AIDS treatment and the novel approaches to anti-HIV therapy in development. We hope that this information will be educational to the layman and stimulating to the researcher, and will contribute to new and creative research projects that will culminate in the development of an effective therapy against HIV and a worldwide eradication of AIDS.

Contents

Contributors

Erik De Clercq, M.D., Ph.D. Professor, Rega Institute for Medical Research, Leuven, Belgium

Ursula Dietrich, Ph.D. Molecular Virology, Georg-Speyer-Haus, Frankfurt am Main, Germany

Patricia E. Fast, M.D., Ph.D. Clinical Research, Aviron, Mountain View, California

Manuel Grez, Ph.D. Group Leader, Georg-Speyer-Haus, Frankfurt am Main, Germany

Dieter Hoelzer, M.D., Ph.D. Medizinische Klinik III, Johann Wolfgang Goethe-Universität, Frankfurt am Main, Germany

Andreas Immelmann, Ph.D. Managing Director, Analysis GmbH, Frankfurt, Germany

Hans Jäger, M.D. KIS–Curatorium for Immunodeficiency, Munich, Germany

Christian Klebba, Dipl.chem. Department of Hematology, Medizinische Klinik III, Johann Wolfgang Goethe-Universität, Frankfurt am Main, Germany

Stefan A. Klein, M.D. Medizinische Klinik III, Johann Wolfgang Goethe-Universität, Frankfurt am Main, Germany

Jörg Kreuter, Ph.D.   Professor and Director, Institute for Pharmaceutical Technology, Biozentrum-Niederursel, Johann Wolfgang Goethe-Universität, Frankfurt am Main, Germany

Marta L. Marthas, Ph.D.   Associate Research Professor, California Regional Primate Research Center, University of California, Davis, California

Stefan Mauss, M.D.   HIV-Specialized Practice, Düsseldorf, Germany

Amanda E. I. Proudfoot, Ph.D.   Senior Scientist, Serono Pharmaceutical Research Institute S.A., Geneva, Switzerland

Peter Ramge   Georg-Speyer-Haus, Frankfurt am Main, Germany

Sally Redshaw, Ph.D.   Roche Discovery Welwyn, Welwyn Garden City, Hertfordshire, England

Helga Rübsamen-Waigmann, Ph.D.   Director of Virus Research, Bayer AG, Wuppertal, and Professor of Biochemistry and Virology, University of Frankfurt, Frankfurt, Germany

Alan M. Schultz, Ph.D.   International AIDS Vaccine Initiative, New York, New York

Gareth J. Thomas, Ph.D.   Roche Discovery Welwyn, Welwyn Garden City, Hertfordshire, England

Alexandra Trkola, Ph.D.   Department of Internal Medicine, University Hospital Zurich, Zurich, Switzerland

Ronald E. Unger, Ph.D.   Department of Pathology, Johannes Gutenberg-Universität Mainz Medical Center, Mainz, Germany

Koen K. A. Van Rompay, D.V.M., Ph.D.   Assistant Research Virologist, California Regional Primate Research Center, University of California, Davis, California

Hagen von Briesen, Ph.D.   Head of Department, Virology/Cell Biology, Georg-Speyer-Haus, Frankfurt am Main, Germany

Timothy N. C. Wells, Ph.D.   Director, Serono Pharmaceutical Research Institute, S. A., Geneva, Switzerland

ANTIVIRALS AGAINST AIDS

1

The Retrovirus Family and the Human Immunodeficiency Virus

Molecular Targets for Therapy and Existing Drugs

Helga Rübsamen-Waigmann
Bayer AG, Wuppertal, and University of Frankfurt, Frankfurt, Germany

I. INTRODUCTION

The retroviruses comprise a large family of viruses, primarily of vertebrates, but they are also found in insects and molluscs. Their genomes of 7–12 Kb contain RNA and are reverse transcribed into DNA during replication. The DNA is subsequently integrated into the genome of the host cell to form the provirus state. As a result of proviral integration, retroviruses cause persistent, lifelong infections.

This family of viruses is associated with a variety of diseases, such as rapidly or slowly developing malignancies, wasting syndromes, neurological disorders, and immunodeficiencies. However, retroviral infection can also lead to lifelong viremia without disease. In addition, retroviruses or parts thereof are found as endogenous genetic elements in humans and other species.

In the 1970s, retroviruses were used to study malignant transformation of cells. This led to the discovery of dominant genes that cause cancer (oncogenes). The first biochemical function of a viral oncogene was found for v-*src*, when Collett and Erikson demonstrated that it was a protein kinase (1). It was then shown that viral mutants, which were temperature sensitive for transformation had a temperature-sensitive v-*src* kinase (2). This among other studies demonstrated that the kinase activity of *src* was essential for its transforming function. A large enzyme family of tyrosine kinases has subsequently been discovered in transforming viruses as well as in normal cells (3). For the viral *src* gene as for most of the other viral oncogenes it has become clear that these genes are related to endogenous human genes of various biochemical classes (called c-*onc* for cellular oncogene), which regulate growth and differentiation. Thus, also in spontaneous tumors of nonviral origin, aberrant forms of these c-*onc* genes have been discovered. Viral oncogenes owe their transforming function either to the acquisition of functional changes compared to their endogenous cellular counterparts or by higher, unregulated levels of the respective oncoprotein.

Another mechanism of cellular transformation by retroviruses is mutagenesis of genes, whose function is to ensure proper DNA replication and cell division. Oncogenic DNA viruses have been found to inactivate tumor suppressor proteins by various mechanisms.

Until the 1980s, retroviruses were thought to be interesting model viruses to study cancer in animals, but they were not considered to be important pathogens for humans. The discovery of the human T- cell leukemia virus (HTLV) in 1980– 1982 (4,5) and later that of the virus causing acquired immunodeficiency syndrome (AIDS)—the human immunodeficiency virus (HIV)—in 1983 (6) has since generated enormous scientific interest in this class of viruses. Retroviruses have evolved over prolonged periods of time with their hosts and, among primate lentiviruses, several transfers between humans and monkeys have occurred over the course of this evolution as have recombinations among related retroviruses (7,8,22,44).

Recently, a retrovirus has been described that has been repeatedly isolated from patients with multiple sclerosis and that has homology to an endogenous human retrovirus, ERV 9 (9). Although its role as etiological agent in this disease remains to be proven, it is likely that an involvement of further retroviruses in human disease will be discovered.

In addition to being studied for their important pathogenic and evolutionary role, derivatives of retroviruses are being intensively studied as tools for gene transfer (10). Because they integrate in their proviral form into the genome of their host cells, retroviruses enable a permanent gene transfer into the target cells and have meanwhile been used as vectors in a variety of gene therapy studies.

Despite the variety of host species and disease manifestations, retroviruses are all similar in their structure and genome organization. The virions are enveloped, are approximately 80 to 100 nm in diameter, and bud from the plasma membrane of the cell. A specific viral enzyme, the reverse transcriptase, which transcribes the viral RNA into DNA, has given the name to this family of viruses. However, reverse transcription is also found in other viruses (e.g., hepatitis B virus) and in cellular transposons and, thus, is not an exclusive property of retroviruses.

II. CLASSIFICATION

Retroviruses are classified into six distinct groups according to the genetic relationship of their reverse transcriptase genes (11,12) (Table 1).The spumaviruses, which had been considered to belong to the retrovirus family, have recently been found to contain DNA, not RNA, as genetic material in the virion (13) and to share several properties with the hepadna viruses (e.g., hepatitis B). These viruses also reverse-transcribe their RNA within the cell and are released as DNA-containing particles. However, in terms of morphology, spumaviruses fit well into the family of retroviruses.

In addition to being classified according to sequence homology, retroviruses are also classified according to the shape of their virions (types A–D, Fig. 1). A-particles were first viewed as immature intracellular forms of the murine mammary tumor virus (MMTV) and the term still denotes strictly intracellular structures, comprising fully formed immature cores of B-type viruses and D-type viruses. Virtually indistinguishable particles are also found in uninfected cell lines derived from a number of rodent species and are products of a high number of endogenous provirus-like particles.

B-particles are the enveloped, extracellular form of MMTV, characterized by an acentric nucleocapsid and prominent surface spikes, formed by the viral envelope (env) proteins.

C-particles are formed by most of the avian and mammalian viruses studied to date. Here, complete intracellular forms are rarely seen, but crescent-shaped budding structures form at the cell membrane. As with B-particles, freshly budded forms have hollow nucleocapsids and need to mature to yield a central, spherical electron-dense structure. In contrast to B-type particles, C-type particles have barely visible surface projections.

D-particles resemble B-types, having a complete intracellular nucleocapsid and an acentric core, but less prominent surface projections.

Bovine leukemia (BLV) virus and HTLV resemble C-type viruses in their mode of budding, but differ in the appearance of their envelope.

Table 1 Classification of Retroviruses

Genus	Example	Genome
1. Avian sarcoma and leukosis viral group	Rous sarcoma virus	Simple
2. Mammalian B-type viral group	Mouse mammary tumor virus	Simple
3. Murine leukemia-related viral group	Moloney murine leukemia virus	Simple
4. Human T-cell leukemia–bovine leukemia viral group	Human T-cell leukemia virus	Complex
5. D-type viral group	Mason-Pfizer monkey virus	Simple
6. Lentiviruses	Human immunodeficiency virus	Complex
7. Spumaviruses[a]	Foamy virus	Complex

[a]Reclassification pending.

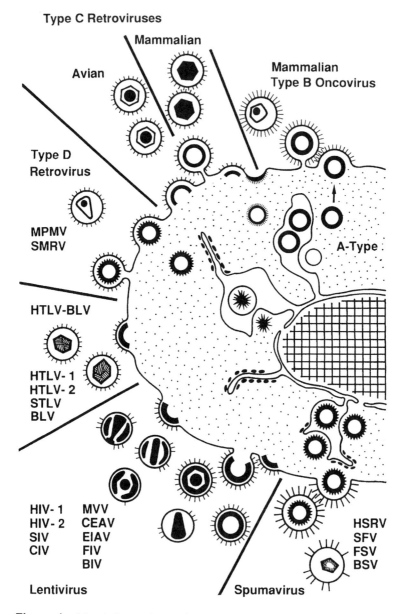

Figure 1   Morphology of retroviruses. (From Hans R. Gelderblom. J AIDS 1991; 5:617–638, with permission of the author and the publisher.)

Lentiviruses, including the human immunodeficiency virus HIV, the caprine encephalitis-arthritis virus CEAV, the equine infectious anemia virus EIAV, the maedi visna virus of sheep (MMV), and the feline immunodeficiency virus (FIV), as well as the bovine immunodeficiency virus BIV also bud like C-type viruses, but the mature virion has a cone-shaped nucleocapsid.

Spumaviruses behave similarly to B-type viruses and preform their nucleo-capsid within the cell, which is condensed to the mature form after release of the virion.

III. GENOME ORGANIZATION

The genome of retroviruses varies between 7000 and 12,300 nucleotides and is unique among viruses in its physical organization, its mode of synthesis, and its way of replication. It is the only diploid virus genome (the two identical RNA molecules are linked at the 5′ end). It is the only viral genome synthesized and processed by the cellular RNA handling machinery with an associated t-RNA to prime replication, and a plus-stranded RNA genome, which does not serve as mRNA upon uncoating in the cell. Genomic retroviral RNA contains a cap and a poly-A sequence. As shown in Figure 2a, the RNA genome is reverse transcribed to form the DNA provirus, which, in turn, serves as template for transcription to RNA by cellular enzymes.

A number of genetic elements are conserved among retroviruses (see Fig. 2). R denotes a terminal redundancy of 20 to 230 bp, which allows the transfer of one nascent DNA during replication from one end of the genome to the other end. U5 contains unique information near the 5′ end and varies between 70 and 240 bp. Some U5 regions are essential for initiation of reverse transcription (14–16). PB is the primer-binding region and is usually 18 bp in length, with complementary bases to the respective t-RNA. The U3 region (190–1200 bp) forms the 5′ portion of the long terminal repeat (LTR) generated at both ends of the DNA provirus after completion of the reverse transcription and contains a number of *cis*-acting signals regulating virus replication.

Figure 2b shows the genomic structures of the major groups of retroviruses with the open reading frames relative to the proviral structure. The first gene 5′ is the *gag* gene in all cases. It yields a precursor protein that is subsequently cleaved into 3 to 5 capsid proteins. The cleavage is a prerequisite for the formation of mature, infectious virions. The three invariant proteins are the matrix protein (MA), the capsid protein (CA), and the nucleic acid binding protein (NC). The pro region encodes the protease (PR), which is necessary for the cleavage of the aforementioned Gag-precursor to generate infectious virus. The *pol* gene encodes two proteins, the reverse transcriptase (RT) and the integrase (IN). Whereas the reverse transcriptase generates a DNA copy of the viral RNA genome upon infection of a

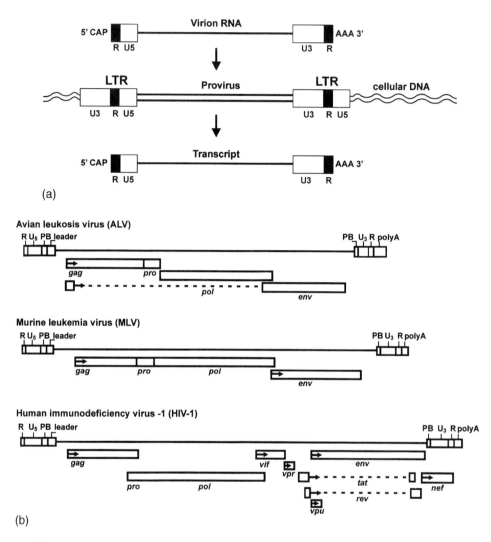

Figure 2 (a) Comparison of the RNA and the DNA forms of the viral genome. Reverse transcription of the RNA genome generates identical structures referred to as long terminal repeats (LTRs) found at both ends of the DNA provirus. Transcription of the provirus between the upstream U3 and downstream U5 regions generates RNA with the same terminal organization as in the parental virus. (R) Terminal direct repeat RNA; (U5) unique regulatory sequences at the 5′ end; (U3) unique regulatory sequences at the 3′ end. (b) Coding regions and regulatory elements of selected retrovirus genomes. Note:The size relations do not represent actual sizes.

cell, the integrase is needed to integrate this copy into the cellular genome to give the proviral state. The *env* gene encodes the two envelope proteins, which are also generated from a large precursor.

In contrast to the first two retrovirus groups in Figure 2b, the human viruses—HTLV and HIV—and the respective animal viruses, contain additional auxiliary genes. The HTLV has two regulatory genes, the transactivator *tax* and the gene *rex*, which is necessary for the expression of structural proteins and partially overlaps *tax* in an alternative reading frame. The HIV, in contrast, contains six auxiliary genes: *tat*, the analogue to *tax*, *vif*, *vpr*, *vpu*, *rev*, and *nef* (see Fig. 2b).

Theoretically, all of the virus-specific structural proteins, enzymes, regulatory proteins, and sequences could be targets of an antiviral chemotherapy, and the design of antiviral agents has profited enormously from the study of their biochemical functions. However, before describing these functions and their role in the replicative cycle in more detail, the degree of sequence variation—and thus functional variation—among retroviruses, and in particular for HIV, should be discussed.

IV. VARIATION AMONG RETROVIRUSES

The rate of genetic variation in any microorganism is the result of three variables: the mutation rate per replication cycle, the number of replication cycles per unit time, and the selective advantage or disadvantage of the mutant.

Generally, genetic diversity of retroviruses can arise as a consequence of point mutations, rearrangements, or recombinations. For oncoretroviruses, such as BLV, a rate for point mutations of 1×10^{-5} bases was estimated as the substitution rate (17,17a). In contrast, the substitution rate for HIV is about 100 times higher ($1–10 \times 10^{-4}$) (18,19,78–81), leading to about three base exchanges in a single reverse transcription of the genome. Similar mutation rates are also found among other lentiviruses.

The high genetic drift, together with recombinations and rearrangements, has led to two major families of the human immunodeficiency virus: HIV-1, first described by Barré- Sinoussi et al. (6), and HIV-2, which was discovered 3 years later (20). The two virus families differ by about 55% to 60% in their nucleic acid sequences.

In contrast to the high divergence on the nucleotide level, however, the genome organization of HIV-1 and HIV-2 is nearly identical and differs only in one auxiliary gene (Fig. 3). The HIV- 1 contains the gene *vpu*, whereas HIV-2 and the simian virus (SIV), are missing *vpu* and contain another gene, *vpx*. Comparison of the sequences between the human immunodeficiency viruses and primate lentiviruses revealed a close evolutionary relationship. The SIV of macaques were found to be related to the HIV-2 family. The closest relative of the HIV-1 family is

HIV-1

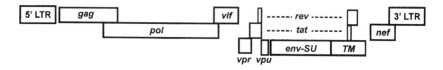

HIV-2 / SIV_MAC

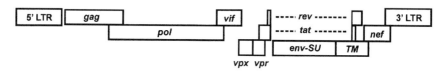

Figure 3   Comparison between the proviral genomes of HIV-1 and HIV-2.

the chimpanzee virus SIVcpz (21,22). Several transmissions between humans and
monkeys have been postulated to explain these relationships (7,8,22,44).

Within each of the HIV families, an extreme genetic heterogeneity exists.
This was first seen at the biological level, when HIV isolates from different patients were found to exhibit very different properties in cell culture (23–25). Subsequent longitudinal analyses of the genetic heterogeneity within a single patient
revealed that a quasispecies of HIV evolves over time, with divergences of up to
6% to 10% in a single individual, concomitant with variations of the replicative
behavior (26). The analysis of biological variation has so far been mainly restricted
to the viruses present in Europe and the United States. However, when studying
HIV worldwide, subtypes have been defined which differ by about 30% on the nucleic acid level. Within the HIV-1 family, two major groups have been discovered:
group M (8,33,34) is composed of the 10 subtypes A through J, and the subgroup
O (for "outliers") denotes isolates from Cameroon, which are a distinct subgroup
(8,35).

Early after infection, not only can cytopathic, syncytium-forming (SI)
viruses be seen in all subtypes studied, but also those that do not form syncytia
(NSI) (27). Normally, a phase follows infection in which the virus is difficult to
isolate from peripheral lymphocytes and only NSI viruses can be obtained (23,26).
This phase is followed by a phase in which SI viruses predominate, concomitant
or shortly before AIDS-related complex (ARC) and full-blown AIDS (28). In pre-
final stage AIDS patients, again, it can be difficult to isolate HIV, and NSI viruses
can be found (29).

The genetic heterogeneity of the HIV quasispecies is also reflected in the host
ranges of the virus. Peripheral lymphocytes, as well as monocytes/macrophages,
are target cells of HIV, and the tropism of the virus can change within an individ-

ual and during transmission (29–31). This results in virus isolates with distinct replication properties in primary lymphocytes and macrophages (7,29,30,30a). As for lymphocytes, growth properties on macrophages differ significantly between various isolates, and biological subtypes of α through δ have been defined based on the formation of multinucleated giant cells and the amount of virus produced (29). Apparently because of the high mutation rate of HIV, the virus adapts to various different host cells (31), which also causes a problem for therapy and even moreso for the development of a protective vaccine. However, host factors such as interleukin (IL)-4 may also be involved in the phenopypic switch (32).

The first wave of HIV from Africa arrived at the end of the 1970s in America through the Caribbean; it continued from there to Europe. The HIV transmission at that time was dominated by subtype B of HIV-1, with rare infections with HIV-2, subtype A in Europe, mostly originating directly from Africa. In contrast, two other HIV-1 subtypes, E and C, have spread from Africa to Thailand and India (36–38); these are currently being transmitted with the highest frequency in the world. The closest relative to the subtype C discovered in India in the early 1990s was an isolate from South Africa (38). Subtype E was first discovered in Thailand along with subtype B infections in drug addicts and is now the predominant subtype spreading in this country. On a worldwide scale, subtype C infections comprised 50% of the HIV-1 infections in 1998. A systematic analysis of subtypes recovered from distinct regions of the world has revealed NSI and SI growth characteristics, also in non-B isolates (27,39). Most recently, an increasing number of non-B subtypes has been seen in Europe and the United States (40). Because of the large amount of international travel, it is anticipated that this trend will continue.

It was long thought that HIV-2 was not spreading throughout the world, although sporadic cases had been found nearly in all countries. However HIV-2 infections were discovered in India in 1990 (41), and the virus has since been spreading along with HIV-1 in many parts of western India (37). It is not unequivocally clear at present how the pathogenicity of HIV-2 compares with HIV-1: All AIDS-defining diseases that have been known for HIV-1 infections have also been found associated with HIV-2 infections (42), as has progressive multifocal leukoencephalopathy as the only AIDS manifestation (43). The transmission rate of HIV-2 appears to be lower compared with HIV-1, and the rate of progression to disease may also be slower.

The discovery of a second subtype of HIV-2, HIVD205 (44), currently denoted as HIV-2 subtype B, has initiated the search for further subtypes within the HIV-2 family (8). Sequences that were characterized from uncultured material yielded evidence for the existence of further subtypes on the genetic level (C to E). However, their biological significance remains to be determined, because it was not possible to grow these viruses.

In India (and other countries such as the Ivory Coast), double infections with HIV-1 and HIV-2 have been demonstrated (37,45,46), but double or even triple infections with several subtypes of HIV-1 or HIV-2 have also been found. Takehisa et al. (47) analyzed a triple infection with the HIV-1 subtypes A, B, and O, which most likely occurred sequentially. It is unclear what the consequences of such superinfections are for the natural course of the disease and for the success of antiretroviral therapy. So far, no indications have been found to suggest that the disease is accelerated by infection with more than one subtype.

Superinfections, however, also lead to the generation of recombinants and pseudotypes: If two viruses infect a single cell simultaneously, it has been shown that multiple recombinations occur between the subtypes. Analysis of HIV recovered from a transfusion patient who had been exposed twice to subtype B not only revealed the two primary viruses, but also recombinants between them (48). Sabino et al. (49) demonstrated for an isolate from Brazil that a double recombination had taken place between the *env* genes of a subtype B virus and a subtype F virus. Similarly Gao et al. (50) isolated an HIV-2 clone, which had resulted from a recombination between two HIV-2 subtypes. Although it has been possible to generate pseudotypes of HIV-1 and HIV-2 in vitro, a recombination between HIV-1 and HIV-2 has not been demonstrated in vivo so far.

In summary, the highly variable nature of HIV, the geographical redistribution of subtypes, and the recombination between them poses significant problems for all areas of AIDS research. Based on this knowledge, the development of a highly effective prophylactic vaccine appears extremely difficult. In contrast, therapeutic antiviral drugs, which target essential enzymes of the virus, have been discovered and are widely used to treat HIV/AIDS. However, emerging drug-resistant variants and subtypes with variable sensitivity to the drugs will be an increasingly significant problem for drug therapy in the future.

V. MOLECULAR TARGETS FOR ANTI-HIV THERAPIES

Knowledge of the molecular mechanisms in each step of the HIV life cycle provides an essential basis for discovering and developing antiviral drugs and therapies aimed at blocking HIV replication and preventing or delaying disease. So far, the most successful approach leading to marketed drugs has been the inhibition of two essential viral enzymes, the reverse transcriptase (RT) and the viral protease (PR) (Fig. 4). Theoretically, any of the other steps in the viral life cycle could be a target of antiretroviral agents as well. This also applies to the regulatory viral proteins Tat, Rev, Vif, Vpr, Vpu/Vpx, and Nef. In the following paragraphs, the different steps in the viral life cycle are discussed.

A. Virion Attachment and Entry

The early phase of the replication cycle begins with the attachment of a virion to the cell surface receptor (see Fig. 4), which is mediated by the extracellular do-

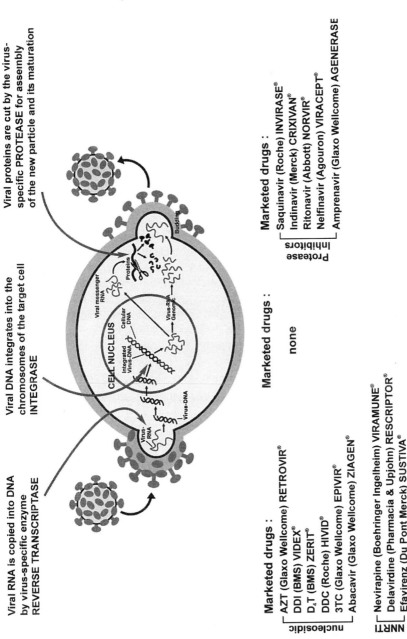

Figure 4 The first enzymatic targets for therapy development against HIV.

main of the envelope glycoprotein gp120 and the cellular receptor CD4. The CD4 is a glycoprotein of 55 kd located on the plasma membranes of helper lymphocytes and macrophages (51,52). It triggers a conformational change in the Env glycoprotein, which is necessary for the fusion of the viral and cellular membrane, and exposes the variable domain V3 to a protease. Cleavage of V3 frees the binding domain of the viral transmembrane protein gp41, which, in turn, interacts with CD4. However, this interaction is not sufficient for viral entry. Experiments trying to infect nonhuman cells expressing CD4 and some CD4-positive human lines failed (53–55), indicating that in vitro CD4 was necessary but not sufficient for viral entry. It was not until 1996 that the coreceptors CCR5 and Fusin (CXCR4), as well as CKR3 and CKR2B, were discovered as coreceptors for the entry of HIV into lymphocytes and macrophages (56,57). In T cells, CXCR4 is used as coreceptor, whereas CCR5 (less frequently CCR3 and rarely CCR2B) is preferred by monocytes/ macrophages (see also chapter 3, Ref. 7). The ligands of CCR5, RANTES, MIP-1 alpha and beta were identified as major HIV-suppressive factors (60).

So far, strategies to block CD4 in order to prevent viral entry into the cell have been effective in vitro but have failed in vivo. Consequently, the coreceptors and the chemokines binding to them are being investigated as potential targets for therapy. It is known that the respective chemokines inhibit HIV replication, most likely by lowering the density of their receptors on the cellular surface (58), without using signal transduction by way of G proteins (58,59). However, the fact that different coreceptors are being used depending on the target cell will make this approach for an anti-HIV therapy very difficult. In addition, previous studies trying to inhibit HIV replication by treatment with a truncated form of the CD4 receptor supposedly coating the virions and thereby rendering them uninfectious, most likely failed in vivo, because HIV can be passed on from cell to cell by membrane fusion and other ways of cellular entry.

B. Reverse Transcription

After uncoating, which is poorly understood, the next step in the viral life cycle consists of reverse transcription of the RNA genome to form a double-stranded DNA molecule. This step has been successfully exploited for the design of antiretroviral therapies. The enzyme, reverse transcriptase (RT), is an RNA-dependent DNA polymerase that synthesizes DNA from RNA as well as from DNA templates (60–62). It also contains an RNAseH activity (63,64), which degrades the RNA after the first DNA strand has been synthesized to allow for the generation of the complementary DNA strand. The RT and RNAseH are indispensable for viral replication. Both enzymes are processed from the gag-pol polyprotein (pro160gag-pol) by the viral protease PR (see later) during virion assembly (65). Subsequently, one subunit of p66 in this homodimer is cleaved by PR near the C-terminus to yield a heterodimer composed of p51 and p66. The heterodimer and the p66 homodimer both display RT and RNaseH activities, whereas p51 alone is not active, although it contains the RT sequence (66,67). However, recently a function in DNA binding could be demonstrated for p51 by mutational analysis of the helix clamp motiv (68).

Although no inhibitor of the RNaseH activity has reached the market, there were six nucleosidic RT inhibitors (AZT, DDI, D4T, DDC, 3TC, and Abacavir) available at mid-1999 and three nonnucleosidic drugs (Nevirapine, Delavirdine, Efavirenz). All nucleosidic drugs are analogues of a DNA-base building block and share a chemical modification that removes the 3´-OH group in the sugar ring (Fig. 5). When they are incorporated into the growing DNA genome of the virus, synthesis stops, because no free 3´-OH group is available for the next nucleotide to be added.

Apart from the nucleosidic inhibitors of the RT, nonnucleosidic inhibitors have been discovered which bind to a hydrophobic pocket close to the active site of the enzyme. The three marketed drugs and some compounds in earlier development are depicted in Figure 6. A map of 3.5 A has been derived from crystals of the RT heterodimer complexed with the nonnucleosidic inhibitor Nevirapine (69). The p51 and p66 subunits interact in a head-to-tail configuration to produce the heterodimer. Four subdomains of p66 are arranged side by side to yield an elongated RT domain, and a connection domain in p66 joins the RT and RNaseH domains. This structure is often compared with a right hand: The subdomains are identified as fingers, palm, and thumb (70). The catalytic site of the RT is a cleft in the palm of the p66 subunit and contains the sequence Tyr183- Met 184- Asp185- Asp186, which is highly conserved in retroviral RTs as well as in other DNA polymerases. Asp110 is also required for catalytic activity. No cleft is evident in the p51 subunit, and amino acid residues in p51 corresponding to the catalytic site of p66 are buried and thus not available for catalysis.

Even though the first generation RT inhibitors of the nonnucleosidic class were disappointing because of their very fast generation of resistance (see later text), drugs such as Nevirapine, Delavirdine, and Efavirenz have reached the market (see Fig. 6). Particularly, a highly active second generation drug such as Efavirenz (71,72), which allows a once daily dosing, is currently being used as an alternative to protease inhibitors in first line regimens. Similarly, GW 420 867, a relative of HBY 097 (see Fig. 6) (73–75) displays nanomolar activity against the virus and has an equally favorable long half life.

The mechanism of resistance development and the type of genetic and phenotypic changes have been studied in great detail. Reverse transcription generally plays a major role in the generation of the diversity of retroviruses (see earlier text) (76). The fidelity of RTs for a variety of retroviruses has been determined in vitro (77) and significant differences were detected between RTs from different retroviruses. The misincorporation rate of HIV-1 RT is between 1 per 1700 and 1 per

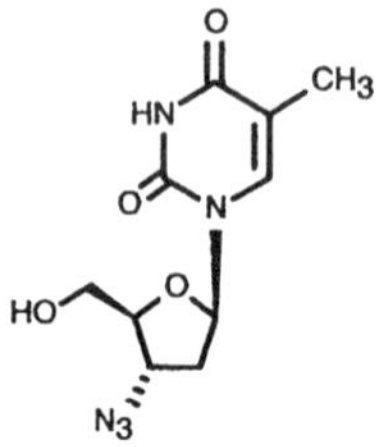

GLAXO WELLCOME
RETROVIR®, Zidovudine*, Azidothymidine, AZT
launched 1987

BIOCHEM / GLAXO WELLCOME
COMBIVIR®, Lamivudine* <u>and</u> Zidovudine*
launched 1998

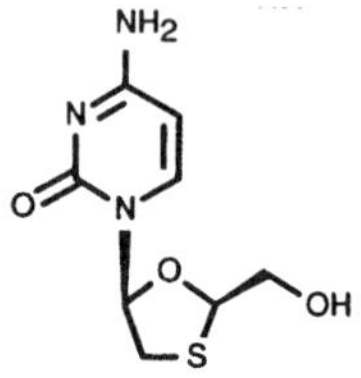

BIOCHEM / GLAXO WELLCOME
EPIVIR®, 3TC®, Lamivudine*
launched 1995

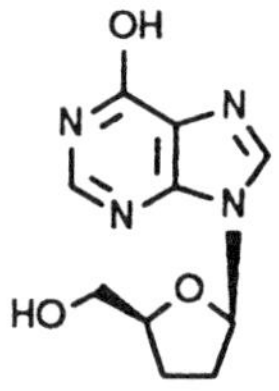

BRISTOL-MYERS-SQUIBB
VIDEX®
DDI, Didanosine,
Dideoxyinosine
launched 1991

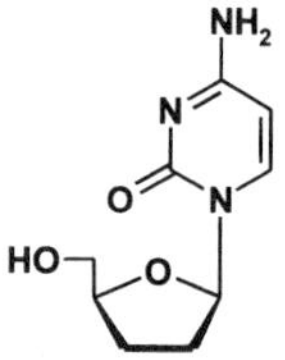

ROCHE
HIVID®
DDC, Zalcitabine,
Dideoxycytidine
launched 1992

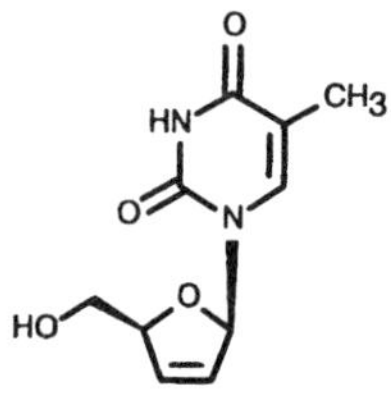

BRISTOL-MYERS-SQUIBB
ZERIT®
D4T, Stavudine
launched 1994

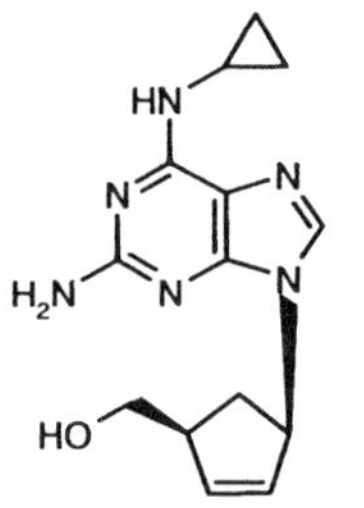

GLAXO WELLCOME
ZIAGEN®
Abacavir
launched January 1999

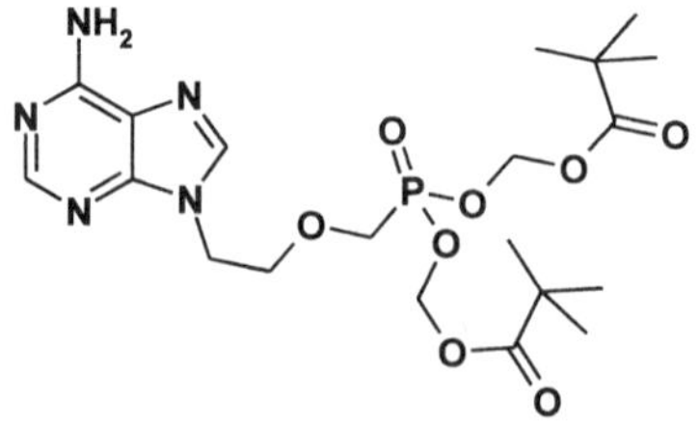

GILEAD SCIENCES
PREVEON®
Adefovir, Dipivoxil
Phase III Clinical Trial

Figure 5 The nucleosidic inhibitors of HIV RT in clinical use up to 1999.

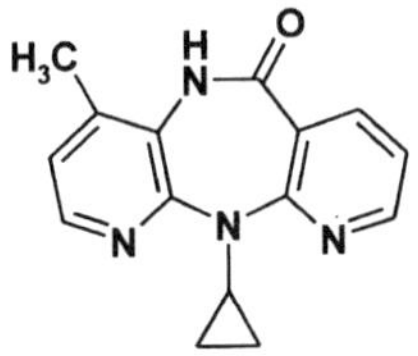

BOEHRINGER INGELHEIM
VIRAMUNE®
Nevirapine (BI-RG 587)
World: launched 1996

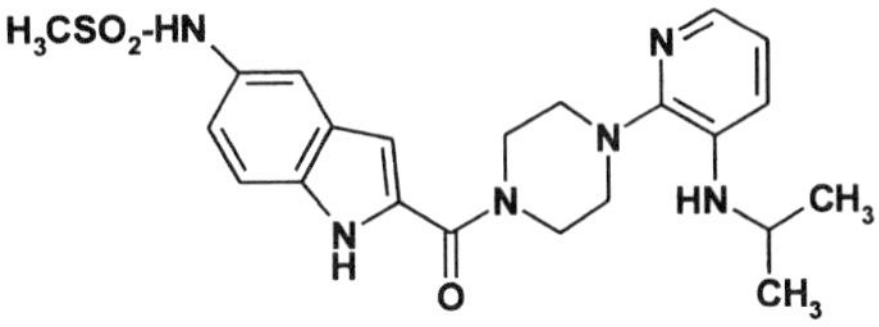

PHARMACIA & UPJOHN
RESCRIPTOR®
Delavirdine mesylate, U 90152 S
World: launched 1997

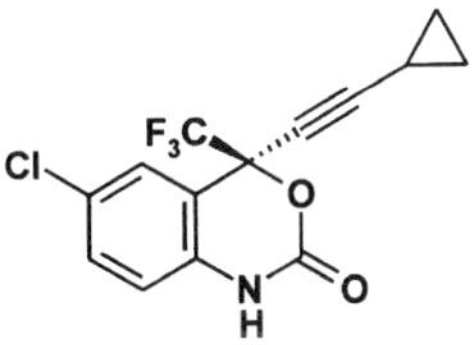

DUPONT MERCK (Licensee)
SUSTIVA®, STOCRIN®
Efavirenz, DMP 266, L - 743726
World: launched 1998

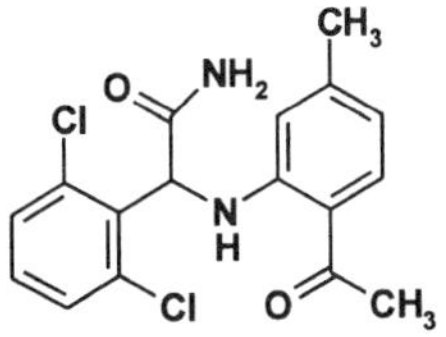

JOHNSON & JOHNSON
Loviride, R 89439
World: Phase II Clinical Trial

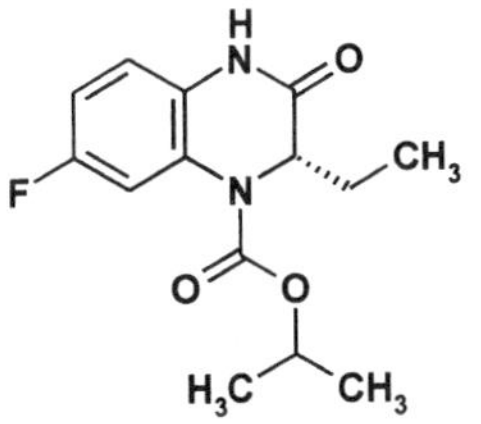

GLAXO WELLCOME
GW 420 867
(formerly HBY 1293A)
(licenced from Bayer / Hoechst)
Phase II

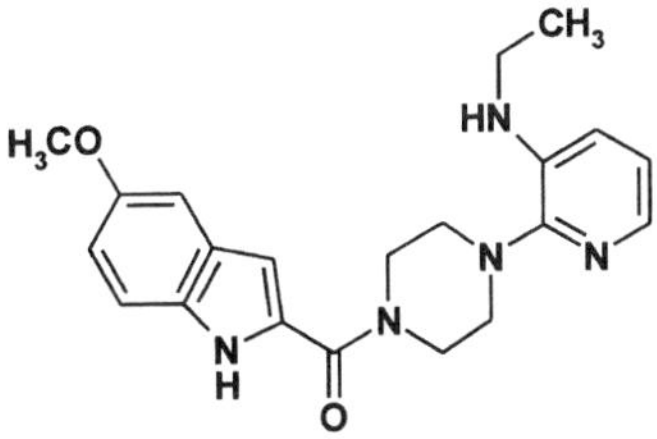

UPJOHN
Atevirdine, U 87201
World: no development reported

Figure 6   The nonnucleosidic inhibitors of HIV-1 RT.

4000 nucleotides (78–80). The rate for other retroviruses is lower, for example, from 1 per 9000 to 1 per 17,000 nucleotides for avian myeloblastosis virus and 1 per 30,000 nucleotides for murine leukemia virus (81). The especially high error rate of HIV-1 RT results in the fast generation of viruses that are resistant against the aforementioned inhibitors. Although prolonged monotherapy with antiretroviral agents has not been efficacious for longer periods of time, a combination of several RT inhibitors and combinations of RT and PR inhibitors have greatly diminished the generation and selection of resistant viruses during prolonged therapy.

VI. THE INTEGRASE

Integrase (IN) is another viral enzyme believed to be essential for a full replicative cycle of HIV in T-cell lines as well as primary lymphocytes and monocytes/macrophages (82–84). It has DNA cleavage as well as DNA-joining or strand-transfer activities (85), integrating the linear double- stranded viral genome into the host cell genome to form the provirus. The IN is cleaved from the C-terminus of the gag-pol precursor as a 32-kd protein. The enzyme contains a highly conserved domain with pairs of His and Cys residues, which adopt a structure similar to the metal finger binding motif in DNA-binding proteins. Its central domain has acidic residues, which are highly conserved in the integrases of retroviruses, retrotransposons, and the transposases of some bacterial transposons. The three- dimensional structure of the catalytic portion, residues 50 through 212, has been determined (86). Multimerization of IN may be essential for integration as well as for incorporation into virus particles. Each molecule of IN has a catalytic site but is thought to have separate binding sites for the ends of linear viral DNA (87).

Cell-free systems with double-stranded oligonucleotides have been used to analyze the steps in the catalytic reaction. These are (a) cleavage of a TT-dinucleotide from the 3′ ends of double-stranded attachment site substrates, (b) cleavage of double-stranded target DNA to produce a staggered 5′ overhang, and (c) strand-transfer activity in which the recessed 3′ end in the substrate DNA is joined to the 5′ phosphoryl group in the target DNA (88,89). Presumably, the conserved amino acids in the active site (Asp64, Asp116, glu152) bind two divalent metal ions, which are involved in the catalytic reaction. In vitro, IN also mediates the reverse reaction, disintegration, and it has been shown that the three amino acids in the active site are essential for all three catalytic activities of the enzyme.

Despite this very detailed knowledge about the catalytic activity of the viral integrase, no compound inhibiting this enzyme has so far reached the market. The most likely reason for this failure is that the in vitro reactions using small oligonucleotides do not adequately reflect the situation within a cell, where cellular factors appear to be involved in the formation of a larger functional complex. However, some interesting molecules have recently been identified (90).

VII. THE VIRAL PROTEASE

The viral protease is essential for the maturation of the virion into an infectious particle (91–93) (see Fig. 4). The mature form of protease (PR) is 99 amino acids in length and displays a molecular weight of 10 k (93). After release from the gag-pol precursor protein, the fully active dimeric PR targets several sites in the gag polyprotein and in the gag-pol precursor protein. The HIV protease is related to cellular proteases on the basis of the conserved amino acids Asp-Thr/Ser-Gly in its active site (94).

Proteases of HIV-1 and HIV-2 have been crystallized and display similar structural features. The HIV-1 PR has specificity for several substrates, which is governed by four amino acids upstream and three amino acids downstream of the cleavage site. Three cleavage sites in the gag-pol precursor fit the consensus sequence Ser-Thr-X-Y-Phe/Try-Pro-Z (cleavage between the Phe/Tyr-Pro linkage). The other cleavages occur at Leu-Ala, Met-Met, Phe-Leu, and Leu-Phe bonds. Inhibitors of PR have been designed on the basis of the oligopeptide substrates of the enzyme. Whereas the first generation inhibitors were peptidomimetics (95) with no or low oral bioavailability and chemically still very close to the natural substrate site (96), improvements enabled the introduction of three first generation protease inhibitors for the therapy of HIV infection, followed by further optimization using molecular design techniques (Fig. 7). These compounds have been very successful in combination regimens to suppress HIV in patients. Their long-term use, however, may be associated with peripheral lipodystrophy, hyperlipidemia, and insulin resistance. Whether this occurs by cross-reactions with human proteins regulating lipid metabolism (97) or because of prolonged lifespan of the patients remains to be determined, because this condition has also been noted in patients who did not receive protease inhibitors. It is to be anticipated that the degree to which this side effect occurs will vary between HIV protease inhibitors and further research will have to determine the optimal regimen.

VIII. THE ACCESSORY AND REGULATORY GENES OF HIV

There are six accessory or regulatory genes in HIV-1: *vif*, *vpr*, *vpu*, *nef*, *tat*, and *rev* (see Fig. 3). Related genes are found in the HIV-2/SIV family, except for *vpx*, which replaces *vpu* (see Fig. 3). Most of these genes are encoded in the middle of the genomes (see Fig. 3), but *nef* and one exon of *tat* and *rev* are located at the 3´ end, within the *env* gene and extending beyond it. Vpr and Vpx are present in the virions, but small amounts of Vif, Vpu, and Nef may be incorporated into viral particles as well.

There has been some conflict in the literature on the function of some of these

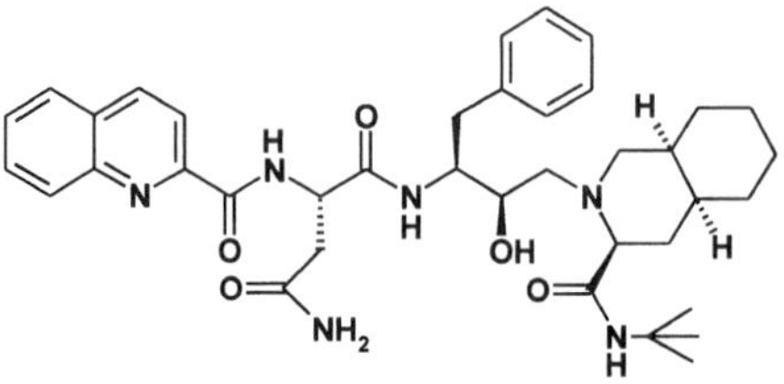

ROCHE
INVIRASE®
Saquinavir, RO-31-8959
launched 1996

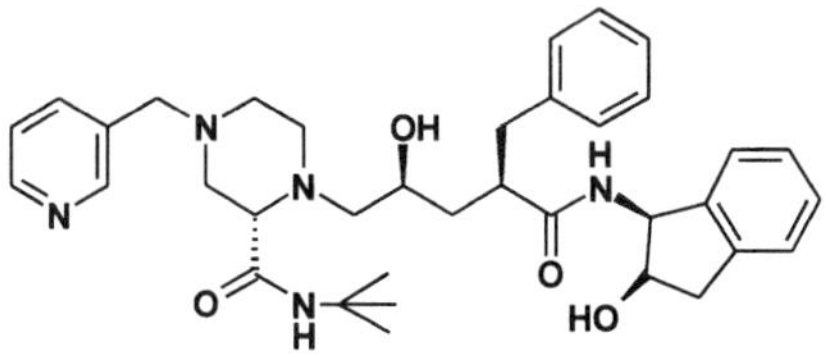

MERCK & CO
CRIXIVAN®
Indinavir, L-735524, MK 639
launched 1996

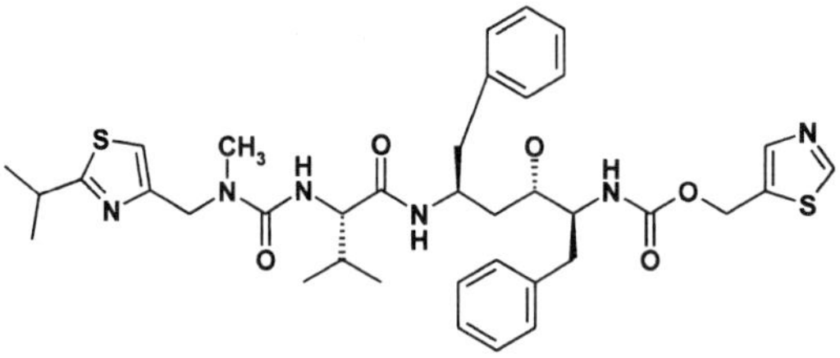

ABBOTT
NORVIR®
Ritonavir, ABT-538
launched 1996

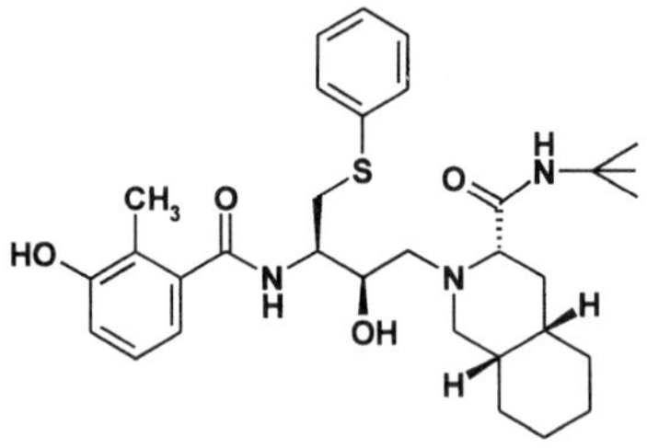

AGOURON
VIRACEPT®
Nelfinavir, AG-1343
launched 1996/97

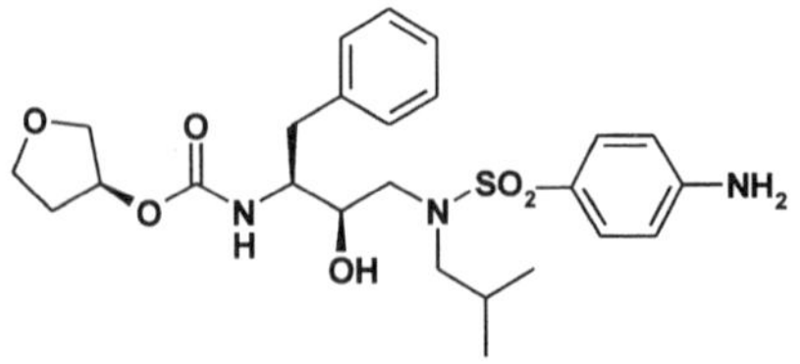

VERTEX PHARMACEUTICALS
Licensee: GLAXO WELLCOME, KISSEI
AGENERASE®
PROZEI®
Amprenavir, VX - 478,
USA : launched May 1999
Japan : Pre-registration

Figure 7 The inhibitors of HIV protease in clinical use up to 1999.

genes, which may partly be due to the fact that these genes are dispensable in tissue culture for viral replication (but modulate replication efficacy). Hence, tissue culture data may not accurately reflect the cell types and physiological conditions that are important for regulating viral replication in vivo. There is no doubt that these genes could potentially be very important targets for drug development if their in vivo function would be better understood. In the following, some generally agreed functions are described.

A. Transcriptional Activator by Way of an RNA Target

Tat is a protein of about 88 amino acids and a potent activator of the HIV-1 long terminal repeat of the nascent chain (LTR) promoter element. Its mechanism is unique in that it acts through binding to an RNA structure called TAR, located immediately 3′ to the LTR transcription start site. This element forms a 59-nucleotide stem-loop structure, to which Tat binds at the U-rich bulge and affects transcriptional elongation. The tat protein has two functional domains, a cofactor-binding domain (close to N-terminus until residue 48) and an arginine-rich RNA binding motive from residue 49 through 58 (98). Activation of the LTR requires the recruitment of cellular factors by Tat to TAR, which bind to the TAR loop.

Although the level of transcription from the LTR is nearly equal in presence and absence of Tat, initiated transcripts are terminated prematurely, within 200 nucleotides of the transcription start site (99), when Tat is missing. This suggests that tat activates the processivity of initiated RNA polymerase II, most likely by enhancing the phosphorylation state of polymerase II (100). It has recently been shown that its function depends on the presence of the human CDK9 kinase and that the interaction is most likely mediated by an associated cyclin, which binds to the TAR loop (101,102).

B. Rev: Nuclear RNA Export Factor

Even though HIV has only a single, genome-length primary transcript, expression of the nine open-reading frames not only requires that this transcript be expressed in the cytoplasm as unspliced RNA (serving as viral genome and as the mRNA for Gag and Pol), but also that the singly spliced RNAs encoding Vif, Vpr, Vpu, and Env and several multiple spliced mRNAs for Tat, Rev, and Nef be generated as well. Splicing of HIV-1 transcripts is entirely performed by cellular proteins. The viral genomes encode 5′ and 3′ splice sites, which lead to the retention of unspliced RNA in the nucleus and preclude expression of proteins from the unspliced mRNA (Gag, Pol) and singly spliced RNA (Env, Vif, Vpr, Vpu). Because the splice sites of HIV-1 are inefficient, a pool of such RNAs accumulates in the nucleus. The function of Rev, a 116-amino acid protein, is to interact with unspliced and singly spliced transcripts and to lead to their efficient nuclear export (103). Because Rev,

Tat, and Nef are encoded by fully spliced HIV-1 mRNAs, these gene products are expressed early after infection. Gag, Pol, Env, Vif, Vpr, and Vpu are dependent on Rev for the transport of their mRNA and, therefore, are expressed late.

The RNA target for Rev is a 234-nucleotide RNA stem-loop structure called RRE (Rev responsive element) encoded within the *env* gene (103). Rev binds, most likely as a monomer, to an RNA bulge within the RRE, then recruits additional monomers. The nuclear export signal in Rev is located between residues 75 and 84 (104). Because Rev contains both an NLS and an NES, it shuttles back and forth between the nucleus and cytoplasm of the cells.

C. Nef: Numerous Effector Functions

Nef is the largest among the auxiliary proteins (206 amino acids) and is expressed at far higher levels than Tat and Rev. Its effect on HIV replication in lymphocytic tumor cell lines was controversial; however, demonstration that it was significantly linked to high virus titers and pathogenicity in macaques (105) revealed its importance in vivo.

In infected cells, Nef has three distinct functions: down regulation of CD4 and MHC I receptors, enhanced virion infectivity, and an effect on cellular signal transduction and activation. Down-regulation of CD4 requires a cluster of leucine and isoleucine residues in the CD4 cytoplasmic tail and occurs by targeting CD4 into clathrin-coated pits, followed by internalization and transport to lysosomes (106). In addition to CD4, Nef also induces the specific down-regulation of cell-surface MHC I receptor, but with lower efficiency (107). This process requires specific residues at the MHC I cytoplasmic tail, including a key tyrosine (107,108). This mechanism inhibits the CTL-mediated lysis of infected cells (109), but apparently is not the only factor contributing to pathogenesis, because CTL responses are mounted by infected individuals.

Although the effect of Nef on virion infectivity is modest in most cultured cells, it increases when primary quiescent cells are infected. Nef is packaged into virions at less than 10 copies per virion and undergoes specific processing by the viral protease. However, the molecular mechanism how infectivity is enhanced by Nef is not well understood and may involve a cellular kinase. Similarly, the effects of Nef on signal transduction in cells is not yet clear. A PXXP motiv in HIV-Nef binds to SH3 domains of some *src* kinases and is required for enhanced growth of Nef[+] viruses (110). However, Nef proteins of distinct HIV-1 or HIV-2 isolates may differ in their binding properties (111). Nef-induced down-regulation of CD4 could liberate the CD4-bound tyrosine kinase lck (112) and thus influence signaling through the TCR/CD3 complex. Nef is also believed to recruit a serine/theronine kinase related to PAK to the plasma membrane (113). Two recent publications shed new light on how Nef may interfere with T-cell signaling. First, Xu et al. (114)

demonstrated that Nef directly interacts with zeta chain of the T-cell receptor, which leads to the up-regulation of FasL. Fackler et al. (114a) showed that Nef interacts with the Vav protein, which is a downstream effector of zeta, leading to the activation of the Nef-associated kinase (p62/NAK) and the jun-N-terminal kinase (JNK). In summary, it appears that Nef stimulates a signaling pathway stemming from the T-cell receptor (114).

D. Vif: Virus Infectivity Factor

In primate lentiviruses, a 5-kb singly spliced vif transcript, which is dependent on rev function, is produced late in the viral replication cycle and results in a protein of 23 to 27 kd (115–117). Early studies of vif function revealed that infectivity of cell-free virus was reduced by a factor of 1000 when vif function was impaired, leading to its name: "virus infectivity factor," although cell-to-cell transmission was comparable to wild-type virus (118,119). Recent studies showed that the requirement for vif also depends on the cell types used so that it appears that, in certain cells, cellular factors are able to complement for vif function. It is currently assumed that vif may govern uncoating or internalization of HIV in restrictive cells, but it could also have a role in virus maturation (120).

E. Vpr: Nuclear Import and G_2 Arrest

The HIV-1, SIVcpz, SIVagm, and SIVmnd each contain only *vpr*, whereas HIV-2 and several other SIV strains (SIVMAC, SIVSMM) contain both vpr and *vpx* (121). On the amino acid levels, Vpr and Vpx are homologous, so that *vpx* may be a duplication of *vpr*. Because the time point for duplication of *vpr* may correlate with the divergence of the HIV-2 group and other primate lentiviruses from a common ancestor, *vpx* may have had a role in the adaptation of the viruses to the primate host species. Nonprimate lentiviruses (FIV, CAEV, BIV, EIAV) do not encode genes for Vpr and Vpx; however, they contain small open-reading frames for proteins which may be functional counterparts (122).

Vpr is a 15-kd virion-associated protein, which is dependent on rev function and thus occurs late in the infection (123,124). It is packaged into the virion nucleocapsid in amounts equivalent to the gag protein. Packaging is mediated by the p6 protein, located at the carboxy terminus of the p55 gag precursor (125). Vpr has a modest effect on enhancing replication of HIV in T-cell lines and primary cells, but a far more pronounced effect on replication in growth-arrested cells such as primary macrophages. It is therefore thought that vpr mediates the nuclear import of preintegration complexes (126). The nuclear localization signal (NLS) of Vpr is distinct from the NLS prototype and leads to accumulation of protein at nuclear pores (127) by interaction with nucleoporins. In addition to its function in nuclear import, vpr induces arrest of cells in the G_2 phase of the cell cycle. This function is mediated by a carboxy terminal domain of about 26 amino acids. Cells expressing vpr contain very low amounts of p34cdc2-cyclin B kinase activity (128).

F. Vpu: Unique to HIV-1

Vpu is an oligomeric integral membrane protein unique to HIV-1 and the closely related SIVcpz. It serves two functions in the viral life cycle: enhancement of virion release from the cells and selective degradation of CD4 in the endoplasmic reticulum (ER). Vpu interacts with a specific target sequence in the cytoplasmic tail of CD4 and targets CD4 to an ER-associated protein degradation pathway. This allows the release of envelope protein from the ER and its incorporation into progeny virus (129,130). Whereas CD4 degradation has been mapped to sequences in the cytoplasmic tail of vpu, enhanced virion release is dependent on the hydrophobic amino-terminal *trans*-membrane domain.

IX. STRUCTURAL PROTEINS

Apart from enzymes and regulatory proteins, structural proteins are also potential targets for drug development. However, because protein–protein interactions are often difficult to inhibit by low molecular weight compounds, a successful drug development has not yet been reported. Rosenwirth et al. (131) have described inhibition of HIV replication by a variant of cyclosporine A, which binds to cyclophilin A, which is incorporated into the virions (132,133). Cyclophilin A may be required to aid the proper folding of gag. Interruption of the interaction between cyclophilin A and gag may thus be another approach for the development of novel antiviral agents. Similarly, disruption of a Zn-finger structure in the nucleocapsid protein has been suggested by Rice et al. (134) as a new approach.

X. SUMMARY AND OUTLOOK

Even though there are numerous targets for inhibiting HIV replication, its intrinsic high variability calls for combining several different drug classes with distinct mechanisms of action. Combining of RT and PR inhibition has been very successful, but resistance is emerging and the pharmacokinetic properties of most drugs are for from being ideal. The search for new antiviral principles that would complement inhibition of RT and PR therefore appears necessary as does the optimization of present drug classes with respect to convenience and tolerability. The HIV research needs to maintain a sense of urgency because the number of infected individuals continues to increase in the industrialized world at a pace of about

+4%/year and exponential growth of the epidemic is still being seen in many developing countries.

ACKNOWLEDGMENTS

The author would like to thank Daniela Cramer for help with the figures and Guy Hewlett for critically reading the manuscript.

REFERENCES

1. Collett MS, Erikson RL. Protein kinase activity associated with avian sarcoma virus src gene product. Proc Natl Acad Sci U S A 1978; 75:2021–2024.
2. Rübsamen H, Friis RR, Bauer H. Src gene product from different strains of avian sarcoma virus: kinetics and possible mechanism of heat inactivation of protein kinase activity from cells infected by transformation-defective, temperature-sensitive mutant and wild-type virus. Proc Natl Acad Sci U S A 1979; 76 (2):967–971.
3. Hunter T. The yin and yang of protein phosphorylation and signaling. Cell 1995; 80: 225–236.
4. Poiesz BJ, Ruscetti FW, Gazdar AF, Bunn PA, Minna JD, Gallo RC. Detection and isolation of type C retrovirus particles from fresh and cultured lymphocytes of a patient with cutaneous T-cell lymphoma. Proc Natl Acad Sci U S A 1980; 77 (12):7415–7419.
5. Yoshida M, Myoshi I, Hinuma Y. Isolation and characterization of retrovirus (ATLV) from cell lines of human adult T-cell leukemia and its implication in the diseases. Proc Natl Acad Sci U S A 1982; 79:2031–2035.
6. Barré-Sinoussi F, Chermann JC, Rey F, Nugeyre MT, Chamaret S, Gruest J, Dauguet C, Axler-Blin C, Brun-Vezinet F, Rozioux C, Rozenbaum W, Montagnier L. Isolation of a T-lymphotropic retrovirus from a patient at risk for acquired immunodeficiency syndrome (AIDS). Science 1983; 220:868–871.
7. Myers G. In: Coffin JM, Hughes SH, Varmus HE, eds. Retroviruses. Cold Spring Harbor, NY: Cold Spring Harbor Laboratory Press, 1997:709–756.
8. Eigen M, Nieselt-Struwe K. How old is the immunodeficiency virus? AIDS 1990; 4: 85–93.
9. Perron H, Garson JA, Bedin F, Beseme F, Paranhos- Baccala G, Komurian-Pradel F, Mallet F, Tuke PW, Voisset C, Blond JL, Lalande B, Seigneurin JM, Mandrand B, The Collaborative Research Group on Multiple Sclerosis. Molecular identification of a novel retrovirus repeatedly isolated from patients with multiple sclerosis. Proc Natl Acad Sci U S A 1997; 94:7583–7588.
10. Miller AD. Development and application of retroviral vectors. In: Coffin JM, Hughes SH, Varmus HE, eds. Retroviruses. Cold Spring Harbor, NY: Cold Spring Harbor Laboratory Press, 1997:709–756.
11. Doolittle RF, Feng DF, McClure MA, Johnson MS. Retrovirus phylogeny and evolution. In: Swanstrom R, Vogt PK, eds. Retroviruses: Strategies of Replication. New York: Springer-Verlag, 1990:1–18.

12. McClure MA. Evolutionary history of reverse transcriptase. In: Skalka AM, Goff SP, eds. Reverse Transcriptase. Cold Spring Harbor, NY: Cold Spring Harbor Laboratory Press, 1993:425–444.
13. Yu SF, Sullivan MD, Linial ML. Evidence that the human foamy virus genome is DNA. J Virol 1999; 73 (2):1565–1572.
13a. Moebes A, Enssle J, Bieniasz PD, Heinkelein M, Lindemann D, Bock M, Mc Clure MO, Rethwilm A. Human foamy virus reverse transcription that occurs late in the viral replication cycle. J Virol 1997; 71 (10):7305–7311.
14. Aiyar A, Cobrinik D, Ge Z, Kung H-J, Leis J. Interaction between retroviral U5 RNA and the TYC loop of the tRNA Trp primer is required for efficient initiation of reverse transcription. J Virol 1992; 66:24604–2472.
15. Aiyar A, Ge Z, Leis J. A specific orientation of RNA secondary structures is required for initiation of reverse transcription. J Virol 1994; 68:611–618.
16. Murphy JE, Goff SP. Construction and analysis of deletion mutations in the U5 region of Moloney murine leukemia virus: effects on RNA packaging and reverse transcription. J Virol 1988; 63:319–327.
17. Mansky LM, Temin HM. Lower mutation rate of bovine leukemia virus relative to that of spleen necrosis virus. J Virol 1994; 68:494–499.
17a. Dougherty JP, Temin HM. Determination of the rate of base-pair substitution and insertion mutations in retrovirus replication. J Virol 1988; 62:2817–2822.
18. Myers G, Pavlaks GN. Evolutionary potential of complex retroviruses. In: Levy JA, ed. The Retroviridae. Vol. I. New York: Plenum Press, 1992:51–105.
19. Takenchi Y, Nagumo T, Hoshino H. Low fidelity of cell-free DNA synthesis by reverse transcriptase of human immunodeficiency virus. J Virol 1988; 62:3900–3902.
20. Clavel FD, Guetard D, Brun-Vezinet F, Chamaret S, Rey MA, Santos-Ferreira MO, Laurent AG, Danguet C, Katlama C, Rosioux C. Isolation of a new human retrovirus from West African patients with AIDS. Science 1986; 233:343–346.
21. Huet T, Cheynier R, Meyerthaus A, Roelants G, Wain-Hobson S. Genetic organization of a chimpanzee lentivirus related to HIV-1. Nature 1990; 345:356–359.
22. Gao F, Bailes E, Robertson DL, Chen YL, Rodenburg CM, Michael SF, Cummins LB, Arthur LO, Peeters M, Shaw GM, Sharp PM, Hahn BH. Origin of HIV-1 in the chimpanzee Pan troglodytes. Nature 1999; 397 (6718):436–441.
23. Rübsamen-Waigmann H, Becker WB, Helm EB, Brodt R, Fischer H, Henco K. Brede HD. Isolation of variants of lymphocytopathic retroviruses from the peripheral blood and cerebrospinal fluid of patients with ARC or AIDS. J Med Virol 1986; 19:335–344.
24. Von Briesen H, Becker WB, Henco K, Helm EB, Gelderblom HR, Brede HD, Rübsamen-Waigmann H. Isolation frequency and growth properties of HIV-variants: multiple simultaneous variants in a patient demonstrated by molecular cloning. J Med Virol 1987; 23:51–66.
25. Fenyö EM, Morfeldt-Manson L, Chiodi F, et al. Distinct replicative and cytopathic characteristics of human immunodefiency isolates. J Virol 1988; 62:4414–4419.
26. Cheng-Mayer C, Seto D, Tateno M, Levy JA. Biologic features of HIV-1 that correlate with virulence in the host. Science 1988; 240:80–82.
27. De Wolf F, Hogervorst E, Goudsmit J, Fenyö E-M, Rübsamen-Waigmann H, Holmes H, Galvao-Castro B, Karita E, Wasi CH, Sempala SDK, Baan E, Zorgdrager F, Lukashov V, Osmanov S, Kuiken C, Cornelissen M, Belsey EM, Heyward W, Esparza J, Vanderperre P, Sempala S, Tugume B, Biryahwaho B, Von Briesen H, Esser

R, Grez M, Newberry A, Ranjbar S, Tomlinson P, Bradac J, McCutchan F, Louwagie J, Hegerich P, Lopezgalindez C, Olivares I, Dopazo J, Mullins JI, Delwart EL, Bachmann HM, Hahn BH, Gao F, Yue L, Saragosti S, Schochetman G, Kalish M, Luo CC, George R, Pau CP, Weber J, Cheingsongpopov R, Kaleebu P, Nara P, Albert J, Myers G, Korber B. Syncytium inducing (SI) and non-syncytium inducing (NSI) capacity of human immunodeficiency virus type 1 (HIV-1) subtypes other than B: phenotypic and genotypic characteristics. AIDS Res Hum Retroviruses 1994; 10, N 11:1387–1400.

28. Spijkerman I, deWolf F, Langendam M, Schuitemaker H, Coutinho R. Emergence of syncytium-inducing human immunodeficiency virus type 1 variants coincides with a transient increase in viral RNA level and is an independent predictor for progression to AIDS. J Infect Dis 1998; 178 (2):397–403.

29. Von Briesen H, Andreesen R, Rübsamen-Waigmann H. Systematic classification of HIV biological subtypes on lymphocytes and monocytes/macrophages. Virology 1990; 178:597–602.

30. Rübsamen-Waigmann H, Willems WR, Bertram U, Von Briesen H. Reversal of HIV-phenotype to fulminant replication on macrophages in perinatal transmission. Lancet 1989; 11:1155–1156.

30a. Kühnel H, von Briesen H, Dietrich U, Adamski M, Mix D, Biesert L, Kreutz R, Immelmann A, Henco K, Meichsner Ch, Andreesen R, Gelderblom H, Rübsamen-Waigmann H. Molecular cloning of two West African human immunodeficiency virus type 2 isolates that replicate well in macrophages: a Gambian isolate, from a patient with neurologic acquired immunodeficiency syndrome and a highly divergent Ghanian isolate. Proc Natl Acad Sci U S A 1989; 86:2383–2387.

31. Levy JA. Pathogenesis of human immunodeficiency virus infection. Microbiol Rev 1993; 57:183–289.

32. Valentin A, Lu WH, Rosati M, Schneider R, Albert J, Karlsson A, Pavlakis GN. Dual effect of interleukin 4 on HIV-1 expression: implications for viral phenotypic switch and disease progression. Proc Natl Acad Sci U S A 1998; 95 (15):8886–8891.

33. Louwagie J, McCutchan F, Mascola J, Eddy G, Fransen K, Peeters M, Van der Groen G, Burke D. Genetic subtypes of HIV-1. AIDS Res Hum Retroviruses 1993; (suppl 1):147S–150S.

34. McCutchan F, Louwagie J, Eddy G, Van der Groen G, Piot P, Myers G, Burke D. Identification of multiple genetic subtypes of HIV-1 and evidence for geographic dispersal. J Acquired Immune Defic Syndr Hum Retrovirol 1993; 6(6):685–685.

35. Gürtler LG, Hauser PH, Eberle J, Von Brunn A, Knapp S, Zekeng L, Tsague JM, Kaptue L. A new subtype of human immunodeficiency virus type 1 (MVP-5180) from Cameroon. J Virol 1994; 68:1581–1585.

36. Ou CY, Takebe Y, Weniger BG. Independent introduction of two major HIV-1 genotypes into distinct high-risk populations in Thailand. The Lancet 1993; 341:1171–1174.

37. Grez M, Dietrich U, Balfe P, Von Briesen H, Maniar JK, Mahambre G, Delwart EL, Mullins JI, Rübsamen-Waigmann H. Genetic analysis of human immunodeficiency virus type 1 and 2 (HIV-1 and HIV-2) mixed infections in India reveals a recent spread of HIV-1 and HIV-2 from a single ancestor for each of these viruses. J Virol 1994; 68:2161–2168.

38. Dietrich U, Grez M, Von Briesen H, Panhas B, Geissendörfer M, Kuhnel H, Maniar J, Mahambre G, Becker WB, Becker MLB, Rubsamen-Waigmann H. HIV-1 strains

from India are highly divergent from prototypic African and United States European strains, but linked to a South African isolate. AIDS 1993; 7(1):23–27.

39. Rübsamen-Waigmann H, Von Briesen H, Holmes H, Björndal A, Körber B, Esser R, Ranjbar S, Tomlinson P, Galvao-Castro B, Karita E, Sempala S, Wasi C, Osmanov S, Fenyö EM, Belsey EM, Heyward W, Esparza J, Vandeperre P, Tugume B, Biryahwaho B, Grez M, Newberry A, Bradac J, McCutchan F, Louwagie J, Hegerich P, Lopezgalindez C, Olivares I, Dopazo J, Mullins JI, Delwart EL, Bachmann HM, Goudsmit J, Dewolf F, Hanh BH, Gao F, Yue L, Saragosti S, Schochetman G, Kalish M, Luo CC, George R, Pau CP, Weber J, Cheingsongpopov R, Kaleebu P, Nara P, Albert J, Myers G. Standard conditions of virus isolation reveal biological variability of HIV-1 in different regions of the world. AIDS Res Hum Retroviruses 1994; 10 N11:1345–1353.

40. Couturie E, Damond F, Rogues P, Fleury H, Barin F, Brunet JB, Brun-Vezinet F, Simon F. HIV-1 diversity in France, 1996–1998. J Infect Dis 2000; 181:470–475.

40a. Weidle PJ, Ganea CE, Irwin KL, Pieniazek D, McGowan JP, Olivio N, Ramos A, Schable C, Lal RB, Holmberg SD, Ernst JA. Presence of human immunodeficiency virus (HIV) type 1, group M, non-B subtypes, Bronx, New York. J Acquir Immune Defic Syndr Hum Retroviral 1998; 18:260–269.

40b. Dietrich U, Ruppach H, Gehring S, Knechten H, Knickmann M, Jäger H, Wolf E, Husak R, Orfanos CE, Brede HD, Rübsamen-Waigmann H, Von Briesen H. Large proportion of non-B HIV-1 subtypes and presence of zidovudine resistance mutations among German seroconvertors. AIDS 1997; 11(12):1532–1533.

41. Rübsamen-Waigmann H, von Briesen H, Maniar JK, Rao PK, Scholz C, Pfützner A. Spread of HIV-2 in India. Lancet 1991; 337(3):550–551.

42. Van der Ende ME, Schutten M, Ly TD, Gruters RA, Osterhaus ADME. HIV-2 infection in 12 European residents: virus characteristics and disease progression. AIDS 1996; 10(14):1649–1655.

43. Rübsamen-Waigmann H, Adamski M, Von Briesen H, Biesert L, Mix D, Unkelbach U, Heusler H, Groener J, Gallenkamp U, Böhm E, Tan KH, Gulotta F. Lethal progressive multifocal leukoencephalopathy in a HIV-2 infected person as the only AIDS manifestation. AIDS-Forschung (AIFO) 1987; 10:572–575.

44. Dietrich U, Adamski M, Kreutz R, Seipp A, Kühnel H, Rübsamen-Waigmann H. A highly divergent HIV-2 related isolate. Nature (London) 1989; 342:948–950.

45. Rayfield M, De CK, Heyward W, Goldstein L, Krebs J, Kwok S, Lee S, McCormick J, Moreau JM, Odehouri K, i.e. Mixed human immunodeficiency virus (HIV) infection in an individual: demonstration of both HIV type 1 and type 2 proviral sequences by using polymerase chain reaction. J Infect Dis 1988; 158:1170–1176.

46. Evans LA, Moreau J, Odehouri K, Seto D, Thomson-Honnebier G, Legg H, Barboza A, Cheng-Mayer C, Levy JA. Simultaneous isolation of HIV-1 and HIV-2 from an AIDS patient. Lancet 1988; 2:1389–1391.

47. Takehisa J, Zekeng L, Miura T, Ido E, Yamashita M, Mboudjeka I, Gürtler L, Hayami M, Kaptue L. Triple HIV-1 infection with group O and group M of different clades in a single cameroonian AIDS patient. J Acquir Immune Defic Syndr Hum Retrovirol 1997; 14:81–82.

48. Diaz RS, Sabino EC, Mayer A, Mosley JW, Busch MP. Dual human immunodeficiency virus type 1 infection and recombination in a dually exposed transfusion recipient. The Transfusion Safety Study Group 1995; 69:3273–3281.

49. Sabino EC, Shpaer EG, Morgado MG, Korber BT, Diaz RS, Bongertz V, Cavalcante S, Galvao-Castro B, Mullins JI, Mayer A. Identification of human immunodeficiency virus type 1 envelope genes recombinant between subtypes B and F in two epidemiologically linked individuals from Brazil. J Virol 1994; 68:6340–6346.

50. Gao F, Yue L, Robertson DL, Hill SC, Hui HX, Biggar RJ, Neequaye AE, Whelan TM, Ho DD, Shaw GM, Sharp PM, Hahn BH. Genetic diversity of human immunodeficiency virus type 2—evidence for distinct sequence subtypes with differences in virus biology. J Virol 1994; 68:7433–7447.

51. Dalgliesh AG, Beverley PCL, Clapham PR, Crawford DH, Greaves MF, Weiss RA. The CD4 (T4) antigen is an essential component of the receptor for the AIDS retrovirus. Nature 1984; 312:763–766.

52. Klatzmann D, Champagne E, Chamaret S, Gruest J, Guétard D, Hercend T, Gluckman JC, Montagnier L. T-lymphocyte T4 molecule behaves as the receptor for human retrovirus LAV. Nature 1984; 312:767–768.

53. Broder CC, Dimitrov DS, Blumenthal R, Berger EA. The block to HIV-1 envelope glycoprotein mediated membrane fusion in animal cells expressing human CD4 can be overcome by human cell components. Virol 1993; 193:483–491.

54. Cheseboro B, Buller R, Portis J, Wehrly K. Failure of human immunodeficiency virus entry and infection in CD4-positive human brain and skin cells. J Virol 1990; 64:215–221.

55. Harrington RD, Geballe AP. Cofactor requirement for human immunodeficiency virus type 1 entry into a CD4-expressing human cell line. J Virol 1993; 67:5939–5947.

56. Feng Y, Broder CC, Kennedy PE, Bergher EA. HIV-1 entry cofactor: functional cDNA cloning of a seven-transmembrane domain, G-protein coupled receptor. Science 1996; 272:872–877.

57. Alkhatib G, Combadiere C, Broder CC, Feng Y, Kennedy PE, Murphy PM, Berger EA. CC-CKR5: a RANTES, MIP-1alpha, MIP-1beta receptor as a fusion cofactor for macrophage-tropic HIV-1. Science 1996; 272:1955–1958.

58. Amara A, Gall SL, Schwartz O, Salamero J, Montes M, Loetscher P, Baggilioni M, Virelitzier JL, Arenzana-Seisdedos F. HIV coreceptor downregulation as antiviral principle: SDF-1α-dependent internalization of the chemokine receptor CXCR4 contributes to inhibition of HIV-replication. J Exp Med 1997; 186(1):139–146.

59. Aramori I, Zhang J, Ferguson SG, Bieniasz PD, Cullen BR, Caron MG. Molecular mechanism of desensitization of chemokine receptor CCR5: receptor signalling and internalization are dissociable from its role as an HIV-coreceptor. EMBO J 1997; 16(15):4604–4616.

60. Cocci F, Devico AL, Garzinodemo A, Arya SK, Gallo RC, Lusso P. Indentification of RANTES, MIP-1 alpha and MIP-1 beta as the major HIV-suppressive factors produced by CD8+ T-cells. Science 1995; 270:1811–1815.

61. Mizutani S, Temin HM. RNA-dependent DNA polymerase in virions of Rous sarcoma virus. Nature 1970; 226:1211–1213 and Baltimore D. RNA-dependent DNA polymerase in virions of RNA tumor viruses. Nature 1970; 226:1209–1211.

62. Skalka AM, Goff SP. Reverse Transcriptase. Cold Spring Harbor, NY: Cold Spring Harbor Laboratory Press, 1993:492.

63. Moelling K, Bolognesi DP, Bauer H, Büsen W, Plassmann HW, Hausen P. Association of the viral reverse transcriptase with an enzyme degrading the RNA moiety of

RNA-DNA hybrids. Nature New Biology 1971; 234:240–243. Comparative Leukemia Research. Bibl Haematol 1973; 39:536–550. And in: Selected Papers in Tumor Virology. Tooze J, Sambrook J, eds. Cold Spring Harbor, NY: Cold Spring Harbor Laboratory Press 1974:815–818.

64. Hansen J, Schulze T, Mellert W, Moelling K. Identification and characterization of HIV-specific RNase H by monoclonal antibody. EMBO J 1988; 7:239–243.

65. Le Grice SFJ. Human immunodeficiency virus reverse transcriptase. In: Skalka AM, Goff SP, eds. Reverse transcriptase. Cold Spring Harbor, NY: Cold Spring Harbor Laboratory Press, 1993:163–191.

66. Hostomsky Z, Hostomska Z, Hudson GO, Woomaw EW, Modes BR. Reconstitution in vitro of RNase H activity by using purified N-terminal and C-terminal domains of human immunodeficiency virus type 1 reverse transcriptase. Proc Natl Acad Sci U S A 1991; 88:1148–1152.

67. Le Grice SFJ, Naas T, Wohlgensinger B, Schatz O. Subunit-selective mutagenesis indicates minimal polymerase activity in heterodimer-associated p51 HIV-1 reverse transcriptase. EMBO J 1991; 10:3905–3911.

68. Maier G, Dietrich U, Panhans B, Schröder B, Rübsamen-Waigmann H, Cellai L, Hermann T, Heumann H. Mixed reconstitution of mutated subunits of HIV-1 reverse transcriptase coexpressed in *Escherichia coli*—two tags tie it up. Eur J Biochem 1999; 261:10–18.

69. Kohlstaedt LA, Wang JM, Friedman JM, Rice PA, Steitz TA. Crystal structure at 3.5 A-resolution of HIV-1 reverse transcriptase complexed with an inhibitor. Science 1992; 256:1783–1790.

70. Kohlstaedt LA, Wang JM, Friedman JM, Rice PA, Steitz TA. The structure of HIV-1 reverse transcriptase. In: Skalka AM,Goff SP, eds. Reverse Transcriptase. Cold Spring Harbor, NY: Cold Spring Harbor Laboratory Press, 1993:223–249.

71. Gazzard BG. Efavirenz in the management of HIV infection. Int J Clin Pract 1999; 53(1):60–64.

72. De Clercq E. Perspectives of non-nucleoside reverse transcriptase inhibitors (NNR-TIs) in the therapy of HIV-1 infection. FARMACO 1999; 54(1-2):26–45.

73. Rübsamen-Waigmann H, Huguenel E, Paessens A, Kleim JP, Wainberg MA, Shah A. Second generation non-nucleosidic reverse transcriptase inhibitor HBY 097 and HIV-1 viral load. Lancet 1997; 9064:1517.

74. Kleim JP, Winkler I, Rösner M, Kirsch R, Rübsamen-Waigmann H, Paessens A, Riess G. In vitro selection for different mutational patterns in the HIV-1 reverse transcriptase using high and low selective pressure of the non-nucleoside reverse transcriptase inhibitor HBY 097. Virology 1997; 231:112–118.

75. Rübsamen-Waigmann H, Huguenel E, Shah A, Paessens A, Ruoff HJ, von Briesen H, Immelmann A, Dietrich U, Wainberg MA. Resistance mutations selected in vivo under therapy with anti-HIV drug HBY 097 differ from resistance pattern selected in vitro. Antiviral Res 1999; 42:15–24.

76. Coffin JM. Genetic diversity and evolution of retroviruses. Curr Top Microbiol Immunol 1992; 176:143–164.

77. Williams KJ, Loeb LA. Retroviral reverse transcriptase: error frequencies and mutagenesis. Curr Top Microbiol Immunol 1992; 176:165–180.

78. Bebenek K, Abbotts J, Roberts JD, Wilson SH, Kunkel TA. Specificity and mecha-

nism of error-prone replication by human immunodeficiency virus-1 reverse transcriptase. J Biol Chem 1989; 264:16948–16956.

79. Preston BD, Poiez BJ, Loeb L. Fidelity of HIV-1 reverse transcriptase. Science 1988; 242:1168–1171.

80. Roberts JD, Bebenek K, Kunkel TA. The accuracy of reverse transcriptase from HIV-1. Science 1988; 242:1171.

81. Roberts JD, Preston BD, Johnston LA, Soni A, Loeb LA, Kunkel TA. Fidelity of two retroviral reverse transcriptases during DNA-dependent DNA synthesis in vitro. Mol Cell Biol 1989; 9:469–476.

82. La Femina RL, Callahan PL, Cordingley MG. Substrate specificity of recombinant human immunodeficiency virus integrase protein. J Virol 1991; 65:624–630.

83. Stevenson M, Haggerty S, Lamonica CA, Meier CM, Welch S-K, Wasiak AJ. Integration is not necessary for expression of human immunodeficiency virus type 1 protein products. J Virol 1990; 64:2421–2425.

84. Wiskerchen M, Muesing MA. Human immunodeficiency virus type 1 integrase: effects of mutations on viral ability to integrate, direct viral gene expression from unintegrated viral DNA templates, and sustain viral propagation in primary cells. J Virol 1995; 69:376–386.

85. Goff SP. Genetics of retroviral integration. Annu Rev Genet 1992; 26:527–544.

86. Dyda F, Hickman AD, Jenkins TM, Engelman A, Craigie R, Davies DR. Crystal structure of the catalytic domain of HIV-1 integrase: similarity to other polynucleotide transferase. Science 1994; 266:1981–1986.

87. Vincent KA, Ellison V, Chow SA, Brown PO. Characterization of human immunodeficiency virus type 1 integrase expressed in *Escherichia coli* and analysis of variants with amino-terminal mutations. J Virol 1993; 67:425–437.

88. Engelman A, Mizuuchi K, Craigie R. HIV-1 DNA integration: mechanism of viral DNA cleavage and DNA strand transfer. Cell 1991; 67:1211–1221.

89. Sherman PA, Fyfe JA. Human immunodeficiency virus integration protein expressed in *Escherichia coli* possesses selective DNA cleaving ability. Proc Natl Acad Sci U S A 1990; 87:5119–5123.

90. Hazuda DJ, Felock P, Witmer M, Wolfe A, Stillmock K, Grobler JA, Espeseth A, Gabryelsk L, Schleif W, Blau C, Miller MD. Inhibitors of strand transfer that prevent integration and inhibit HIV-1 replication in cells. Science 2000; 287:646–650.

91. Kohl NE, Emini EA, Schleif WA, Davis LJ, Heimbach JC, Dixon RA, Scolnick EM, Sigal IS. Active human immunodeficiency virus protease is required for viral infectivity. Proc Natl Acad Sci U S A 1988; 85:4686–4690.

92. Loeb DD, Swanstrom R, Everitt L, Manchester M, Stamper SE, Hutchison CA. Complete mutagenesis of the HIV-1 protease. Nature 1989; 340:397–400.

93. Katz RA, Skalka AM. The retroviral enzymes. Annu Rev Biochem 1994; 63:133–173.

94. Loeb DD, Hutchinson CA, Edgell MH, Farmerie WG, Swanstrom R. Mutational analysis of human immunodeficiency virus type 1 protease suggests functional homology with aspartic proteases. J Virol 1989; 63:111–121.

95. Kempf DJ. Design of symmetry-based, peptidomimetic inhibitors of human immunodeficiency virus protease. In: Kuo LC, Shafer JA, eds. Retroviral Proteases. San Diego: Academic Press, 1994:334–354.

96. Vaca P. Design of tight-binding human immunodeficiency virus type 1 protease inhibitor. In: Kuo LC, Shafer JA, eds. Retroviral proteases. San Diego: Academic Press, 1994:311–334.
97. Car A, Samaras K, Chisholm DJ, Cooper DA. Pathogenesis of HIV-1 protease inhibitor-associated peripheral lipodystrophy, hyperlipidaemia, and insulin resistance. Lancet 1998; 351:1881–1883.
98. Cullen BR. Regulation of HIV gene expression. AIDS 1995; 9:19–32.
99. Kao S-Y, Calman AF, Luciw PA, Peterlin BM. Antitermination of transcription within the long terminal repeat of HIV-1 by tat gene product. Nature 1987; 330:489–493.
100. Yang X, Herrmann CH, Rice AP. The human immunodeficiency virus tat proteins specifically associate with TAK in vivo and require the carboxyl-terminal domain of RNA polymerase II for function. J Virol 1996; 70:4576–4584.
101. Zhu Y, Pe'ery T, Peng J, Ramanathan Y, Marshall N, Marshall T, Amendt B, Mathews MB, Price DH. Transcription elongation factor P-TEFb is required for HIV-1 tat transactivation in vitro. Genes Dev 1997; 11:2622–2632.
102. Wei P, Garber ME, Fang S-M, Fischer WH, Jones KA. A novel CDK9-associated C-type cyclin interacts directly with HIV-1 tat and mediates its high-affinity, loop-specific binding to TAR RNA. Cell 1998; 92:451–462.
103. Malim MH, Hauber J, Le S-Y, Maizel JV, Cullen BR. The HIV-1 rev trans-activator acts through a structured target sequence to activate nuclear export of unspliced viral mRNA. Nature 1989; 338:254–257.
104. Fisher U, Huber J, Boelens WC, Mattaj IW, Lührmann R. The HIV-1 Rev activation domain is a nuclear export signal that accesses an export pathway used by specific cellular RNAs. Cell 1995; 82:475–483.
105. Kestler HW, Ringler DJ, Mori K, Panicali DL, Sehgall PK, Daniel MD, Desrosiers RC. Importance of the nef gene for maintenance of high virus loads and for development of AIDS. Cell 1991; 65:651–662.
106. Aiken C, Konner J, Landau NR, Lenburg ME, Trono D. Nef induces CD4 endocytosis: requirement for a critical dileucine motif in the membrane-proximal CD4 cytoplasmic domain. Cell 1994; 76:853–864.
107. Le Gall S, Erdtmann L, Benichou S, Berlioz-Torrent C, Liu L, Benarous R, Heard J-M, Schwartz O. Nef interacts with the μ subunit of clathrin adaptor complexes and reveals a cryptic sorting signal in MHC I molecules. Immunity 1998; 8:483–495.
108. Greenberg ME, Iafrate AJ, Skowronski J. The SH3 domain-binding surface and an acidic motif in HIV-1 Nef regulate trafficking of class I MHC complexes. EMBO J 1998; 17:2777–2789.
109. Collins KL, Chen Bk, Kalams SA, Walker BD, Baltimore D. HIV-1 Nef protein protects infected primary cells against killing by cytotoxic T-lymphocytes. Nature 1998; 391:397–401.
110. Saksela K, Cheng G, Baltimore D. Proline-rich (PxxP) motifs in HIV-1 Nef bind to SH3 domains of a subset of Src kinases and are required for the enhanced growth of Nef⁺ viruses but not for down-regulation of CD4. EMBO J 1995; 14:484–491.
111. Karn T, Hock B, Holtrich U, Adamski M, Strebhardt K, Rübsamen-Waigmann H. Nef proteins of distinct HIV-1 or -2 isolates differ in their binding properties for HCK: isolation of a novel Nef binding factor with characteristics of an adaptor protein. Virology 1998; 246:45–52.

112. Salghetti S, Mariani R, Skowronski J. Human immunodeficiency virus type 1 Nef and p56^{lck} protein-tyrosine kinase interact with a common element in CD4 cytoplasmic tail. Proc Natl Acad Sci U S A 1995; 92:349–353.

113. Sawai ET, Khan IH, Montbriand PM, Peterlin BM, Cheng-Mayer C, Luciw PA. Activation of PAK by HIV and SIV Nef: Importance for Aids in rhesus macaques. Curr Biol 1996; 6:1519–1527.

114. Xu XN, Laffert B, Screaton GR, Kraft M, Wolf D, Kolanus W, Mongkolsapay J, McMichael AJ, Baur AS. Induction of Fas ligand expression by HIV involves the interaction of Nef with the T-cell receptor zeta chain. J Exp Med 1999; 189 (9):1489–1496.

114a. Fackler OT, Luo W, Geyer M, Alberts AS, Peterlin BM. Activation of Vav by Nef induces cytoskeletal rearrangements and downstream effector functions. Mol Cell 1999; 3(6):729–739.

115. Kann NC, Franchini G, Wong-Staal F, Du Bois GC, Robey WG, Lautenberger JA, Papas TS. Identification of HTLV-III/LAV sor gene product and detection of antibodies in human sera. Science 1986; 231:1553–1555.

116. Lee TH, Coligan JE, Allan JS, McLane MF, Groopman JE, Essex M. A new HTLV-III/Lav protein encoded by a gene found in cytopathic retroviruses. Science 1986; 231:1546–1549.

117. Sodroski JG, Goh WC, Rosen CA, Tarter A, Portetelle D, Burny A, Haseltine WA. Replication and cytopathic potential of HTLV-III/LAV with sor gene deletions. Science 1986; 231:1549–1553.

118. Fisher AG, Ensoli B, Ivanoff I, Chamberlain M, Petteway S, Ratner L, Gallo RC, Wong-Staal F. The sor gene of HIV-1 is required for efficient virus transmission in vitro. Science 1987; 237:888–893.

119. Strebel K, Daugherty D, Cohen D, Folks T, Martin M. The HIV "A" (sor) gene product is essential for virus infectivity. Nature 1987; 328:728–730.

120. Hoglund S, Ofverstedt L-G, Nilsson A, Lundquist P, Gelderblom H, Ozel M, Skoglund U. Spatial visualization of the maturing HIV-1 core and its linkage to the envelope. AIDS Res Hum Retroviruses 1992; 8:1–7.

121. Myers G, Korber B, Wain-Hobson S, Jeang KT, Henderson LE, Pavlakis GN. Human retroviruses and AIDS. A compilation and analysis of nucleic acid and amino acid sequences. Los Alamos, NM: Los Alamos National Laboratory, 1994.

122. Clements JE, Wong-Staal F. Molecular biology of lentiviruses. Semin Virol 1992; 3: 137–146.

123. Garrett ED, Tiley LS, Cullen BR. Rev activates expression of the human immunodeficiency virus type 1 vif and vpr gene products. J Virol 1991; 65:1653–1657.

124. Schwartz S, Felber BK, Pavlakis GN. Expression of human immunodeficiency virus type 1 vif and vpr mRNA is rev-dependent and regulated by splicing. Virology 1991; 183:677–686.

125. Paxton W, Connor RI, Landau NR. Incorporation of Vpr into human immunodeficiency virus type 1 virions: requirement for the p6 region of gag and mutational analysis. J Virol 1993; 67:7229–7237.

126. Heinzinger NK, Bukrinsky MI, Haggerty SA, Ragland AM, Kewalramani V, Lee M-A, Gendelman HE, Ratner L, Stevenson M, Emerman M. The Vpr protein of human immunodeficiency virus type 1 influences nuclear localization of viral nucleic acids in nondividing host cells. Proc Natl Acad Sci U S A 1994; 91:7311–7315.

127. Vodicka MA, Koepp DM, Silver PA, Emerman M. HIV-1 Vpr interacts with the nuclear transport pathway to promote macrophage infection. Genes Dev 1998; 12:175–185.

128. Ree F, Braaten D, Franke EK, Luban J. Human immunodeficiency virus type 1 Vpr arrests the cell cycle in G_2 by inhibiting the activation of p34^{cdc2}-cyclin B. J Virol 1995; 69:6859–6864.

129. Willey RL, Maldarelli F, Martin MA, Strebel K. Human immunodeficiency virus type 1 Vpu protein induces rapid degradation of CD4. J Virol 1992; 66:7193–7200.

130. Margottin F, Mour SP, Durand H, Selig L, Benichou S, Richard V, Thomas D, Strebel K, Benarous R. A novel human WD protein, h-βTrCP, that interacts with HIV-1 Vpu connects CD4 to the ER degradation pathway through an F-box motif. Mol Cell 1998; 1:565–574.

131. Rosenwirth B, Billich A, Datema R, Donatsch P, Hammerschmid F, Harrison R, Hiestand P, Jaksche H, Mayer P, Peichl P, Quesniaux V, Schatz F, Schuurmann HJ, Traber R, Wenger R, Wolff B, Zenke G, Zurini M. Inhibition of human immunodeficiency virus type 1 replication by SDZ NIM 811, a nonimmunosuppressive cyclosporine analog. Antimicrob Agents Chemother 1994; 38:1763–1772.

132. Franke EK, Yuan HEH, Luban J. Specific incorporation of cyclophilin A into HIV-1 virions. Nature 1994; 372:359–362.

133. Thali M, Bukovsky A, Kondo E, Rosenwirth B, Walsh CT, Sodroski J, Gottlinger HG. Functional association of cyclophilin A with HIV-1 virions. Nature 1994; 372:363–365.

134. Rice WG, Supko JG, Malspeis L, Buckheit RW, Clanton D, Bu M, Graham L, Schaeffer CA, Turpin JA, Domagala J, Gogliotti R, Bader JP, Halliday SM, Coren L, Sowder RC, Arthur LO, Henderson LE. Inhibitors of HIV nucleocapsid protein zinc fingers as candidates for the treatment of AIDS. Science 270:1194–1197.

2
Antiretroviral Treatment of HIV Infection

Stefan Mauss
HIV-Specialized Practice, Düsseldorf, Germany

Hans Jäger
KIS—Curatorium for Immunodeficiency, Munich, Germany

I. INTRODUCTION

Since 1995, a dramatic change in the incidence of human immunodeficiency virus (HIV)-associated diseases and deaths has occurred (Fig. 1). This change is due to the introduction of new antiretroviral medicaments, particularly the HIV protease inhibitors, and the introduction of antiretroviral combination regimens in clinical practice (1–3). In addition, a new instrument for monitoring the efficacy of individual treatment, the HIV viral load assay, became widely available. This chapter gives an overview of the clinically available antiretroviral agents and current treatment strategies, starting with data from monotherapy trials, which reflect optimal safety and efficacy for a specific medicament. However, monotherapy can no longer be considered as the standard of care for HIV infection. Following the presentation of individual agents, current treatment strategies are discussed.

II. INHIBITORS OF REVERSE TRANSCRIPTASE

Dosages, dose adjustments, and interactions of nucleoside reverse transcriptase inhibitors and nonnucleoside reverse transcriptase inhibitors are shown in Tables 1 and 2.

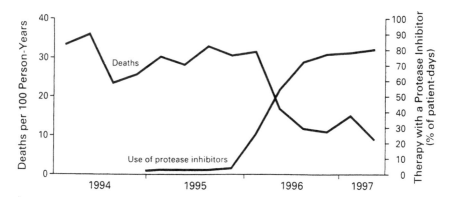

Figure 1 Mortality rate in a cohort of 1255 HIV- seropositive patients with less than 100 CD4+ cells/mm^3 and the frequency of use of protease inhibitors. (From Ref. 3.)

A. Zidovudine (Azidothymidine)

Studies conducted in 1987 demonstrated that zidovudine, the first antiretroviral agent, at a dose of 1500 mg per day was able to reduce the frequency of HIV-associated diseases and deaths in HIV-positive patients with acquired immunodeficiency syndrome (AIDS)-related complex of AIDS (4). However, this beneficial effect was accompanied by considerable side effects (5); in about one third of the patients, severe anemia or leukopenia developed, and approximately half reported nausea or headache.

Consequently, subsequent studies with zidovudine had two aims: the first to reduce the dose of zidovudine to diminish the incidence of side effects and the second to assess whether HIV-positive patients with less advanced disease would benefit from treatment. In 1990, two studies were published showing that a dose of 1200 mg (6) and even 500 mg per day (7) was as effective as higher doses. The same studies tested the efficacy of zidovudine in patients with less advanced disease: AIDS-related complex (6), asymptomatic HIV infection (7), and moderate cellular immunosuppression. The observation period in both studies was approximately 2 years. During this period, a reduction in the frequency of HIV-associated diseases but not deaths was observed. This effect could only be demonstrated for HIV-positive patients with less than 500 CD4+ cells/μL. These studies led to the recommendation in the United States that minor symptomatic or asymptomatic HIV-positive patients with less than 500 CD4+ cells/μL should be given zidovudine monotherapy.

In the following years, two important studies stimulated a vivid controversy about the role of zidovudine monotherapy in the treatment of HIV infection. Both studies compared an immediate treatment with zidovudine with a deferred therapy following the occurrence of an HIV-associated disease or an immunological progression. In the first study from 1992 (8), mildly symptomatic HIV-positive patients with 200 to 500 CD4+ cells were treated with a high-dose regimen of zidovudine (1500 mg per day) either immediately following the occurrence of an AIDS-defining event or after a decrease in CD4+ cells below 200/μL while receiving placebo. After an observation period of 4 years, the group receiving immediate zidovudine treatment demonstrated a significant benefit with regard to the incidence of HIV-associated diseases but not with regard to number of deaths. These results were in contrast to the outcome of the European Concorde study (9). The Concorde study had essentially the same design as the American study except that the dosage of zidovudine was 1000 mg per day. The observation period in this study was 3.5 years. Only during the first year did a trend in favor of the immediate treatment group seem to exist, although no statistical significance was reached. The effect vanished in the second and third year of the study. In addition, a small but durable increase in CD4+ cells over the whole study period in the immediately treated group was not translated into clinical benefit. Thus, the value of CD4+ cells as a predictor of treatment success was brought into question. Retrospectively, it is clear that the overall increase in the CD4+ cells was too low to change the natural course of the HIV infection.

The results from the Concorde and the Australian-European study (10), which assessed the efficacy of zidovudine monotherapy in asymptomatic patients with more than 500 CD4 cells, led to the conclusion that zidovudine monotherapy was only beneficial over a limited period of about 1 year. The HIV-positive patients with less advanced disease showed a reduction only in morbidity of AIDS-defining diseases, not in mortality rate.

The main side effects of zidovudine are headache, nausea, anemia, neutropenia, and a rarely occurring myopathy caused by interference with mitochondrial metabolism.

The oral bioavailability is 60%. It is metabolized to azidothymidine-glucoronide in the liver and excreted renally. The penetration in the cerebrospinal fluid is approximately 50% of the serum concentration; the intracellular half-life is 3 hours. Mutations associated with in vitro resistance are at codons 41, 67, 70, 151, 215, 219 of the reverse transcriptase. The codon 215 mutation was shown to be associated with a negative clinical outcome (11–13).

B. Didanosine (ddI)

After initial studies investigating safety and tolerance of didanosine (ddI) (14–16), a comparative study between didanosine and zidovudine was conducted (17) in antiretroviral naive patients. The mortality rate in the didanosine group was about 30% higher than that in the group receiving zidovudine monotherapy. This finding is in contrast with the result of the ACTG 175 study in which didanosine was shown to have at least the same clinical efficacy as zidovudine monotherapy (18).

The next approach was the assessment of the efficacy of didanosine in zidovudine-treated patients. After a pretreatment period with zidovudine of at least 6 months, the patients were either switched to didanosine 500 mg per day or kept

Table 1 Dosages, Intake Requirements, and Drug Interactions of the Approved Nucleoside Reverse Transcriptase Inhibitors

Medicament	Trade name and manufacturer	Daily dosage	Intake modalities	Drug interactions
Abacavir (ABC)	Ziagen Glaxo Wellcome	2 × 1 tbl @ 300 mg	With or without food	Plasma level-↑ of methadone (+15%) ABC ↑ with ethanol (100 mg) (+41%)
Didanosine (ddI) Dideoxyinosine	Videx Bristol Myers Squibb	1 × 4 tbl @ 100 mg or 1 × 2 tbl @ 150 mg liquid (10 mg/ml): 1 × 40 mL	On an empty stomach (at least 2 hours after or ⅓ hour before a meal)	Increased risk of pancreatitis when coadministered with pentamidine intravenously or in patients with chronic alcoholism May increase neurotoxicity of isoniazide, vincristine, zalcitabine, stavudine Methadone inhibits uptake of didanosine by 60% Ganciclovir increases uptake of didanosine by 70%
Lamivudine (3TC) Dideoxy-3'-thiacytidine	Epivir Glaxo Wellcome	2 × 1 tbl @ 150 mg	With or without food	Not in combination with zalcitabine (inhibition of phosphorylation)
Stavudine (d4T) Didehydro-dideoxythymidine	Zerit Bristol Myers Squibb	2 × 1 caps ≦ 60 kg: @ 30 mg > 60 kg: @ 40 mg	With or without food	May increase neurotoxicity of didanosine, zalcitabine, isoniazide, vincristine Not in combination with zidovudine (inhibition of phosphorylation of stavudine)

Zalcitabine (ddC) Dideoxycytidine	Hivid	Hoffman-La Roche	3 × 1 tbl @ 0.75 mg	With or without food	May increase neurotoxicity of didanosine, stavudine, isoniazide, vincristine, dapsone. Not in combination with lamivudine (inhibition of phosphorylation)
Zidovudine (ADV) Azidothymidine (AZT)	Retrovir	Glaxo Wellcome	2 × 1 caps @ 250–300 mg	With or without food	Increased bone marrow toxicity when coadministered with ganciclovir, doxorubicin, and other myelosuppressive medicaments. Not in combination with stavudine due to inhibition of phosphorylation of stavudine. Not in combination with ganciclovir due to inhibition of phosphorylation of zidovudine. In vitro antagonistic effects of ribavirin on antiretroviral efficacy of ZDV
Zidovudine + lamivudine (AZT + 3TC) (fixed combination)	Combivir	Glaxo Wellcome	2 × 1 tbl @ 300 mg AZT + 150 mg 3TC	With or without food	See zidovudine and lamivudine

Table 2 Dosages, Intake Requirements, and Drug Interactions of the Approved Nonnucleoside Reverse Transcriptase Inhibitors

Medicament	Trade name and manufacturer	Daily dosage	Intake modalities	Modified dosage in antiretroviral combination	Drug interactions
Delavirdine (DLV)	Rescriptor Pharmacia & Upjohn	3 × 4 tbl @ 100 mg	With or without food	With IDV DLV: no dose modification IDV: 3 × 600 mg With RTV no dose modification With SQV-hgc/sgc no dose modification With NFV DLV: 3 × 600 mg NFV: no dose modification	DLV ↓ with anticonvulsants (carbamazepine, phenobarbital, phenytoin), rifabutin or rifampicin for this combination not recommended DLV-absorption ↓ with H$_2$-receptor-antagonists (cimetidine, famotidine, nizatidine, ranitidine) Plasma level-↑ of saquinavir (.50%), IDV (+50%–100%), clarithromycine (≈ +100%), phenytoin, quinidine, dapsone, phenprocoumon, warfarin, trimethoprim, sulfamethoxazole, methadone Sildenafil levels may be increased Contraindications: tranquilizer/sedatives (benzodiazepines (alprazolam, midazolam, triazolam)), amphetamines, antihistamines (terfenadine, astemizole), anticonvulsants (carbamazepine, phenobarbital, phenytoin), calcium channel blockers (dihydropyridines), antiarrhythmics (amiodarone); prokinetics (cisapride); tuberculostatics (rifabutin, rifampicin)
Efavirenz (EFV)	Sustiva DuPont Pharma	1 × 3 caps @ 200 mg	With or without food, before bedtime	With IDV EFV: no dose modification IDV: 3 × 1000 mg	EFV ↑ with RTV (+ 21%), APV (+15%), fluconazole (+16%) EFV ↓ with rifampicine (−26%), FTV (−12%) Plasma level-↓ of IDV (−31%), FTV (−61%), APV (−36%), methadone

| Nevirapine (NVP) | Viramune Boehringer Ingelheim | 1 × 1 tbl for 14 days; thereafter 2 × 1 tbl @ 200 mg | With or without food | With IDV
NVP: no dose modification
IDV: 3 × 1000 mg
With RTV
no dose modification, no safety data
With NFV
no dose modification
Combination with SQV-hgc (INV) not recommended | NVP ↑ with cimetidine (+21%), macrolides (+12%)
Plasma level-↓ of IDV (−28%), SQV (−27%), ketoconazole (−63%), rifabutin (−16%), rifampicin (−37%), possibly of methadone, oral contraceptives
Alternative contraceptive methods recommended in addition to oral contraceptives
Contraindications: SQV-hgc (INV), ketoconazole |

With RTV
EFV: no dose modification
RTV: dose reduction may be necessary
Combination with SQV hard-gel capsule (hgc) (INV) and SQV soft-gel capsule (sgc) (FTV) as single PI not recommended

Clarithromycin: rash (about 50%) because of plasma level-↑ of active metabolites (+34%); alternative drug: azithromycin
Contraindications: sedatives (midazolam, triazolam), antihistamines (terfenadine, astemizole), prokinetics (cisapride), ergotamine derivatives

on zidovudine. The study participants were HIV-positive patients with AIDS-related complex and less than 300 CD4+ cells/μL or asymptomatic HIV-positive patients with less than 200 CD4+ cells/μL. In these patients, didanosine reduced the incidence of HIV-associated disease and mortality compared to zidovudine (19). The results of this study were corroborated by the findings of two identically designed studies (20,21). In both studies, the switch from zidovudine to didanosine resulted in fewer AIDS-defining events as compared with the groups continuing on zidovudine.

The main side effects of didanosine are nausea, dry mouth, an elevation in liver enzymes, and peripheral polyneuropathy. A rare but serious side effect is the occurrence of acute pancreatitis, the frequency being higher in patients with a history of pancreatitis. Acute abdominal pain in patients given didanosine should lead to prompt withdrawal of medication and the exclusion of acute pancreatitis.

To date, didanosine is available as a tablet, which can be chewed or dissolved in water. A powder-based solution that requires refrigerated storage is also approved for children.

The bioavailability of didanosine is 40%, and about 50% of the drug is excreted renally. Penetration into the cerebrospinal fluid is responsible for 20% of the serum concentration. It has a long intracellular half-life of 25 to 40 hours. Mutations associated with in vitro drug resistance are at codons 65, 74, 151, and 184 of the reverse transcriptase. There is partial in vitro cross-resistance to zalcitabine and lamivudine.

C.   Hydroxyurea and Didanosine

One option to increase the intracellular phosphorylation of didanosine is the concomitant administration of hydroxyurea, a drug approved for treatment of chronic myeloic leukemia. Treatment with hydroxyurea is thought to deplete the cellular nucleotide-3-phosphate pool and to improve the phosphorylation of nucleotide or nucleoside analogues especially from the purine type (22). In a placebo-controlled comparative study, hydroxyurea was able to achieve a greater reduction in viral load in combination with stavudine and didanosine compared to stavudine and didanosine as double combination treatment (23). However, at the end of the study period of 12 weeks, the increase in the CD4+ cell count in the double nucleoside combination group was higher than in the group receiving the combination with hydroxyurea because of the lymphopenic effects of the latter. In patients in the early stages of HIV-infection receiving a triple combination with stavudine and indinavir, the increase in the CD4+ cell count seems to be greater (24,25). This may be due to the initial higher CD4+ cell counts in these patients and to the additional use of an HIV protease inhibitor.

Hydroxurea itself has no effect on HIV replication (26). The main side effects of hydroxyurea are an increase in liver enzymes, myalgia, and lymphopenic leukopenia.

D. Zalcitabine (ddC)

At the same time that the first clinical endpoint study with didanosine was conducted, a study compared zalcitabine (ddC) with zidovudine as monotherapy for first line treatment in HIV infection (27). After 1 year, significantly more participants had died in the zalcitabine group. For this reason, zalcitabine was not considered a suitable first line treatment.

The efficacy of zalcitabine after at least 6 months of treatment with zidovudine was assessed in two other studies (28, 29). In contrast to didanosine, in neither trial could a benefit be shown for a switch from zidovudine to zalcitabine as compared to continuation of zidovudine therapy.

However, in patients with advanced disease and prolonged periods of zidovudine monotherapy, zalcitabine seemed to be at least as effective as didanosine (30). This study led to the approval of zalcitabine for antiretroviral treatment of zidovudine-pretreated patients.

Frequent side effects of zalcitabine are peripheral polyneuropathy, aphthous stomatitis, and nonallergic rash. The two latter conditions usually appear during the first weeks of treatment and can be treated without withdrawing therapy. Because there have been reports of liver failure in patients with chronic hepatitis B, such patients should not be given zalcitabine or should at least be closely monitored. In the case of peripheral polyneuropathy, zalcitabine must be stopped, particularly if the neurological examination indicates axonal neuropathy.

The oral bioavailability of zalcitabine is 85%. About 20% of the drug is excreted renally. Approximately 20% of the serum concentration is found in the cerebrospinal fluid. In vitro resistance is associated with mutations at codons 65, 69, 74, and 184 of the reverse transcriptase. Cross-resistance to ddI is reported from in vitro data.

E. Lamivudine

Lamivudine is a reverse transcriptase inhibitor with rapid development of resistance in monotherapy, resulting in swift loss of clinical efficacy (31,32). Resistance occurs at codon 184 of the reverse transcriptase gene and is found in almost all patients exposed to lamivudine. The 184 mutation results in a moderate in vitro cross-resistance to didanosine, abacavir, and zalcitabine.

In monotherapy, lamivudine was not considered a promising antiretroviral agent, but it has proven to be an effective partner in combination therapy. Its tolerability is extraordinarily good. Only few side effects can be attributed to lamivudine, consisting of rash, headache, nausea, or an increased frequency in leukopenia in combination with zidovudine.

The bioavailability of lamivudine is 85%. It is eliminated unchanged by way of renal excretion. The concentration in the cerebrospinal fluid is approximately 6% of the serum concentration. The intracellular half-life is 12 hours.

F. Stavudine

In a larger clinical trial, stavudine was compared with zidovudine monotherapy in zidovudine-pretreated patients. After only 7 weeks of zidovudine pretreatment, a switch to stavudine appeared to be beneficial, resulting in a more pronounced and longer lasting increase in the CD4+ cell count and a significant reduction in the frequency of AIDS-defining diseases and mortality (33–35). This trial led to the approval of stavudine as antiretroviral treatment for zidovudine-pretreated patients. More recent data from combination therapy trials with nucleoside reverse transcriptase inhibitors showing equivalence to zidovudine resulted in its approval for primary treatment of HIV infection.

The main side effect of stavudine is peripheral polyneuropathy, usually occurring after several months of treatment. Increased liver enzymes may also be observed.

The bioavailability of stavudine is 85%; about 50% is excreted renally. The concentration in the cerebrospinal fluid is about 10% to 40% of the serum concentration. The intracellular half life is 3.5 hours. Mutations associated with resistance in vitro are found at codons 50 and 75. The mutation at codon 75 confers in vitro to cross-resistance to didanosine, zalcitabine, and lamivudine.

G. Nevirapine

Nevirapine, a nonnucleoside reverse transcriptase inhibitor, was one of the first medicaments with antiretroviral activity to be tested in humans. However, as with lamivudine, within a few weeks, nevirapine led to a rapid development of resistance associated with a loss in clinical efficacy (36). Even in double combination with zidovudine or didanosine, efficacy was limited by the prompt appearance of resistance caused by one-step mutation at codon 106 or 181 of the reverse transcriptase gene (21,37). Only its use in triple combination (as discussed later) allowed this agent a place with drugs used for treatment of HIV infection (38,39).

The main side effect of nevirapine is the appearance of rashes, which are toxic in nature and can be reduced in frequency by initiating therapy with half the daily dose for the first 2 weeks. A few cases of Steven-Johnsons syndrome have been reported (40). Other side effects include anorexia, nausea, and hepatotoxic reactions. Because hepatic failure has been reported, a marked increase in alanine transaminase (ALT) or bilirubin should prompt therapy withdrawal.

The bioavailability of nevirapine is 90% and it is metabolized by the cytochrome P-450 system in the liver. Its concentration in the cerebrospinal fluid is about 45% of the serum level.

Mutations associated with resistance to nevirapine in vitro are described at codons 103, 106, 108, 181, 188, and 190 of the reverse transcriptase. In vitro cross-resistance to delavirdine and efavirenz exists.

H. Delavirdine

Delavirdine is a nonnucleoside transcriptase inhibitor. It has never been extensively studied as monotherapy. Its only indication is in combination therapy with other antiretroviral agents, as discussed later. The main side effects of delavirdine include rashes, sometimes severe, nausea, loss of appetite, insomnia, and strange dreams.

The bioavailability of delavirdine is 60% to 80%, and it is metabolized by the hepatic cytochrome P-450 system. The concentration in the cerebrospinal fluid is 0.5% of the serum concentration. Mutations of the reverse transcriptase associated with in vitro resistance are at codons 103, 181, and 236. In vitro cross-resistance to nevirapine and efavirenz exists.

I. Efavirenz (DMP 266)

Efavirenz is another nonnucleoside transcriptase inhibitor that was approved in 1998. In studies using dosages ranging from 200 to 600 mg per day, efavirenz achieved a marked reduction in HIV viral load during the first weeks and an increase in the CD4+ cell count equivalent to that seen with protease inhibitors. In a direct comparison over a period of 48 weeks, efavirenz in combination with zidovudine and lamivudine achieved as least as favorable results (CD4+ cell count, HIV-RNA) as the combination containing indinavir (41). As known with other agents of this class, resistance develops by a one-step mutation at codon 103 and less frequently at codons 188 and 190 (42). Monotherapy experience with efavirenz is limited to a study period of 12 weeks, in which efavirenz-resistant HIV strains developed in the first patients.

One of the main side effects of evafirenz is dizziness; therefore, it is recommended that the once daily dosage be taken before retiring. In addition, rashes, usually mild, are seen in a considerable number of patients. More severe cutaneous reactions have also been reported (43,44).

J. Abacavir (1592U89)

A recently approved agent for first line treatment of HIV-positive patients is the nucleoside reverse transcriptase inhibitor abacavir. In a monotherapy trial over 12 weeks, abacavir achieved a marked viral load reduction of almost 2 logs, which is comparable to the results reported from HIV protease inhibitors (45). All other studies with abacavir were designed as combination therapy trials. Recently, reported trials showed a strong initial effect on viral load and CD4+ cell count for the triple nucleoside reverse transcriptase inhibitor combination of abacavir plus zidovudine plus lamivudine, which was sustained for 48 weeks (46–49).

In contrast to the impressive efficacy of abacavir in antiretroviral naive patients, the effect in HIV-positive patients given multiple nucleoside transcriptase inhibitors seems to be much reduced (50–52). In the compassionate use program, only approximately 25% of the patients who started a new combination treatment including abacavir reached a viral load reduction greater than 0.5 log. The effect of abacavir is adversely correlated with the presence of phenotypically resistant viral isolates before treatment. In patients in whom a phenotypic resistance of more than eightfold was observed, no viral load reduction was reported. In those with a less than fourfold phenotypic resistance against abacavir, however, approximately 30% responded with a reduction in viral load of at least 0.5 log. Even in the positively selected population, the benefit of abacavir seems to be limited (50).

The most important side effect of abacavir is a hypersensitivity reaction with fever, nausea, elevated liver enzymes, and rash, with more than 90% of these events occurring during the first 6 weeks of treatment. It should be noted that rash does not appear consistently and may occur a few days after the onset of the other symptoms. Patients judged to be hypersensitive against abacavir should not be rechallenged, because shock and death have been reported in these patients. Other less severe side effects include nausea and headache.

K. Adefovir

Adefovir is a nucleotide analogue that was filed for approval in the United States in 1999, with a moderate effect on viral load in treatment-naive patients (53). Interestingly, it may have a stronger effect in patients in whom resistance to lamivudine or lamivudine plus zidovudine has already developed (54). These results, however, should be regarded with caution in that other trials do not support the role of adefovir in the therapy of pretreated patients (55,56). Adefovir depletes the body of carnitine, requiring a daily supplement of 500 mg (57). In addition, it causes a renotubular dysfunction, resulting in the loss of phosphate and bicarbonate in up to 40% of patients after 6 months of treatment with 125 mg per day (58). The reversibility of this Fanconi-like syndrome may be incomplete. In conclusion, the role of adefovir, which is under investigation at a dose of 60 mg per day, remains to be determined.

III. REVERSE TRANSCRIPTASE INHIBITORS IN CLINICAL STUDIES

Reverse transcriptase inhibitors, which are being investigated in clinical phase I or phase II studies, include FTC and bis-POM-PMPA.

FTC is a lamivudine analogue that has a markedly higher activity than lamivudine in vitro, although it shares a complete cross-resistance (59).

Bis-POM-PMPA is a nucleoside analogue that completely inhibited infection in monkeys when given prior to 24 hours after exposure to HIV (60). Studies performed in HIV-seropositive humans showed a dose-dependent response, allowing a once daily dosage (61).

IV. COMBINATION THERAPY WITH REVERSE TRANSCRIPTASE INHIBITORS (CONVERGENT COMBINATION THERAPY)

Beginning in the late 1980s, the first trials investigating the effect of combining two nucleoside reverse transcriptase inhibitors were conducted (62,63). Small pilot studies indicated a more pronounced effect on surrogate markers in the combination treatment groups. These observations stimulated the design of an ACTG-study comparing monotherapies of zidovudine and of zalcitabine with a combination of both agents (29).

All patients had a history of at least 6 months pretreatment with zidovudine monotherapy. At the end of the study, there was no difference between the three treatment groups with respect to AIDS-defining events or mortality. However, after stratification of the patients according to their CD4+ cell counts, which was not planned in the original protocol, the group of patients with more than 150 CD4 cells/μL had a statistically significant reduction in the frequency of AIDS-defining events during the first 12 months of the study (zidovudine = 14%, zalcitabine = 12%, zidovudine + zalcitabine = 5%, $P < 0.02$).

The first study that compared a treatment of zidovudine monotherapy with zidovudine plus zalcitabine and zidovudine plus didanosine in antiretroviral naive patients was presented by Schooley in 1994. After 72 weeks of treatment, patients on zidovudine monotherapy showed a decrease in their CD4+ cell counts below baseline, whereas patients in both combination therapy groups had CD4+ cell counts above baseline. The difference was highly statistically significant. With respect to the clinical outcome, there was a trend in favor of the combination therapy groups.

Two milestone studies assessing the effect of combination therapy with two nucleosides versus monotherapy were the American ACTG 175 study and the European Delta study (18,64).

The American ACTG 175 study compared zidovudine and didanosine monotherapies with the combinations of zidovudine plus zalcitabine and zidovudine plus didanosine. After a median observation period of about 2 years, both combination therapy groups and the didanosine monotherapy group were superior to zidovudine monotherapy [AIDS-defining events and deaths: ZDV, 32 (12%); ZDV + ddI, 20 (8%); ZDV + ddC, 16 (6%); ddI, 23 (9%)] in antiretrovirally non-pretreated patients. In antiretrovirally pretreated patients the combination of zidovudine plus didanosine—or didanosine alone—showed a significant reduction in the frequency of AIDS-defining events and deaths compared with zidovudine monotherapy: [ZDV, 64 (18%); ZDV + ddI, 45 (13%); ZDV + ddC, 60 (17%); ddI, 48 (14%)]. The data from antiretroviral naive patients are comparable to the data from the European Delta study. In the Delta study there was a significant reduction of AIDS-defining diseases and mortality in both combination therapy groups compared to zidovudine monotherapy [mortality: zidovudine, 16 (5%); zidovudine + zalcitabine, 11, (6%); zidovudine + didanosine, 9 (6%); $p < 0.001$]. The design of the Delta study did not include a didanosine monotherapy group.

In contrast to the results from the ACTG 175 study, in the Delta study, zidovudine-pretreated patients had no statistically significant benefit from both combination therapies as compared to zidovudine monotherapy (mortality: zidovudine, 26%; zidovudine + zalcitabine, 26%; zidovudine + didanosine, 23%, p = nonsignificant). This contradiction may be explained by the higher rate of discontinuation of study medication in the Delta study (75%) as compared with the ACTG 175 study (52%).

Zidovudine plus lamivudine was the third double nucleoside reverse transcriptase inhibitor combination to show superiority over zidovudine monotherapy. In four trials, two European and two from the United States, a marked and sustained increase in CD4+ cell count and reduction in viral load were shown for the combination therapy as compared with zidovudine monotherapy (65–67). This effect was found in antiretroviral naive patients and was less pronounced in antiretrovirally pretreated patients.

A large clinical endpoint study—the Caesar trial (68)—demonstrated conclusively the translation of the positive influence on surrogate markers into clinical benefit. In antiretroviral naive patients, the frequency of AIDS-defining diseases and deaths were 20% in the zidovudine monotherapy group as compared with 9% for zidovudine plus lamivudine ($p < 0.01$). The study contained a triple therapy group receiving zidovudine plus lamivudine plus loviride, a nonnucleoside reverse transcriptase inhibitor; it showed, however, no benefit over the double combination of zidovudine plus lamivudine. Incidence of death and AIDS-defining diseases was the same as that with the double combination.

An interesting second antiviral activity of lamivudine is its efficacy against the hepatitis B virus (69), which might offer interesting therapeutic options in HIV-positive patients with a chronic hepatitis B virus co-infection (70).

A trial that compared the combinations of zidovudine plus lamivudine with stavudine plus lamivudine was reported (71). In this trial, both combinations showed equivalent efficacy with regard to the CD4+ cell count and HIV viral load over an observational period of 1 year. Another combination widely used in clinical practice is stavudine plus didanosine, which seems to have a comparable efficacy as indicated by surrogate markers (72,73).

In contrast, zidovudine plus stavudine is a combination that should not be used in antiretroviral treatment. Two ACTG studies investigated the efficacy of this combination in comparison with other nucleoside reverse transcriptase inhibitors.

Its effect of the double combination was even less than that of stavudine monotherapy (74). This is due to an inhibition of the phosphorylation of stavudine by zidovudine, which can be demonstrated in vitro (75).

The first trial demonstrating the superiority of a convergent triple combination consisting of two nucleoside reverse transcriptase inhibitors and one nonnucleoside reverse transcriptase inhibitor was the INCAS trial (38). This trial was designed to assess the efficacy of two double combinations (zidovudine plus didanosine, zidovudine plus nevirapine) and two triple combinations consisting of zidovudine plus didanosine plus nevirapine. The study population consisted of antiretroviral naive HIV-positive patients with modest immunosuppression (median CD4+ cell count 415/μL). After an observation period of 1 year, patients in the zidovudine plus nevirapine group showed neither an increase in the CD4+ cell count nor a reduction in viral load to below 20 copies/mL. In the group receiving the double combination of zidovudine plus didanosine, after 1 year, the increase in the CD4+ cell count was still above baseline but less than with the triple combination. The viral load after 1 year of treatment was less than 20 copies/mL in 12% of the patients given zidovudine plus didanosine as compared to 51% in the triple combination group. Only very few clinical events occurred during the study period. No difference in clinical benefit was observed between the treatment groups. These results were supported by the Atlantic study, which showed persistent effects of two convergent (stavudine + didanosine + nevirapine/lamivudine) and one divergent regimen (stavudine + didanosine + indinavir) on HIV viral load and the CD4+ cell count over 24 weeks (76).

In the ACTG study, 241 zidovudine pretreated patients (n = 398) were randomized to zidovudine plus didanosine or zidovudine plus didanosine plus nevirapine (39). The sequential triple combination with nevirapine was superior in viral load decrease and CD4+ cell count increase, but after 48 weeks, both surrogate markers were below baseline even in the triple combination. This demonstrates the limited efficacy of nevirapine as the second newly added drug in a sequential triple combination.

Delavirdine was licensed as part of a combination therapy with zidovudine. In combination with zidovudine, it showed a moderate effect on HIV viral load with a reduction of less than 1 log naive or zidovudine-pretreated patients (77). A study in 367 predominantly treatment-naive patients comparing a triple combination of zidovudine plus lamivudine plus delavirdine to two double combination regimens, zidovudine plus lamivudine and zidovudine plus delavirdine, demonstrated a more durable viral load suppression in the triple combination group after 24 weeks. A viral load of fewer than 40 copies/mL after 24 weeks was found in 60% of the patients under triple combination compared to 1% (zidovudine plus lamivudine) and 5% (zidovudine plus delavirdine), respectively (78,79). No clinical endpoint studies have been conducted with this drug.

Abacavir has been studied in a triple combination with zidovudine plus lamivudine. The data from these studies indicate a longer lasting synergistic effect of the three drugs (46,47). In an add-on strategy, abacavir has only limited efficacy (80).

The pivotal study concerning efavirenz demonstrated that, after 48 weeks, the combination of efavirenz plus zidovudine plus lamivudine was at least as effective when compared to an indinavir-containing triple treatment (41). The activity of efavirenz in heavily pretreated patients seems to depend on the activity of the agents used in the combination (52). Another nonnucleosidic inhibitor that was analyzed in clinical studies in combination with nucleosidic drugs is L697, 661 (52a).

V. HIV PROTEASE INHIBITORS

The availability of HIV protease inhibitors dramatically changed the clinical course of the HIV epidemic in the western world. In association with the increased use of the HIV protease inhibitors, a reduction in the incidence of HIV-associated opportunistic infections and mortality has been reported (1–3).

The introduction of a new class of antiretroviral drugs, however, started not only a revolution in antiretroviral therapy of uncertain duration but also complicated HIV therapy by increasing the number of drug interactions. Most of the interactions are based on the interference with the drug metabolism by the cytochrome 450 isoenzyme system in the liver. All the available HIV protease inhibitors are inhibitors of the cytochrome 450 pathway, blocking, to a greater or lesser extent, some of the isoenzymes. The strongest inhibitor is ritonavir, followed by indinavir, nelfinavir, amprenavir, and saquinavir. The drug interactions are listed in detail in Table 3.

A recently reported adverse effect of the protease inhibitors appears to be a change in the distribution of body fat known as lipodystrophy syndrome. This syndrome results in an increase in fat in the abdomen and neck region, whereas the fat mass in the face, the limbs and the buttocks is decreased (81–83). Recently, however, this effect was also discussed in context with nucleosidic inhibitors, in particular, stavudine. The pathophysiological mechanism may be attributable to interference with mitochondrial functions. The second class of side effects reported for HIV protease inhibitors are increased incidences of hyperglycemia (84,85) and hyperlipidemia (86, for review: 87), as well as diarrhea.

A. Saquinavir

The first HIV protease inhibitor approved for the treatment of HIV infection was saquinavir. The approval was granted for a study with a now outdated design in which a combination therapy of zalcitabine plus saquinavir proved to be superior to monotherapy with either zalcitabine or saquinavir in zidovudine pretreated patients. The double combination achieved a reduction in the frequency of AIDS-defining diseases and mortality compared to the monotherapy groups (88).

A study with a more relevant design was the ACTG 229 study (89), which showed a superior effect on surrogate markers (CD4+ cell count, HIV viral load) for the triple combination consisting of zidovudine plus zalcitabine plus saquinavir compared to the two double combination groups (zidovudine plus saquinavir, zidovudine plus zalcitabine). The study was too small to demonstrate a clinical benefit. For this reason, a large study aiming at clinical endpoints was initiated with the same design. In the early phase of the trial, a zidovudine monotherpay group was included as a fourth subgroup. At the end of 1995, because of the results of the ACTG 175 and the Delta studies, participants in the zidovudine monotherapy group were switched to the triple combination. This study enrolled 3485 patients with a maximum of 16 weeks of zidovudine pretreatment. After a median observation period of 17 months, the triple therapy group showed a statistically significant reduction in the combined number of AIDS-defining diseases and deaths: 76 cases compared to 216 cases under treatment with zidovudine plus saquinavir and 142 cases under zidovudine plus zalcitabine ($p < 0.001$) (90).

Saquinavir is generally tolerated well. The most common side effects are dose-dependent diarrhea, meteorism, nausea, and fatigue.

On the other hand, the bioavailability of saquinavir in the commercial formulation called "hard gel capsules" is poor. Because of metabolism by the hepatic cytochrome P450 system and because of great variability in intestinal absorption, the average bioavailability is only 4% with substantial intraindividual variation. The plasma level of saquinavir is increased by intake of food with the medicament and by the concomitant administration of grapefruit juice or ketoconazole, which are inhibitors of the cytochrome P450 system. The strongest inhibitor of the metabolism of saquinavir, however, is ritonavir, a characteristic that is currently used in antiretroviral treatment strategies (discussed later). The concentration of saquinavir in the cerebrospinal fluid is less than 1% of the serum concentration, but in animal models (rat), a marked concentration of saquinavir was found in the brain tissue, which is attributed to the lipophilic nature of the drug (Jan Mous, personal communication).

The plasma levels of saquinavir "hard gel capsule" can be increased by increasing the dosage (91). But even this approach could not guarantee a clinically sufficient plasma concentration among the whole study population. This major shortcoming led to the development of a formulation with superior bioavailability, the so-called soft-gel capsule. The bioavailability of this formulation is 10% to 20%. Despite the favorable pharmacokinetic profile, the manufacturer's recommended daily dosage (3600 mg/day) is twice as high as for the less bioavailable "hard-gel capsule" (1800 mg/day).

A small study comparing a triple combination of zidovudine plus lamivudine plus soft-gel saquinavir with zidovudine plus lamivudine plus indinavir

Table 3 Dosages, Intake Requirements, and Drug Interactions of the Approved HIV Protease Inhibitors

Medicament	Trade name and manufacturer	Daily dosage	Intake modalities	Modified dosage in antiretroviral combination	Drug interactions
Amprenavir (APV)	Agenerase Glaxo Wellcome	2 × 8 caps @ 150 mg	If possible without food	With RTV APV: 2 × 450 mg RTV: 2 × 400 mg (preliminary data) With NFV no dose modification With rifabutin APV: no dose modification rifabutin: 1 × 150 mg	APV ↑ with IDV (+26%), clarithromycin (+18%), ketoconazole (+32%) APV ↓ with FTV (−38%), EFV (−36%), rifabutin (−14%), rifampicin (−82%) Plasma level-↓ of IDV (−38%), FTV (−19%) Contraindications: antihistamines (terfenadine, astemizole), ergotamine derivatives, prokinetics (cisapride), sedatives (midazolam, triazolam), tuberculostatics (rifampicin)
Indinavir (IDV)	Crixivan Merck Sharp & Dohme	3 × 2 caps @ 400 mg on an empty stomach	On an empty stomach or with a light meal (2 hours after or 1 hour before a protein- and fat-rich meal—not necessarily in combination with ritonavir)	With RTV IDV: 2 × 400 mg RTV: 2 × 400 mg With NVP IDV: 3 × 1000 mg NVP: no dose modification With EFV IDV: 3 × 1000 mg EFV: no dose modification With DLV IDV: 3 × 600 mg DLV: no dose modification	IDV-↑ with β-blockers, calcium channel blockers, antiarrhythmics, RTV (+480%), NFV (+51%), clarithromycin (+29%), clindamycin, itraconazole, ketoconazole (+68 IDV-↓ with APV (−38%), NVP (−27%), EFV (−24%), fluconazole (−19%), grapefruit juice (−26%), possible with dexamethasone, carbamazepine, phenytoin, phenobarbital, rifabutin Plasma level-↑ of NFV (83%), d4T (+21%), AZT (+17%), APV (+26%), methadone (+30%), rifabutin (+100%), clarithromycin (+53%), sildenafile (careful dosage, lack of

Nelfinavir (NFV) Viracept Agouron distribution in Europe: Hoffman-La Roche	2 × 5 tbl @ 250 mg or 3 × 3 tbl @ 250 mg	With a protein- and fat-rich meal	With rifabutin IDV: 3 × 1000 mg rifabutin: 1 × 150 mg With ketoconazole IDV: 3 × 600 mg ketoconazole: no dose modification With SQV-sgc (FTV) NFV: no dose modification FTV: 2 × 1200 mg With RTV NFV: 2 × 500–750 mg RV: 2 × 400 mg Wiht NVP NFV: eventual increase of dosage (3 × 1000 mg or 2 × 1500 mg) NVP: no dose modification With EFV no dose modification With rifabutin NFV: no dose modification rifabutin: 1 × 150 mg	experience, increase of plasma level probable), streptomycin Plasma level-↓ of oral contraceptives, alterantive contraceptive methods recommended in addition to oral contraceptives Contraindications: terfenadine, astemizole, triazolam, midazolam, cisapride, rifampicin, ergotamine derivatives NFV-↑ with ketoconazole (+35%), SQV (+18%), IDV (+83%) and RTV (+152%) NFV-↓ with: some anticonvulsants (carbamazepine, phenobarbital, phenytoin), with rifabutin (−32%), rifampicin (−82%) Plasma level-↑ of IDV (AUC +51%), SQV (AUC + 392%), rifabutin (+207%), methadone Plasma level-↓ ZDV (−35%), rifampicin (−82%), terfenadine, oral contraceptives (ethinyl estradiol (−47%), norethindrone (−18%); alternative contraceptive methods recommended in addition to oral contraceptives) Contraindications: some antihistamines (terfenadine, astemizole), rifampicin, benzodiazepines (triazolam, midazolam), cisapride

Table 3 Continued

Medicament	Trade name and manufacturer	Daily dosage	Intake modalities	Modified dosage in antiretroviral combination	Drug interactions
Ritonavir (RTV)	Norvir Abbott	2 × 6 caps @ 100 mg or 2 × 7.5 mL liquid solution (8 mg/mL) contains 43% ethanol	Liquid solution has to be taken with a protein- and fat-rich meal; capsules can be taken without a meal, but absorption is increased if taken with food	With SQV hard get capsule (hgc) and SQV soft gel capsule (sgc) RTV: 2 × 400 mg SQV: 2 × 400–600 mg With IDV RTV: 2 × 400 mg IDV: 2 × 400 mg With NFV RTV: 2 × 400 mg NFV: 2 × 1000 mg (preliminary data) With NVP no dose modification With EPV RTV: eventual dose reduction EFV: no dose modification	RTV-↑ with fluconazole (+15%), with fluoxetine (+19%) RTV-↓ with rifampicin (−35%), probably with phenobarbital, carbamazepine, dexamethasone, phenytoin Plasma level-↑ of SQV (20-fold), NLV (2-fold); clarithromycin, erythromycin, mefloquine (3-fold), ondansentron, sildenafil (10-fold), carbamazepine, corticosteroids, cyclosporines; amprenavir (AUC +800%), methadone (2-fold), amphetamines (2- to 3-fold), fluoxetin, ecstasy (2- to 3-fold), β-blockers, calcium channel blockers (nifedipine, nicardipine, nimodipine, nisoldipine, nitrendipine), anticonvulsants (carbamazepine (3-fold), phenytoin, phenobarbital), oral anticoagulants (phenprocoumon), rifabutin (3-fold), rifampicin

Plasma level-↓ of morphine derivatives (−50%), heroin (−50%); oral contraceptives (ethinyl estradiol −41%), alternative contraceptive methods recommended

Contraindications: sedatives (aprazolam, clorazepate, diazepam, estazolam, flurazepam, triazolam, zolpidem), antidepressants (bupropion), antiarrhythmics (amiodarone, encainide, flecainide, propafenon, quinidine), antihypertensives (bepridil), neuroleptics (clozapine, pimozide), analgetics (pethidine, piroxicam, propoxyphene), antihistamines (terfenadine, astemizole), ergotamines, dihydroergotamines, cisapride, rifabutin

Alternatives to contraindicated medications: sedatives (temazepan, lorazepam), antidepressants (fluoxetine, desiprimine), analgetics (paracetamol, oxycodone, codeine, tramadol, acetylsalicyclic acid), antihistamines (loratadine, cetirizine), anticonvulsants: valproic acid, antimycobacterials (clarithromycin, ethambutol), gastrointestinal prokinetics (domperidone)

Table 3 Continued

Medicament	Trade name and manufacturer	Daily dosage	Intake modalities	Modified dosage in antiretroviral combination	Drug interactions
Saquinavir—hard gel capsule (SQV-hgc or INV)	Invirase Hoffman-La Roche	Due to poor bioavailability, only recommended in combination with 2 × 100–600 mg ritonavir: 2 × 2–3 caps @ 200 mg	In combination with ritonavir (2 × 200–600 mg): with a protein- and fat-rich meal	Due to poor bioavailability, only recommended in combination with RTV, e.g.: INV: 2 × 400–600 mg RTV: 2 × 400 mg	SQV ↑ with: RTV (20-fold), NLV (4- to 5-fold), DLV (4- to 5-fold), ketoconazole (200 mg/day; +130%); grapefruit juice (+50–100%) SQV ↓: NVP (−24%), rifabutin (−43%), rifampicin (−84%), phenytoin, phenobarbital, carbamazepine, clonazepam, dexamethasone (combinations not recommended) Plasma level-↑ of clindamycin, calcium channel blockers, dapsone, antiarrhythmics, β-blockers, sildenafil (careful dosage) Plasma level-↓ of DLV (−15) Contraindications: rifampicin, terfenadine, astemizole, cisapride, ergotamines

| Saquinavir— soft gel capsule (SQV-sgc or FTV) | Fortovase Hoffman-La Roche | 3 × 6 caps @ 200 mg
FTV has to be stored in the refrigerator | With a protein- and fat-rich meal | With RTV
FTV: 2 × 400–600 mg
RTV: 2 × 400 mg
With NFV
FTV: 3 × 800 mg or 2 × 1200 mg
NFV: no dose modification
With NVP
FTV: 3 × 1400 mg
NVP: no dose modification
Combination with EFV not recommended (SQV-sgc ↓ 62%) | SQV (single dose of 1200 mg)-↑ with IDV (+364%), NFV (+392%)
SQV (2 × 400 mg)-↑ with RTV (+121%), compared to SQV-sgc 3 × 1200 mg)
SQV-↑ with clarithromycin (+177%)
SQV ↓ with EFV (−62%), APV (−18%), anticonvulsants (carbamazepine, phenobarbital, phenytoin)
Plasma level-↑ of NFV (AUC +18%), terfenadine (+368%, metabolite +120%; with SQV-single dose of 800 or 1200 mg), sildenafil (+210%)
Effect of clarithromycin may be altered (clarithromycin ↑, active metabolite ↓)
No change in RTV plasma level
Contraindications: terfenadine, astemizole, cisapride, some sedatives (midazolam, triazolam), ergotamine derivatives |

showed a comparable effect of both triple combinations on viral load and a more pronounced increase in the CD4+ cell count in the soft-gel saquinavir group after 24 weeks (92).

According to the first bioavailability study, the main side effects are diarrhea, nausea, and, less commonly, an increase in liver transaminases (ALT, AST) (93). On this basis, at the end of 1997, the soft-gel preparation of saquinavir was approved in the United States for treatment of HIV infection.

Antiretroviral agents with the interesting potential to increase the bioavailability of saquinavir, soft gel and hard gel, include ritonavir, which increases saquinavir levels about 20-fold, and nelfinavir and delavirdine, which both produce a five-fold increase (94–97).

B. Ritonavir

Ritonavir demonstrated its clinical efficacy in a large controlled trial involving 1090 patients with advanced HIV infection and a CD4 cell count below 100/µL. All patients were pretreated with nucleoside reverse transcriptase inhibitors, and ritonavir was added to the current treatment regimen. After a median observation period of 6 months, 36 patients (4.8%) had died in the ritonavir group compared to 64 patients (8.4%) in the placebo group ($p < 0.01$). The combined number of AIDS-defining events and deaths was significantly lower among those receiving ritonavir (n = 69, 12.7%) compared to placebo (n = 149, 27.3%) (98). The maximal mean CD4+ cell count was 78 cells/µL at week 16 compared to 31/µL at baseline. The maximal decrease of the viral load was 1.3 log at week 4 (99).

The effect of ritonavir in combination with two nucleoside reverse transcriptase inhibitors for treatment of antiretroviral naive patients is equivalent to that for other HIV protease inhibitors. For example, in one smaller study, the combination of ritonavir plus zidovudine plus zalcitabine in antiretroviral naive patients, CD4+ cell count increased from a median of 156/µL to 303/µL at month 6. The median HIV-RNA was reduced from 70,000 copies/mL to 900 copies/mL (100).

In addition to the increase of the absolute number of the CD4+ cells, ritonavir increased the number of CD8+ cells and improved the ability of the CD4+ cells to proliferate in vitro (101). Similar effects have meanwhile been shown for several HIV protease inhibitor–containing regimens (102–107).

The side effects of ritonavir are frequent and consist of nausea, vomiting, diarrhea, loss of appetite, taste perturbation, and perioral paresthesias. In addition, increases in triglycerides, liver enzymes, and cholestatic enzymes occur frequently. To reduce the side effects, a stepwise dosage escalation from 300 mg b.i.d. over the first 4 to 6 days to a final dose of 400 to 600 mg b.i.d. is recommended.

The bioavailability of ritonavir is about 70%, and the intake of the medication, particular of the liquid formulation, with meals increases serum levels. Ritonavir is predominantly metabolized in the liver by the cytochrome P450 isoenzyme 3A4.

In animal models, no penetration of the substance into the spinal fluid or the brain has been found. Even so, in a small study in 13 patients given a combination of ritonavir and saquinavir, the viral load in the spinal fluid of 12 of 13 patients was below the detection limit of 400 copies/mL (108).

Ritonavir is a strong inhibitor of the cytochrome P450 system, particularly the cytochrome isoenzymes 3A4 and 2D6. Clinically relevant interactions are listed in Table 2. An interesting phenomenon is the change caused in the pharmacokinetic profile of other concomitant antiretroviral agents while that of ritonavir remains unchanged. Two therapeutically relevant interactions are the observed increases in the plasma levels of saquinavir (109) or indinavir (110). The dosages of both drugs can be halved when coadministered with ritonavir.

Because of the possible decrease in metabolism, a dose reduction of ritonavir is recommended in patients with liver cirrhosis.

C. Indinavir

Indinavir was first tested in a set of pilot studies containing indinavir monotherapy groups. These studies showed marked median increases of the CD4+ cell count of about 60 to 100 cells/μL from a baseline of 110 to 300 cells/μL. The maximal decrease in HIV viral load ranged from 1.5 to 2.3 log, comparable to results obtained with ritonavir and nelfinavir (111–115). After observation periods ranging from 6 to 12 months, triple combinations consisting of two nucleosides and indinavir demonstrated a longer lasting decrease in HIV viral load compared to indinavir monotherapy (100,111,115). For example, in one study comparing the effect of indinavir monotherapy with a double combination of zidovudine plus lamivudine and a triple combination of all these agents, after 24 weeks, 90% of the participants in the triple group, 43% of patients receiving indinavir monotherapy, and none of the patients in the double nucleoside combination group had a viral load less than 500 copies/mL (115).

The first clinical endpoint study demonstrating a clinical benefit for indinavir was the ACTG 320 trial (116). A total of 1156 patients were enrolled and randomized to either a nucleoside reverse transcriptase inhibitor group zidovudine plus lamivudine or to a group receiving a triple combination containing indinavir. All patients were zidovudine pretreated but had no pretreatment with lamivudine or an HIV-protease inhibitor. In the triple combination group, the frequency of AIDS-defining diseases and deaths was 6% versus 11% under the double nucleoside combination ($p < 0.01$) In accordance with these results, a longer lasting CD4+ cell count response and viral load reduction under the triple combination was observed.

One side effect of indinavir is the occurrence of renal stones and crystalluria, the latter being observed in up to 20% of patients in initial trials (111,112). The incidence was decreased by increased fluid intake (more than 1.5L/day). After this precaution, the incidence of kidney stones in the compassionate use program was about 5%. Another common side effect seen with indinavir is increased bilirubin unaccompanied by other signs of liver cell damage. In addition, nausea, dry skin, pruritus, diarrhea, elevated liver enzymes (ALT, AST), and paronychia have also been reported as indinavir related.

Bioavailability of indinavir is reported to be 40% to 60% in humans and is reduced by fat and protein-rich meals (117). There is as yet no data concerning the concentration of the drug in the spinal fluid or brain tissue.

Indinavir is predominantly metabolized through cytochrome P-450 3A4. The resulting drug interactions are listed in Table 3. Possible interactions of therapeutic interest are an increase in indinavir plasma levels by delavirdine (two-fold) and ritonavir (five-fold) (110). The concomitant administration of ritonavir showed a stable pharmacokinetic profile in HIV-seronegative volunteers, enabling twice daily dosage.

A European study assessed twice daily dosing of indinavir (118), proving that low trough levels result in an increased rate of virological failure (119).

Because of its hepatic metabolism, a dose reduction of indinavir is recommended in patients with liver cirrhosis and decreased liver function.

D. Nelfinavir

Nelfinavir is the most recent HIV protease inhibitor approved for the treatment of HIV infection. This approval was granted exclusively on surrogate marker data.

The largest completed study enrolled 297 antiretroviral naive patients who were treated with a double combination of zidovudine plus lamivudine or a triple combination adding nelfinavir to these two agents (120). Nelfinavir was tested in two different doses, 500 mg b.i.d. versus 750 mg b.i.d. The mean CD4 cell count was $283/\mu L$ and the mean HIV viral load was 80,000 copies/mL. The mean increase in CD4+ cells in the triple therapy groups was 155 cells/μL compared to approximately 90 cells/μL in the patients receiving the double combination. After 24 weeks, more than 80% of subjects in the triple combination groups exhibited a viral load of less than 500 copies/mL, whereas only 25% in the double combination group were below this threshold. Both differences were statistically significant (p < 0.01). Comparison of the two nelfinavir treatment groups revealed no statistical difference. However, when only patients with an HIV viral load of more than 100,000 copies/mL or a CD4 cell count with less than 300 cells/μL were evaluated, the treatment group with the higher nelfinavir dose was statistically superior to the low dose group. After 12 months, 60% of the patients in the twice daily 500-mg group were below 500 copies/mL as compared to 80% in the 750-mg group.

In conclusion, the effect of nelfinavir in triple combination therapy is comparable to the efficacy of indinavir, ritonavir, or soft-gel saquinavir. However, in patients with evidence of HIV protease inhibitor failure, the efficacy of nelfinavir appears to be limited (121).

The most frequent side effects of nelfinavir are gastrointestinal, including loose stools, diarrhea, meteorism, abdominal pain, and nausea. Rash is a less frequent side effect.

The bioavailability of nelfinavir is 20% to 80% and is higher when the drug is taken with food. It is metabolized via the cytochrome P-450 system, predominantly inhibiting the cytochrome P450 3A isoenzyme system. Ritonavir and indinavir increase the concentration of nelfinavir or its active metabolite. Nelfinavir increases the plasma level of saquinavir about four-fold (95).

Nelfinavir has a plasma half-life of about 5 hours, the longest half-life of all protease inhibitors. For this reason, twice daily dosing seems possible. According to an interim analysis of an ongoing study, a dosage of 1250 mg twice daily seems to have the same efficacy as 750 mg thrice daily (122).

VI. HIV PROTEASE INHIBITORS IN CLINICAL TRIALS

Amprenavir (141W94) is an HIV protease inhibitor currently in phase III clinical studies. After the completion of pharmacokinetic studies demonstrating a plasma half-life of 7 to 10 hours, a dosage of 1200 mg b.i.d. was selected for the phase II and III trials. A trial containing a monotherapy group showed a loss of effect on HIV viral load within 12 weeks, which could be explained by rapid development of resistance against amprenavir (1). In a study with a duration of 24 weeks, amprenavir in combination with abacavir or zidovudine plus lamivudine exhibited a viral load reduction similar to that of other triple regimens containing a protease inhibitor (1). Amprenavir is metabolized by the cytochrome P-450 pathway. Its potential for drug interactions is estimated to be in the range of indinavir. Side effects include diarrhea or loose stools, rash, and headache (123). The mutations induced by amprenavir differ from those of other protease inhibitors (124). Whether the different mutation profile translates into clinical benefit and less cross-resistance with the other HIV protease inhibitors remains to be determined (125).

ABT-378 is a protease inhibitor with a 10-fold higher activity compared to ritonavir in vitro. It seems to be active against ritonavir-resistant HIV strains (126). In combination with low-dose ritonavir (50–100 mg), twice daily dosage is possible (83,127).

Protease inhibitors in preclinical development include KNI-272, DMP-450, and PNU-140690, the latter being a nonpeptidomimetic compound.

VII. THE DOUBLE COMBINATION OF HIV PROTEASE INHIBITORS

The combinations of ritonavir plus saquinavir, ritonavir plus indinavir, and nelfinavir plus saquinavir have the potential of increasing the efficacy of at least one of the drugs or having a more convenient dosage regimen.

The combination of ritonavir plus saquinavir has been evaluated in larger clinical trials (128). In a dose of 400 to 600 mg twice daily, ritonavir increases the saquinavir concentration about 20-fold (94). According to the manufacturer, no difference in pharmacokinetics has been found between saquinavir hard-gel capsule and the soft-gel formulation when coadministered with ritonavir.

The study by Cameron and coworkers (128) demonstrated in HIV protease inhibitor naive patients that ritonavir, 400 to 600 mg twice daily, and saquinavir, 600 mg twice daily, achieved superior results with respect to the effect on surrogate markers and tolerance. After an observation period of 12 months, 90% of the evaluable 109 participants had a viral load of less than 200 copies/mL.

Although larger controlled studies are needed, the combination of ritonavir plus indinavir at a dosage of 400 mg b.i.d. for each compound or 100 mg b.i.d. for ritonavir and 800 mg b.i.d. for indinavir has found a widespread use in daily practice (129). The dosages were recommended on the basis of pharmacokinetic studies with HIV-negative volunteers (130).

To date, the combination of ritonavir and saquinavir is widely used in salvage regimens in combination with reverse transcriptase inhibitors and considered as a suitable first line treatment by some investigators, particularly for patients with high HIV viral load.

VIII. DIVERGENT COMBINATION THERAPY

The most frequently used triple therapies in 1997 were divergent combination regimens consisting of two nucleoside reverse transcriptase inhibitors and one HIV protease inhibitor. The single use of one HIV protease inhibitor cannot be recommended because reduced efficacy and early development of resistance were demonstrated in several clinical trials (1,100,115). Divergent triple combination has been shown to be clinically superior to convergent double combinations with two nucleoside reverse transcriptase inhibitors in several studies (90,116). Although the demonstration of clinical efficacy was limited to trials with patients with moderate to advanced immunosuppression, in patients with less advanced stages of the HIV infection, only a benefit concerning HIV viral load and CD4+ cell count in the direct comparison of double versus triple combinations has been shown so far.

In 1998, following the impressive results of the efavirenz and abacavir studies, together with the results from the Atlantic study, the easier to take convergent regimens consisting of three reverse transcriptase inhibitors became increasingly popular. Combination of three medicaments is not necessarily an endpoint: two Dutch studies (131,132) demonstrated that, compared to a triple combination, a quadruple or quintuple combination seems to be more effective at least over the short term with regard to the reduction of viral load. Long-term data, however, reflecting the tolerance of the quadruple or quintuple regimens are not yet available.

IX. NEW ANTIRETROVIRAL TARGETS

Among agents with new antiretroviral targets that are currently in clinical studies are the fusion inhibitors, such as T 20, which is administered intravenously and shows a marked dose-dependent depression of HIV viral load (133–135).

Integrase inhibitors are currently in their preclinical development phase (136).

Another class of agents in phase I studies are zincfinger inhibitors (137). However, it is too early to make judgments concerning the possible clinical role of these substances.

X. MAJOR OBSTACLES IN CURRENT ANTIRETROVIRAL TREATMENT STRATEGIES

Major obstacles in successful antiretroviral treatment in daily practice are the considerably lower response rates to HIV protease inhibitor treatment as compared to the results from clinical trials (138,139). Although this may be explained by reduced compliance of patients outside clinical studies, other possible reasons include the existence of phosphorylation interactions, which may interfere with the efficacy of nucleoside reverse transcriptase inhibitor treatment (140), and different primary susceptibilities of different HIV genotypes to antiretroviral agents (141). In addition, resistant viruses are increasingly transmitted (142–144).

Another major problem is the development of resistance and cross-resistance as a result of prolonged treatment with antiretroviral agents. There seems to be specific cross-resistance between some nucleoside reverse transcriptase inhibitors whereas nonnucleoside reverse transcriptase inhibitors and at least peptidomimetic HIV protease inhibitors seem to suffer from cross-class resistance. In vitro resistance developed to nelfinavir and saquinavir did not lead to extensive cross-resistance to indinavir or ritonavir, but in vivo results suggest that at least long-term treatment with both medicaments does result in clinically relevant cross-resistance to ritonavir and indinavir (74). Therefore, only an early switch of therapy after an increase in viral load under treatment with nelfinavir or saquinavir may circumvent the development of cross-resistance to indinavir or ritonavir. This practice, however, is based only on in vitro findings, which must be validated in clinical trials.

There seems to be a complete cross-resistance between nevirapine and delavirdine, whereas efavirenz may be able to overcome a partial cross-resistance caused by nevirapine or delavirdine (145). These findings are based on in vitro data, which must be confirmed in vivo.

XI. CURRENT TREATMENT STRATEGIES

Since the introduction of HIV viral load testing into clinical practice in 1996, treatment decisions are no longer based on CD4+ cell count only but have become more and more viral load dependent. In decisions concerning the change of treatment, the HIV viral load is considered to be the most important factor in clinical practice.

In 1996, when David Ho presented his model of viral kinetics and predicted that an eradication of HIV would be possible within years, a considerable number of physicians started treating everyone who was HIV-positive. The slogan accompanying this attitude was "Hit hard and early!" Even David Ho, however, had to admit that the eradication might not be achievable with current regimens (Chicago 1998, oral presentation); consequently, the current guidelines take a more conservative standpoint (146, International AIDS Society Guidelines, 147).

In general, treatment is considered feasible in patients with acute HIV infection, in which a reduction of the viral burden and a restoration of the immune system can be expected (148). However, the necessary duration of antiretroviral treatment in patients with acute HIV infection is unknown. Antiretroviral treatment is not recommended for patients without acute HIV infection and a viral load of less than 10,000 copies/mL and a CD4+ cell count greater than 500/µL. Treatment with antiretroviral therapies is recommended for patients with less than 500 CD4+ cells or an HIV viral load of more than 10,000 copies/mL. The impact of these guidelines on clinical practice, however, may not be too strong, as shown by a survey among leading HIV clinicians concerning their antiretroviral treatment strategies (149).

A recent increasing trend is not to use HIV protease inhibitor–containing regimens as first line therapies. This is due to the long-term side effects such as lipodystrophy syndrome or hyperglycemia, which went unnoticed during the pivotal clinical studies but which are now being reported following the broad use of these drugs in clinical practice. Most physicians are using triple combinations containing two nucleoside reverse transcriptase inhibitors and one nonnucleoside reverse transcriptase inhibitor or hydroxyurea (146). Another reason for avoiding HIV protease inhibitors is the loss of efficacy of the second HIV protease inhibitor–containing regimen (150–152), which has led some physicians to tend to save this drug group for second line therapy.

An interesting approach is the so-called induction-maintenance strategy. In the induction phase with a multiple antiretroviral combination regimen, the HIV viral load is maximally suppressed. This "hit hard" regimen is followed by a regimen with two drugs, which are convenient to take and are used to sustain the maximal viral load suppression. In the first two trials assessing this approach, however, a viral rebound occurred significantly more frequently in patients in the double combination groups as compared to patients who maintained their triple combination (74,153), although this could be explained by an inadequate study design that did not include ultrasensitive HIV viral load assays as qualification criteria. Further trials using stricter criteria are ongoing.

The most widely used salvage strategy for patients treated with a failing regimen containing an HIV protease inhibitor is a combination of saquinavir and ritonavir in addition to two nucleoside reverse transcriptase inhibitors. This approach achieves a reduction of the viral load below the detection limit of 200 to 500 copies/mL in 40% to 60% of the participants (150,154–156). Preliminary data indicate that regimens containing six and more drugs may be more effective in achieving a reduction of viral load, but the tolerance problems accompanying these regimens may hamper long-term efficacy (157).

In conclusion, the introduction of antiretroviral combination therapy and particularly the HIV protease inhibitors has opened a new era in the HIV epidemic. In the western world, a dramatic decline in the incidence of HIV-associated diseases and mortality rate has occurred. However, the durability of this effect can in no way be guaranteed. Failures of HIV protease inhibitors–containing regimens are being reported more and more frequently. This may not necessarily translate into rapid clinical worsening of the patient, in that the immunological improvement provides protection against development of the disease for a certain amount of time (60). In the long run, however, these individuals will experience clinical progression of their HIV infection. Thus, at least in patients with moderate immunosuppression and moderate levels of viral load, alternative treatment strategies not containing an HIV protease inhibitor are warranted to spare the effect of these powerful antiretroviral medicaments.

Although new therapeutic agents with a new therapeutic approach such as integrase inhibitors, fusion inhibitors, or zincfinger inhibitors are currently entering preclinical and clinical trials, they will not be available for general use in the near future. Current treatment strategies have to be based on the available classes of drugs and their shortcomings. There is thus an urgent need for strategic trials assessing the best method of sequencing with currently available antiretroviral medicaments in combination therapy.

ACKNOWLEDGMENTS

We are grateful for the stimulating discussions with Eva Wolf during the preparation of the manuscript, the secretarial assistance of Illa Chrubasik and Sigrid

Detschey, and the final editing by Dianne Lydtin. This contribution is dedicated to Professor Dr. Georg Strohmeyer on the occasion of his 70th birthday.

REFERENCES

1. Murphy R, El-Sadr W. Impact of protease inhibitor containing regimens on the risk of developing opportunistic infections and mortality in the CPCRA 034/ACTG 277 study (abstr). 5th Conference on Retroviruses and Opportunistic Infections. 1998, Abstr. No. 181:113.
2. Robert Koch-Institut, Bundesinstitut für Infektionskrankheiten und nicht übertragbare Krankheiten (ed.). 128. Bericht des AIDS-Zentrums im Robert Koch-Institut über aktuelle epidemiologische Daten (Quartalsbericht IV/97).
3. Pallela FJ Jr, Delaney KM, Moorman AC, Loveless MO, Fuhrer J, Statten GA, Aschman DJ, Holberg SD. Declining morbidity and mortality among patients with advanced human immunodeficiency virus infection. N Engl J Med 1998; 338:853.
4. Fischl MA, Richman DD, Grieco MH, et al. The efficacy of azidothymidine (AZT) in the treatment of patients with AIDS and AIDS-related complex. N Engl J Med 1987; 317:185–191.
5. Richmann DD, Fischl MA, Grieco MH, et al. The toxicity of azidothymidine (AZT) in the treatment of patients with AIDS and AIDS-related complex. N Engl J Med 1987; 317:192–197.
6. Fischl MA, Richman DD, Hansen N, et al. The safety and efficacy of zidovudine (AZT) in the treatment of patients with mildly symptomatic HIV-infection. A double blind, placebo controlled trial. The AIDS Clinical Trials Group. Ann Intern Med 1990; 112:727–737.
7. Volberding PA, Lagakos SW, Koch MA, et al. Zidovudine in asymptomatic human immunodeficiency virus infection. A controlled trial in persons with fewer than 500 CD4-positive cells per cubic millimeter. The AIDS Clinical Trial Group of the National Institute of Allergy and Infectious Diseases. N Engl J Med 1990; 322:941–949.
8. Hamilton JD, Hartigan PM, Simberkoff MS, et al. A controlled trial of early vs late treatment with zidovudine in symptomatic human immunodeficiency virus infection—results of the Veterans Affairs Cooperative Study. N Engl J Med 1992; 326: 437–443.
9. Concorde Coordinating Committee. MRC/ANRS randomised double-blind controlled trial of immediate and deferred zidovudine in symptom-free HIV infection. Lancet 1994; 343:871–881.
10. Cooper DA, Gatell DM. Zidovudine in persons with asymptomatic HIV infection and CD4+ cell count greater than 400 per cubic millimeter. N Engl J Med 1993; 329:297–303. In: DAH, Antiretrovirale Therapie der HIV-Infektion, Stand: 6/95.
11. Rey D, Pi T, Hughes M, Merigan TC, Katzenstein DA. Plasma codon 215 mutations in subjects treated with zidovudine in ACTG 175. 4th Conference on Retroviruses and Opportunistic Infection. Jan 22–26 1997. Abstr. No. 584.
12. Merigan TC, Hirsch RL, Fisher AC, Meyerson LA, Goldstein G, Winters MA. The prognostic significance of serum viral load, codon 215 reverse transcriptase mutation and CD4+ T cells on progression of HIV disease in a double-blind study of thymopentin. AIDS 1996; 10(2):159–165.

13. Kozal MJ, Shafer RW, Winters MA, Katzenstein DA, Aguiniga E, Halpern J, Merigan TC. HIV-1 syncytium-inducing phenotype, virus burden, codon 215 reverse transcriptase mutation and CD4 cell decline in zidovudine-treated patients. J Acquired Immune Defic Syndr Hum Retrovirol 1995; 9(1):101–102.

14. Yarchoan R, Mitsuya H, Thomas RV, Pluda JM, Hartman NR, Perno C-F, Marczyk KS, Allain J-P, Johns DG, Broder S. In vivo activity against HIV and favorable toxicity profile of 2′, 3′-dideoxyinosine. Science 1989; 245:412–415.

15. Connolly KJ, Allan JD, Fitch H, Jackson-Pope L, McLaren C, Canetta R, Groopman JE. Phase I study of 2′- 3′-dideoxyinosine administered orally twice daily to patients with AIDS or AIDS-related complex and hematologic intolerance to zidovudine. Am J Med 1991; 91(5):471–478.

16. Lambert JS, Mindell S, Reichman RC, Plank CS, Laverty M, Morse GD, Knupp C, McLaren C, Pettinelli C, Valentine FT, Dolin R. 2′,3′-dideoxyinosine (ddI) in patients with the acquired immunodeficiency syndrome or AIDS-related complex. N Engl J Med 1990; 322:1333–1340.

17. Dolin R, Amato DA, Fischl MA, Pettinelli C, Beltangady M, Liou SH, Brown MJ, Cross AP, Hirsch MS, Hardy WD. Zidovudine compared with didanosine in patients with advanced HIV type 1 infection and little or no previous experience with zidovudine. Arch Intern Med 1995; 155(9):961–974.

18. Hammer S, Katzenstein D, Hughes M, et al. A trial comparing nucleoside monotherapy with combination therapy in HIV- infected adults with CD4 cell counts from 200 to 500 per cubic millimeter. N Engl J Med 1996; 335:1081–1090.

19. Kahn JO, Lagakos SW, Richmann DD, et al. A controlled trial comparing continued zidovudine with didanosine in human immunodeficiency virus infection. N Engl J Med 1992; 327:581–587.

20. Spruance SL, Pavia AT, Peterson D, et al. Didanosine compared with continuation of zidovudine in HIV-infected patients with signs of clinical deterioration while receiving zidovudine. Ann Intern Med 1994; 120:360–368.

21. Myers MW, Montaner JG, The Incas Study Group. Italy, Netherlands, Canada, Australia, and USA. A randomized, double-blinded comparative trial of the effects of zidovudine, dindanosine and nevirapine combinations in antiviral naive, AIDS-free, HIV- infected patients with CD4 counts 200–600/mm^3. XI International Conference on AIDS. Vancouver, July 7–12, 1996. Abstr. No. Mo.B.294.

22. Gao WY, Cara A, Gallo RC, Lori F. Low levels of deoxynucleotides in peripheral blood lymphocytes: a strategy to inhibit human immunodeficiency virus type 1 replication. Proc Nat. Acad Sci U S A 1993; 90:8925–8928.

23. Rutschmann OT, Opravil M. ddI + d4T ± hydroxyurea for HIV-1 infection (abstr). 5th Conference on Retroviruses and Opportunistic Infections. Chicago, IL, Feb 1–5, 1998, Abstr. No. 656:203.

24. Lori F, Jessen H, Clerici M, Lieberman J, Lisziewicz J. Consistent, sustained HIV suppression without rebound by hydrxyurea, ddI and a protease inhibitor prevents loss of immunologic functions. 5th Conference on Retroviruses and Opportunistic Infections. Chicago, Feb 1–5, 1998, Abstr. No. 655:203.

25. Jessen H, Clerici M, Liebermann J, Lisziewicz J, Lori F. Hydroxyurea, ddI and a protease inhibitor repress HIV in different compartments and reconstitute immunologic functions. 6th European Conference on Clinical Aspects and Treatment of HIV-Infection. Hamburg, Oct 11–15, 1997, Abstr. No. 130.

26. Rossero R, McKinsey D. Open label combination therapy with stavudine, didanosine and hydroxyurea in nucleoside experienced HIV-1 infected patients. 5th Conference on Retroviruses and Opportunistic Infections. Chicago, Feb. 1–5, 1998, Abstr. No. 653:202.

27. Follansbee S, Drew L, Olson R, et al. The efficacy of zalcitabine (ddC) vs zidovudine (ZDV) as monotherapy in ZDV naive patients with advanced HIV disease. IX International Conference on AIDS. Berlin, 1993, PO-B26-2113.

28. Fischl MA, Olson RM, Follansbee SE, et al. Zalcitabine compared with zidovudine in patients with advanced HIV-1 infection who received previous zidovudine therapy. Ann Intern Med 1993; 118:762–769.

29. Fischl MA, Stanley K, Collier AC, et al. Combination and monotherapy with zidovudine and zalcitabine in patients with advanced HIV disease. Ann Intern Med 1995; 122:24–32.

30. Abrams DI, Goldman AI, Launer C, et al. A comparative trial of didanosine or zalcitabine after treatment with zidovudine in patients with human immunodeficiency virus infection. N Engl J Med 1994; 330:657–662.

31. Pluda J, Cooley T, Montaner J, et al. Phase I/II study of 3TC (GR 109714X) in adults with ARC or AIDS. IX International Conference on AIDS. Berlin, 1993, WS-B26-2.

32. Boucher CAB. HIV development of drug resistance. In: Jäger H. HIV-Medizin: Möglichkeiten der individualisierten Therapie. 4. Münchner AIDS-Tage. ecomed. München 1994:41–43.

33. Friedland G. D4T current status. In: Jäger H. HIV-Medizin: Möglichkeiten der individualisierten Therapie. Münchner AIDS-Tage. ecomed. München 1994:299–300.

34. Pavia AT, Gathe J, BMS-019 Study Group Investigators. Clinical efficacy of stavudine (d4T, Zerit®) compared to zidovudine (ZDV, Retrovir®) in ZDV-pretreated HIV positive patients (abstr). 35th Interscience Conference on Antimicrobial Agents and Chemotherapy, 1995:235.

35. Bristol-Myers Squibb Company, Princeton, NJ. Stavudine (Zerit™) also known as d4T. Final results of the study BMS-019 (AI455-019) Phase III comparative trial. Princeton, Bristol-Myers Squibb Company, 1995.

36. Richman DD. Loss of nevirapine activity associated with the emergence of resistance in clinical trials. IIX International Conference on AIDS. Amsterdam, 1992, Abstr. No. PoB 3576.

37. Cheeseman SH, Havlir D, McLaughlin MM, et al. Phase I/II evaluation of nevirapine alone and in combination with zidovudine for infection with human immunodeficiency virus. J AIDS 1995; 8:141–151.

38. Montaner JSG, Reiss P, Cooper D, et al. A randomized, double-blind trial comparing combinations of nevirapine, didanosine and zidovudine for HIV-infected patients. JAMA 1998; 279(12):930–938.

39. D'Aquilla RT, Hughes MD, Johnson VA, Fischl MA, Sommadossi J-P, Liou S-h, Timpone J, Myers M, Basgoz N, Niu M, Hirsch MS. Nevirapine, zidovudine and didanosine compared with zidovudine and didanosine in patients with HIV-1 infection. Ann Intern Med 1996; 124:1019–1030.

40. Warren KJ, Boxwell DE, Kim N, et al. Nevirapine-associated Stevens-Johnson syndrome. Lancet 1998; 351(9102):567.

41. Tashima K, Staszewski S, Stryker R, Johnson P, Nelson M, Morales-Ramirez J, Manion DJ, Farina D, Labriola D, Ruiz N, the Study 006 Investigator Team. A phase III,

multicenter, randomized, open-label study to compare the antiretroviral activity and tolerability of efavirenz + indinavir, versus EFV + zidovudine + lamivudine, versus IDV + ZDV + 3TC at 48 weeks. 6th Conference on Retroviruses and Opportunistic Infections. Chicago, Jan 31–Feb 4, 1999, Abstr. No. LB 16.

42. Mayers D, Riddler S, Bach M, et al. Durable clinical anti-HIV-1 activity and tolerability for DMP 266 in combination with indinavir (IDV) at 24 weeks. 37th Interscience Conference on Antimicrobial Agents and Chemotherapy, Toronto, Canada, Sept 28–Oct 1, 1997, Abstr. No. I-175.

43. Wagner, et al. 8th Eur Cong Clin Microbiol Inf Dis. Lausanne, May 1997, Abstr. No. 3043.

44. Hicks C, Haas D, Seekins D, Cooper R, Gallant J, Carpenter C, Ruiz NM, Manion DM, Plougham LM, Labriola DF. A phase II, double blind, placebo-controlled, dose-ranging study to assess the activity and safety of DMP 266 (Efavirenz, Sustiva™) in combination with open-label zidovudine (ZDV) with lamivudine (3TC). 6th European Conference on Clinical Aspects and Treatment of HIV-Infection. Hamburg, Germany, Oct 11–15, 1997, Abstr. No. 920.

45. Sonnerborg A, Lancaster D, Torres R, et al. The safety and the antiviral effect of 1592U89, alone and in combination with zidovudine in HIV-infected patients with 200–500 cell/μl. 3rd International Congress on Drug Therapy in HIV Infection. Birmiham, UK, Nov. 3–7, 1996, Abstr. No. OP4.1.

46. Fischl M, Greenberg S, Clumeck N, Peters B, Rubio R, Gould J, Boone G, West M, Spreen B, Lafon S. Ziagen (abacavir, ABC, 1592) combined with 3 TC & ZDV is highly effective and durable through 48 weeks in HIV-1 infected antiretroviral-therapy-naive subjects (CNAA3003). 6th Conference on Retroviruses and Opportunistic Infections. Chicago, Jan 31–Feb 4, 1999, Abstr. No. 19.

47. Staszewski S, Keiser P, Gathe J, Haas D, Montaner J, Hammer S, Delfraissy J-F, Cutrell A, Lafon S, Thorborn D, Pearce G, Spreen W, Tortell S, the CNA3005 International Study Team. Ziagen/combivir is equivalent to indinavir/combivir in antiretroviral therapy naive adults at 24 weeks. 6th Conference on Retroviruses and Opportunistic Infections. Chicago, Jan 31–Feb 4, 1999, Abstr. No. 20.

48. Staszewski S, Katlama C, Harrer T, Massip P, Yeni P, Cutrell A, Tortell SM, Steel HM, Lanier ER, Pearce G. Preliminary long-term open-label data from patients using abacavir (1592) containing antiretroviral treatment regimens. 5th Conference on Retroviruses and Opportunistic Infections. Chicago, Feb 1–5, 1998. Abstr. No. 658.

49. Torres R, Saag M, Lancaster D, Sonnerborg A, Feinberg J, Thompson M, Lang W, Schooley R, Mulder J, D'Aquila R, Santin M, Lafon S, Antiviral effects of abacavir (1592) following 36 weeks of therapy. 5th Conference on Retroviruses and Opportunistic Infections. Chicago, Feb 1–5, 1998, Abstr. No. 659.

50. Lanier ER, Stone C, Griffin P, Thomas D, Lafon S. Phenotypic sensitivity to 1592 (abacavir) in the presence of multiple genotypic mutations: correlation with viral load response. 5th Conference on Retroviruses and Opportunistic Infections. Chicago, Feb. 1–5, 1998, Abstr. No. 686.

51. Mellors JW, Hertogs K, Peeters F, Lanier R, Miller V, Graham N, Larder B, Stoffels P, Pauwels R. Susceptibility of clinical HIV-1 isolates to 1592U89. 5th Conference on Retroviruses and Opportunistic Infections. Chicago, Feb. 1–5, 1998, Abstr. No. 687.

52. Eron J, Falloon J, Masur H, Ait-Khaled M, Thomas D, Manion D, Rogers M for the CNAA2007 Study Team. Activity of combination abacavir/amprenavir/efavirenz

therapy in HIV-1 infected subjects failing their current protease inhibitor containing regimen. 4th International Congress on Drug Therapy in HIV Infection. Glasgow, Nov 8–12, 1999 Abstr. No. OP5.2.

52a. Staszewski S, Massari FE, Kober A, Göhler R, Durr S, Anderson KW, Schneider CL, Waterbury JA, Bakshi KK, Taylor VI, Hildebrand CS, Kreisl C, Hoffstedt B, Schleiff WA, von Briesen H, Rübsamen-Waigmann H, Calandra GB, Ryen JR, Stille W, Emini EA, Byrnes VW. Combination therapy with zidovudine prevents selection of human immunodeficiency virus type 1 variants expressing high-level resistance to L-697,661 a nonnucleoside reverse transcriptase inhibitor. J Infect Dis 1995; 171:1159–1165.

53. Deeks S, Collier A, Lalezari J, Pavia A, Rodrigue D, Jaffe HS, Toole J, Kahn J. A randomized double-blind, placebo-controlled study of bis-POM PMEA in HIV-infected patients. Third Conference on Retroviruses and Opportunistic Infections. Washington, DC, Jan 28–Feb 1, 1966, Abstr. No. 407.

54. Miller M, Anton K, Mulato A, Lamy P, Cherrington M. HIV-1 expressing the 3TC-associated M184V mutation in reverse transcriptase (RT) shows increased sensitivity to Adefoivir and PMPA as well as decreased replication capacity in vitro. 12th World AIDS Conference. Geneva, Jun 28–Jul 3, 1998, Poster 41214.

55. Hammer S, Squires K, Degruttola V, Fischl M, Bassett R, Demeter L, Hertogs K, Larder B, the ACTG 372B Study Team. Randomized trial of abacavir and nelfinavir in combination with efavirenz and adefovir dipivoxil as salvage therapy in patients with virologic failure receiving indinavir. 6th Conference on Retroviruses and Opportunistic Infections. Chicago, Jan 31–Feb 4, 1999, Abstr. No. 490.

56. Fisher E, Brosgart C, Cohn D, Chaloner K, Pulling C, Alston B, Schmetter B, El-Sadr W. Placebo-controlled, multicenter trial of adefovir dipivoxil in patients with HIV disease. 6th Conference on Retroviruses and Opportunistic Infections. Chicago, Jan 31–Feb 4, 1999, Abstr. No. 491.

57. De Simone C, Famularo G, Tzantzoglou S, Trinchieri V, Moretti S, Sorice F. Carnitine depletion in peripheral blood mononuclear cells from patients with AIDS: Effect of oral carnitine. AIDS 1994; 8:655–660.

58. Barriere S, Winslow D, Coakley D, Rooney J. Safety of adefovir dipivoxil in the treatment of HIV-infection. 12th World AIDS Conference. Geneva Jun 28–Jul 3, 1998, Abstr. No. 12386.

59. Pottage J, Thompson M, Kahn J. Delehanty J, McCreedy B, Rousseau F. Potent antiretroviral efficacy of low dose FTC, initial results from a phase I/II clinical trial. 5th Conference on Retroviruses and Opportunistic Infections. Chicago, Feb 1–5, 1998, Abstr. No. LB9 (224).

60. Tsai CC, Follis KE, Sabo A, Beck TW, Grant RF, Bischofberger N, Benveniste RE, Black R. Prevention of SIV infection in macaques by (R)-9-(2-phosphonyl-methoxypropyl)adenine. Science 1995; 270:1197.

61. Deeks SG, Barditch-Crovo P, Lietman PS, Collier A, Safrin S, Coleman R, Cundy KC, Kahn JO. The safety and efficacy of PMPA prodrug monotherapy: preliminary results of a phase I/II dose-escalation study. 5th Conference on Retroviruses and Opportunistic Infections. Chicago, Feb 1–5, 1998, Abstr. No. LB8.

62. Meng T-C, Fischl MA, Boota AM, et al. Combination therapy with zidovudine and dideoxycytidine in patients with advanced human immunodeficiency virus infection. A phase I/II study. Ann Intern Med 1992; 116:13–20.

63. Yarchoan R, Perno CF, Thomas RV, et al. Phase I studies of 2´,3´-dideoxycytidine in severe human immunodeficiency virus infection as a single agent and alternating with zidovudine (AZT). Lancet 1988; 1:76–81.

64. Delta Coordinating Committee. Delta: a randomized double-blind controlled trial comparing combinations of zidovudine plus didanodine or zalcitabine with zidovudine. Lancet 1996; 348:283–291.

65. Eron JJ, Benoit SL, Jemsek J, MacArthur RD, Santana J, Quinn JB, Kuritzkes DR, Fallon MA, Rubin M. Treatment with lamivudine, zidovudine, or both in HIV-positive patients with 200 to 500 CD4+ cells per cubic millimeter. N Engl J Med 1995; 333(25):1662–1669.

66. Staszewski S, Loveday C, Picazo JJ, Dellamonica P, Skinhoj P, Johnson MA, Danner SA, Harrigan PR, Hill AM, Verity L, McDade H for the Lamivudine European HIV working group. Safety and efficacy of lamivudine-zidovudine combination therapy in zidovudine experienced patients. JAMA 1996; 276:111–117.

67. Katlama C, Ingrand D, Loveday C, Clumeck N, Mallolas J, Staszewski S, Johnson M, Hill AM, Pearce G, McDade H. Safety and efficacy of lamivudine-zidovudine combination therapy in antiretroviral-naive patients. A randomized controlled comparison with zidovudine monotherapy. Lamivudine European HIV working group. JAMA 1996; 276(2):118–125.

68. Caesar Coordinating Committee. Randomised trial of addition of lamivudine or lamivudine plus loviridine to zidovudine-containing regimens for patients with HIV-1 infection: the Caesar trial. Lancet 1997; 349(9063):1413–1421.

69. Furman PA, Davis M, Liotta DC, et al. The anti-hepatitis B virus activities, cytotoxities, and anabolic profiles of the (-) and (+) enantiomers of cis-5-fluoro-1-[2-(hydroxymethyl)-1,3-oxathiolan-5-yl] cytosine, Antimicrob Agents Chemother 1992; 36(22):2686–2692.

69a. Deres K, Rübsamen-Waigmann. Development of resistance and perspectives for future therapies against hepatitis B infections: lessons to be learned for HIV. Infection 1999; 27(suppl 2):545–555.

70. Cooper D, Montaner J, Katlama C, et al. The Caesar trial: final results. 4th Conference on Retroviruses and Opportunistic Infections. Washington, DC, Jan 22–26, 1997, Abstr. No. 367.

71. Kuritzkes DR, Marschner IC, Johnson VA, Bassett RL, Eron JJ, Fischl MA, Bone G, Skovronski J, Wood K, Bell DL, Pettinelli CB, Sommadossi JP, ACTG 306 Study Team. A randomized, double-blind, placebo-controlled trial of lamivudine (3TC) in combination with zidovudine (ZDV), stavudine (d4T), or didanosine (ddI) in treatment naive patients. 5th Conference on Retroviruses and Opportunistic Infections. Chicago, Feb. 1–5, 1998, Abstr. No. 1.

72. Raffi F, Auger S, Billaud E, Besnier JM, Chennebault JM, Michelet C, Perre P, Lafeuillade A, May T, Arvieux C, Paillant C, Barin F, Billaudel S. Antiviral effect and safety of didanosine-stavudine combination therapy in HIV-infected subjects: interim results of a pilot trial. 4th Conference on Retroviruses and Opportunistic Infections (United States). Jan 22–26, 1997, Abstr. No. 554.

73. Durant J, Rahelinirina V, Delmas B, Dupre F, Carmagnolle MF, Halfon P, Van PN, Dellamonica P. A pilot study of the combination of stavudine (d4T) and didanosine (ddI) in patients with less than 350 CD4/µl and who are not eligible for a treatment

with ZDV. 4th Conference on Retroviruses and Opportunistic Infections (United States). Jan 22–26, 1997, Abstr. No. 553.

74. Havlir DV, Marschner IC, Hirsch MS, Collier AC, Tebas P, Bassett RL, Ioannidis JPA, Holohan MK, Leavitt R, Boone G, Richman DD. Maintenance antiretroviral therapies in HIV-infected subjects with undetectable plasma HIV RNA after triple-drug therapy. N Engl J Med 1998; 339:1261.

75. Hoggard PG, Kewn S, Barry MG, Khoo SH, Back DJ. Effects of drugs in 2′,3′-dideoxy-2′,3′- didehydrothymidine phosphorylation in vitro. Antimicrob Agents Chemother 1997; 41(&):1231–1236.

76. Carr A, Cooper D, Thorisdottir A, et al. Prevalence and severity of protease inhibitor induced lipodystrophy and insulin resistance. 12th World AIDS Conference. Geneva Jun 28–Jul 3, 1998, Abstr. No. 12462.

77. James JS. Delavirdine (Rescriptor) approved. AIDS Treatment News 1997; 269:1–3.

78. Wathen L, Freimuth W, Getchel L, Greenwald C, Crampton D. Use of HIV-1 RNA PCR in patients on Rescriptor (DLV) + Retrovir (ZDV) + Epivir (3TC), ZDV + 3TC or DLV + ZDV allowed early differentiation between treatment groups. 5th Conference on Retroviruses and Opportunistic Infections. Chicago, Feb. 1–5, 1998, Abstr. No. 694.

79. Sargent S, Green S, Para M, Freimuth W, Wathen L, Getchel L, Greenwald C. Sustained plasma viral burden reductions and CD4 increases in HIV-1 infected patients with Rescriptor (DVL) + Retrovir (ZDV) + Epivir (3TC). 5th Conference on Retroviruses and Opportunistic Infections. Chicago. Feb. 1–5, 1998, Abstr. No. 699.

80. Rozenbaum W, Delphin N, Katlama C, Massip P, Bentata M, Mamet JP, Sturge G, for the CNAB3009 team. Treatment intensification with ziagen in HIV infected patients with previous 3TC/ZDV antiretroviral treatment-CNAB3009. 6th Conference on Retroviruses and Opportunistic Infections. Chicago, Jan 31–Feb 4, 1999, Abstr. No. 377.

81. Carr A, Samaras K, Burton S, et al. A syndrome of peripheral lipodystrophy, hyperlipidemia and insulin resistance in patients receiving HIV protease inhibitors. AIDS 1998; 12:F51–F58.

82. Carr A, Samaras K, Chilson DJ, et al. Pathogenesis of HIV-1-protease inhibitor associated peripheral lipodystrophy, hyperlipidaemia and insulin resistance. Lancet 1998; 351:1881–1883.

83. Murphy R, King M, Brun S, Orth K, Hicks C, Eron J, Thommes J, Gulick R, Thompson M, White C, Benson C, Hammer S, Kessler H, Bertz R, Hsu A, Kempf D, Sun E, Japour A, for the M97-720 Study Group. ABT-378/ritonavir therapy in antiretroviral-naive HIV-1 infected patients for 24 weeks. 6th Conference on Retroviruses and Opportunistic Infections. Chicago, Jan 31–Feb 4, 1999, Abstr. No. 15.

84. Walli R, Herfort O, Michl GM, et al. Treatment with protease inhibitors associated with peripheral insulin resistance and impaired glucose tolerance in HIV-1 infected patients. AIDS 1998, 12:F167–F173.

85. Mauss S, Wolf E, Jaeger H. Impaired glucose tolerance in patients receiving and those not receiving protease inhibitors. Ann Intern Med 1999, 130:162–163.

86. Henry K, Melroe H, Huebesch J, et al. Atorvastatin and gemfibrozil for protease-inhibitor-related lipid abnormalities. Lancet 1998; 352:1031–1032.

87. Flexner C. Pharmacologic causes of treatment failure. 5th Conference on Retroviruses and Opportunistic Infections. 1998, Abstr. No. S47.
88. Salgo MP, Mikklos BP, Beattie D, et al. Saquinavir (invirase, SQV) vs. Hivid (zalcitabine, ddC), vs. combination as treatment for advanced HIV infection in patients discontinuing/unable to take retrovir (zidovudine, ZDV), Xi International Conference on AIDS. Vancouver, Canada, Jul 7–12, 1996, Abstr. No. MO.B.410.
89. Collier AC, Coombs RW, Schoefeld DA, et al. Treatment of human immunodeficiency virus infection with saquinavir, zidovudine, and zalcitabine. N Engl J Med 1996; 334:1011–1017.
90. Stellbrink HJ, on behalf of the Invirase International Phase III Trial (SV-14604). Clinical and survival benefit of saquinavir (SQV) in combination with zalcitabine (ddC) and zidovudine (ZDV) in untreated/minimally treated HIV-infected patients. 6th European Conference on Clinical Aspects and Treatment of HIV-Infection. Hamburg, Germany, Oct 11–15, 1997, Abstr. No. 212.
91. Schapiro JM, Winters MA, Stewart F, Efron B, Norris J, Kozal MJ, Merigan TC. The effect of high-dose saquinavir on viral load and CD4+ T-cell counts in HIV-infected patients. Ann Intern Med 1996; 124:1039–1050.
92. Borleffs JC. First Comparative Study of Saquinavir Soft Gel Capsules versus indinavir as part of triple therapy regimen (CHEESE). 5th Conference on Retroviruses and Opportunistic Infections. Chicago, Feb 1–5, 1998.
93. Gill MJ, Beall G, Beatti D, et al. Safety of saquinavir soft gel capsule (SQV-SGC) in combination with other antiretroviral agents: multicenter study NV15182: 24 week analyses. Interscience Conference on Antimicrobial Agents and Chemotherapy. Toronto, Sep 28–Oct 1, 1997, Abstr. No. I-90.
94. Merry C, Barry MG, Mulcahy F, Ryan M, et al. Saquinavir pharmacokinetics alone and in combination with ritonavir in HIV-infected patients. AIDS 1997; 11:F29–F33.
95. Kravcik S, Sahai J, Kerr B, et al. Nelfinavir mesylate (NFV) increases saquinavir-soft gel capsule (SQV-SGC) exposure in HIV+ patients. 4th Conference on Retroviruses and Opportunistic Infections. Washington, DC, Jan 22–26, 1997, Abstr. No. 371.
96. Cox SR, Ferry JJ, Batts DH, et al. Delaviridine and marketed protease inhibitors (PIs): pharmacokinetic studies in healthy volunteers. 4th Conference on Retroviruses and Opportunistic Infections. Washington, DC, Jan 22–26, 1997, Abstr. No. 372.
97. Buss N, on behalf of the Fortovase® Study Group, Roche Products Ltd. Saquinavir soft gel capsule (Fortovase®): Pharmacokinetics and drug interactions. 5th Conference on Retroviruses and Opportunistic Infections. Chicago, Feb 1–5, 1998, Abstr. No. 354 (145).
98. Cameron B, Heath-Chiozzi M, Kravcik S, Mills R, et al. Prolongation of life and prevention of AIDS in advanced HIV immunodeficiency with ritonavir. 3rd Conference on Retroviruses and Opportunistic Infections. Washington, DC, 1996, Abstr. No. LB6a.
99. Heath-Chiozzi M, Leonad J, Henry D, et al. Anti HIV activity and lymphocyte surrogate marker response dynamics to retonavir therapy in advanced HIV immunodeficiency. 3rd Conference on Retroviruses and Opportunistic Infections. Washington, DC, 1996, Abstr. No. LB6b.

100. Mathez D, De Truchis P, Gorin I, et al. Ritonavir, AZT, DDC as a triple combination in AIDS patients. 3rd Conference on Retroviruses and Opportunistic Infections. Washington, DC, 1996, Abstr. No. 285.

101   Kelleher A, Carr A, Zaunders J, Cooper DA. Immunologic effects of ritonavir, a HIV protease inhibitor. 3rd Conference on Retroviruses and Opportunistic Infections. Washington, DC, 1996, Abstr. No. 232.

102. Jaramillo A, Zaunders J, Kelleher T, Cooper DA. Improvement in T-cell receptor BV perturbations following combination therapy with indinavir and nucleoside RT inhibitors. 5th Conference on Retroviruses and Opportunistic Infections. Chicago, Feb. 1–5, 1998, Abstr. No. 153.

103. Gorochov G, Neumann AU, Kereveur A, Parizot C, Li T, Katlama C, Karmochkine M, Raguin G, Autran B, Debre P. Disordering of CD4 and CD8 T-cell repertoires during progression to AIDS and restoration of the CD4 repertoire under antiviral therapy. 5th Conference on Retroviruses and Opportunistic Infections. Chicago, Feb 1–5, 1998, Abstr. No. 154.

104. Lantz O, Martinon F, Peguillet I, Taoufik Y, Lefebvre P, Bellissant E, Goujard C, Michelet C, Guillet JJ, Delfrissy JF. Longitudinal study of cytokine gene expression and TCR Vb repertoire on patients after initiation of ritonavir plus saquinavir therapy (ANRS 069). 5th Conference on Retroviruses and Opportunistic Infections. Chicago, Feb 1–5, 1998, Abstr. No. 155.

105. Weiss L, Girard PM, Roux A, Ancuta P, Tessey C, Kazatchkine MD, Haeffner-Cavaillon N. Changes in immunological status of HIV-infected patients receiving triple combination antiretroviral therapy. 5th Conference on Retroviruses and Opportunistic Infections. Chicago, Feb. 1–5, 1998, Abstr. No. 156.

106. Hengel RL, Jones BM, Kennedy SM, Hubbard MS, McDougal JS. Reconstitution of "naive" (CD45RA+CD62L+CD4+ T-cells after potent anti-HIV-1 therapy. 5th Conference on Retroviruses and Opportunistic Infections. Chicago, Feb 1–5, 1998, Abstr. No. 157.

107. Wilkinson J, Zaunders J, McQueen P, Delaney S, Cooper DA. CD8 T cell-mediated suppression of HIV-1 is enhanced in patients receiving stavudine/indinavir therapy. 5th Conference on Retroviruses and Opportunistic Infections. Chicago, Feb. 1–5, 1998, Abstr. No. 164.

108. Farthing C, Japour A, Cohen C, et al. Cerebrospinal fluid (CSF) and plasma HIV RNA suppression with ritonavir (RIT)-saquinavir (SQV) in protease inhibitor naive patients. 37th Interscience Conference on Antimicrobial Agents and Chemotherapy. Toronto, Ontario, Canada, Sept 28–Oct 1, 1997, LB-3.

109. Kempf D, Marsh K, Denissen J, et al. Coadministration with ritonavir enhances the plasma levels of HIV protease inhibitors by inhibition of cytochrome P450. 3rd Conference on Retroviruses and Opportunistic Infections. Washington, DC, 1996, Abstr. No. 143.

110. Hsu A, Granneman GR, Japour A, Cao G, Locke C, Carothers L, Dennis S, El-Shourbagy T, Leonard J, Sun E. Evaluation of potential ritonavir and indinavir combination BID regimens. 37th Interscience Conference on Antimicrobial Agents and Chemotherapy.

111. Massari F, Staszewski S, Berry P, Kahn J, Frank I, Heath-Chiozzi M, Sampson J, Eron J, Eyster E, Teppler H, Schleif W, Condra J, Leavitt R, Emini E. A double-blind,

randomized trial of indinavir (MK-639) alone or with zidovudine in naive patients. 35th Interscience Conference on Antimicrobial Agents and Chemotherapy. San Francisco, 1995, Abstr. No. LB-6.

112. Massari F, Conant M, Mellors J. A phase II open-label, randomized study of the triple combination of indinavir, zidovudine and didanosine versus indinavir alone and zidovudine/didanosine in antiretroviral naive patients. 3rd Conference on Retroviruses and Opportunistic Infections. Washington, DC, 1996, Abstr. No. 200.

113. Mellors J, Steigbigel RT, Gulick R, et al. Antiretroviral activity of the oral protease inhibitor, MK-639, in p24 antigenemic, HIV-1 infected patients with <500 CD4/mm³. 35th Interscience Conference on Antimicrobial Agents and Chemotherapy. San Francisco, 1995, Abstr. No. 172.

114. Steigbigel RT, Berry P, Mellors J, McMahon D, et al. Efficacy and safety of the HIV protease inhibitor indinavir sulfate (Mk 639) at escalating dose. 3rd Conference on Retroviruses and Opportunistic Infections. Washington, DC, 1996, Abstr. No. 146.

115. Gulick R, Mellors J, Havlir D, et al. Treatment with indinavir, zidovudine and lamivudine in adults with human immunodeficiency virus infection and prior antiretroviral therapy. N Engl J Med 1997; 337:734–739.

116. Hammer S, Squires K, Hughes M, et al. A controlled trial of two nucleoside analogues plus indinavir in persons with human immunodeficiency virus infection and CD4 counts of 200 per cubic millimeter or less. N Engl J Med 1997; 337:725–733.

117. Lin JH, Chiba M, Balani SK, et al. Species differences in the pharmacokinetics and metabolism of indinavir, a potent human immunodeficiency virus protease inhibitor. Drug Metab Dispos 1996; 24(10):1111–1120.

118. Protocol 069, data from Merck & Co.

119. Acosta EP, Henry K, Weller D, Page LM, Bacon L, Rhame F, Gilson I, Rosenstein H, Schacker T. Indinavir pharmacokinetics between exposure and antiviral effect. Interscience Conference on Antimicrobial Agents and Chemotherapy. Toronto, Sep 28–Oct 1, 1997, Abstr. No. A-15.

120. Petersen AK, Gersten M, Knowles, et al. Long-term virological and immunological response to treatment with Viracept (nelfinavir mesylate) in combination with zidovudine and lamivudine. 6th European Conference on Clinical Aspects and Treatment of HIV-Infection. Hamburg, Germany, Oct 11–15, 1997, Abstr. No. 210.

121. Ballard C, Toerner JG, Colwell B, et al. Early CD4, viral load, and quality of life response to salvage treatment with nelfinavir: the UCSD Owen Clinic Nelfinavir Expanded Access experience. 37th Interscience Conference on Antimicrobial Agents and Chemotherapy. Toronto, Ontario, Canada, Sept 28–Oct 1, 1997, Abstr. No. I-192.

122. Johnson M, Petersen A, Winslade J, Clendeninn N. Comparison of BID and TID dosing of Viracept (nelfinavir, NFV) in combination with stavudine (d4T) and lamivudine (3TC). 5th Conference on Retroviruses and Opportunistic Infections. Chicago, Feb 1–5, 1998, Abstr. No. 373.

123. Schooley RT, the 141W94 International Study Group. Preliminary data from a phase I/II study on the safety and antiviral efficacy of the combination of 141W94 and 1592U89 in HIV-infected patients with 150 to 400 cell/mm³. 4th Conference on Retroviruses and Opportunistic Infections. Washington, DC, 1997, Abstr. No. LB3.

124. Partaledis JA, et al. In vitro selection and characteristics of human immunodeficiency

virus type 1 isolates with reduced sensitivity to hydroxyethilamino sulfonamide inhibitors of HIV-1. J Virol 1995; 69:5228–5235.

125. Tisdale M, Myers RE, Harrigan PR, et al. Analyses of HIV genotype and phenotype during 4 weeks dose-escalating monotherapy with the HIV protease inhibitor 141W94 in HIV-infected patients with CD4 counts 150–400 mm^3. 4th Conference on Retroviruses and Opportunistic Infections. Washington, DC, 1997, Abstr. No. 593.

126. Japour A. Future prospects in protease inhibitor therapy. Satellite symposium: optimizing the use of protease inhibitors. 6th European Conference on Clinical Aspects and Treatment of HIV-Infection. Hamburg, Germany, Oct 11, 1997, Abstr. Book No. 24-27.

127. Lal R, Hsu A, Chen P, et al. single dose pharmacokinetics of ABT-378 in combination with ritonavir. 37th Interscience Conference on Antimicrobial Agents and Chemotherapy. Toronto, Ontario, Canada, Sept 28–Oct 1, 1997, Abstr. No. I-194.

128. Cameron DW. HAART: Maximizing synergies. Satellite symposium: HAART: tailoring therapy to the individual. 6th European Conference on Clinical Aspects and Treatment of HIV-Infection. Hamburg, Germany, Oct 12, 1997, oral presentation.

129. Rockstroh JK, Bermann F, Wiesel W, et al. Efficacy and safety of BID firstline ritonavir/indinavir plus double nucleoside combination therapy in HIV-infected individuals. 6th Conference on Retroviruses and Opportunistic Infections. Chicago, Jan 31–Feb 4, 1999, Abstr. No. 631.

130. Saah AJ, Winchell G, Seniuk M, et al. Multiple-dose pharmacokinetics (PK) and tolerability of indinavir (IDV) ritonavir (RTV) combinations in healthy volunteers. 6th Conference on Retroviruses and Opportunistic Infections. Chicago, Jan 31–Feb 4, 1999, Abstr. No. 362.

131. de Wolf F, Lukashov VV, Danner SA, Goudsmit J, Lange JMA. Clearance of HIV-1 following treatment with three, four and five anti-HIV drugs. 5th Conference on Retroviruses and Opportunistic Infections. Chicago, Feb 1–5, 1998, Abstr. No. 384.

132. Prins J, Jurriaans S, Roos M, de Wolf F, Miedema F, Lange J. An attempt at maximally suppressive anti-HIV therapy. 5th Conference on Retroviruses and Opportunistic Infections. Chicago, Feb 1–5, 1998, Abstr. No. 385.

133. Dezube BJ, Wong TK, Dahl TA, Chapman B, Ono M, Gillies SD, Chen LB, Crumpacker CS. A fusion inhibitor (FP-21399) for the treatment of HIV infection: a phase I study. 5th Conference on Retroviruses and Opportunistic Infections. Chicago, Feb 1–5, 1998, Abstr. No. 650.

134. Hopkins S, Lambert MD, Rency MR, Johnson MR, Saag M. Pentafuside (T-20), a novel inhibitor of HIV-1 fusion: pharmacokinetics in rodents, monkeys and man. 4th Conference on Retroviruses and Opportunistic Infections. Washington, DC, Jan 22–25, 1997, Abstr. No. 224.

135. Lalezari J, Eron J, Carlson M, Arduino R, Goodgame J, Cohen C, Jones L, Gleavy A, Dusek A, Venetta T, Dimassimo E, Hopkins S, for the TRI-003 Study Group. Safety, pharmacokinetics, and antiviral activity of T-20 as a single agent in heavily pre-treated patients. 6th Conference on Retroviruses and Opportunistic Infections. Chicago, Jan 31–Feb 4, 1999, Abstr. No. LB13.

136. Gogliotti RD, Ellsworth EL, Holler TP, Hupe D, Foltin SK, Kennedy RM, Sanchez JP, Domagala JM. Quinolones as novel HIV integrase inhibitors. 5th Conference on Retroviruses and Opportunistic Infections. Chicago, Feb 1–5, 1998, Abstr. No. 641.

137. Hendersen LE, Chertova E, Ott D, Hewess M, Cases-Finet JR, Kane B, Johnson DG, Sowder II RC, Rossio J, Lifson J, Arthur LO, NCI-FCRDC, SAIC-Frederick, Frederick MD. In vitro and in vivo activity of antiretroviral compounds attacking NC zinc fingers. 5th Conference on Retroviruses and Opportunistic Infections. Chicago, Feb 1–5, 1998, Abstr. No. 7.

138. Deeks S, Loftus R, Cohen P, Chin S, Grant R. Incidence and predictors of virologic failure to indinavir (IDV) or/and ritonavir (RTV) in an urban health clinic. 37th Interscience Conference on Antimicrobial Agents and Chemotherapy. Toronto, Ontario, Canada, Sept 28–Oct 1, 1997, Abstr. No. LB-2.

139. Fätkenheuer G, Theisen A, Rockstroh J, et al. Virological treatment failure of protease inhibitor therapy in an unselected cohort of HIV-infected patients. AIDS 1997; 11:113–116.

140. Sommadossi JP, Zhou XJ, Moore J, Havlir DV, Friedland G, Tierney C, Smeaton L, Fox L, Richman D, Pollard R, the ACTG 290 team. Impairment of stavudine (d4T) phosphorylation in patients receiving a combination of zidovudine (ZDV) and d4T (ACTG 290). 5th Conference on Retroviruses and Opportunistic Infections. Chicago, Feb. 1–5, 1998, Abstr. No. 3.

141. Descamps D, Collin G, Letourneur F, Apetrei C, Damond F, Loussert-Ajaka I, Simon F, Saragosti S, Brun-Vezinet F. Susceptibility of human immunodeficiency virus type 1 group O isolates to antiretroviral agents: in vitro phenotypic and genotypic analyses. J Virol 1997; 71(11):8893–8898.

142. Dietrich U, Ruppach H, Gehring S, Knechten H, Knickmann M, Jäger H, Wolf E, Husak R, Orfanos CE, Brede HD, Rübsamen-Waigmann H, von Briesen H. Large proportion of non-B HIV-1 subtypes and presence of AZT-resistance mutations among German seroconvertors. AIDS 1997; 11:1532–1533.

143. Boden D, Hurley A, Zhang L, Yunzhen Cao, Yong G, Jones E, Tsay J, Ip J, Farthing C, Limoli K, Parkin N, Markowitz M. HIV-1 drug resistance in newly infected individuals. JAMA 1999; 282:1135–1141.

144. Little SJ, Daar ES, D'Aquila RT, Keiser PH, Connick E, Whitcomb JM, Hellmann NS, Petropoulos CJ, Sutton L, Pitt JA, Rosenberg ES, Koup RA, Walker BD, Richman DD. Reduced antiretroviral drug susceptibility among patients with primary HIV infection. JAMA 1999; 282:1142–1149.

145. Jeffrey S, Baker D, Tritch R, Rizzo C, Logue K, Bacheler L. A resistance and cross-resistance for SUSTIVA™ (Efavirenz, DMP 266). 5th Conference on Retroviruses and Opportunistic Infections. Chicago, Feb. 1–5, 1998, Abstr. No. 702.

146. DHHS proposes new HIV-AIDS treatment guidelines. Public Health Rep. 1997; 112(5):359–360.

147. German-Austrian guidelines for antiretroviral therapy of HIV infection. Eur J Med Res 1997; 2:535–542.

148. Walker BD. HIV infection: the body fights back. 5th Conference on Retroviruses and Opportunistic Infections. Chicago, Feb. 1–5, 1998, Abstr. No. L4.

149. Treatment Issues' second survey of physicians' treatment practice. Treatment Issue 1997/98; 12(1):3–17.

150. Tebas P, Royal M, Fichtenbaum C, Blutman J, Arens M, Horgan M, Powderly W. Relationship between adherence to HAART and disease state. 5th Conference on Retroviruses and Opportunistic Infections. Chicago, Feb. 1–5, 1998, Abstr. No. 149.

151. de Truchis P, Force G, Zucman D, Leclerc V, Rouveix E, Simonpoli AM, Berthe H. Effects of a "salvage" combination therapy with ritonavir + saquinavir in HIV-infected patients previously treated with protease-inhibitors (PI). 5th Conference on Retroviruses and Opportunistic Infections. Chicago, Feb. 1–5, 1998, Abstr. No. 425.

152. Lawrence J, Schapiro J, Winters M, Montoya J, Zolopa A, Pesano R, Winslow D, Merigan TC. Salvage therapy with indinavir plus nevirapine in patients previously treated with two other protease inhibitors and multiple reverse transcriptase inhibitors. 5th Conference on Retroviruses and Opportunistic Infections. Chicago, Feb. 1–5, 1998, Abstr. No. 422:158.

153. Pialoux G, Raffi F, Brun-Vezinet F, Meiffrédy V, Flandre P, Gastaut J-A, Dellamonica P, Yeni P, Delfraissy J-F, Aboulker J-P. A randomized trial of three maintenance regimens given after three months of induction therapy with zidovudine, lamivudine and indinavir in previously untreated HIV-1-infected patients. N Engl J Med 1998; 339:1269.

154. Puig T, Bonjoch A, Ruiz L, Arno A, Sirera G, Romeu J, Clotet B. Usefulness of ritonavir and saquinavir combination therapy for HIV-advanced patients failing on indinavir. 37th Interscience Conference on Antimicrobial Agents and Chemotherapy. Toronto, Ontario, Canada, Sept. 28–Oct. 1, 1997, Abstr. No. I-201:281.

155. Henry K, Kane E, Melroe H, Simpson J, Patick A, Winslow D. Experience with a ritonavir/saquinavir based regimen for the treatment of HIV-infection in subjects developing increased viral loads while receiving nelfinavir. 37th Interscience Conference on Antimicrobial Agents and Chemotherapy. Toronto, Ontario, Canada, Sept. 28–Oct 1, 1997, Abstr. No. I-204:282.

156. Batisse D, Salmon-Seron D, Karmpochkine M, Ginsburg C, Castiel P, Raguin G, Weiss L, Sicard D, Kazatchkine MD. Efficacy and safety of ritonavir and saquinavir in combination in protease inhibitors-experienced patients. 37th Interscience Conference on Antimicrobial Agents and Chemotherapy. Toronto, Ontario, Canada, Sept. 28–Oct 1, 1997, Abstr. No. I-206:281.

157. Workman C, Mussen R, Sullivan J, Fitzroy St. Salvage therapy using six drugs in heavily pretreated patients. 5th Conference on Retroviruses and Opportunistic Infections. Chicago, Feb. 1–5, 1998, Abstr. No. 426.

3
Antivirals and Resistance

Ursula Dietrich
Georg-Speyer-Haus, Frankfurt am Main, Germany

Andreas Immelmann
Analysis GmbH, Frankfurt, Germany

I. INTRODUCTION

Soon after the discovery of the retrovirus HIV (human immunodeficiency virus) as the causative agent of the acquired immunodeficiency syndrome (AIDS) (1), early concepts of AIDS-therapy focused on the specific inhibition of the retroviral life cycle. Consequently, the first target for antiretroviral therapy against HIV was a viral enzyme, reverse transcriptase (RT), which specifically catalyzcs the retrotranscription of the viral RNA genome into DNA. Zidovudine (AZT), a nucleoside analogue that competitively inhibits RT, was the first antiviral drug approved for HIV therapy (2). Although AZT treatment of HIV-positive persons resulted in clinical benefit for the patients, this benefit was only of limited duration. It soon became clear that viruses rapidly develop resistance for AZT, resulting in drug failure and clinical deterioration. This was shown by isolated virus from patients receiving AZT for more than 6 months, showing reduced susceptibility for AZT as compared with the pretreatment isolates from the same patients (3). Furthermore, in elegant in vitro studies, specific amino acid exchanges within RT were shown to be responsible for AZT resistance (4).

Numerous clinical trials and in vitro studies have shown that the development of resistance under treatment is not unique to AZT, but is the major limitation of a sustained antiviral effect of any HIV drug tested so far. This occurs regardless of the antiviral target and the mode of action of the drug. Resistance mutations have not only been identified for all RT inhibitors known to date (this volume, chapter on RT inhibitors) (5–9) but also for all inhibitors of a second enzyme, the function of which is essential for the production of infectious virus progeny, the viral protease (this volume, chapter on protease inhibitors) (10–13).

The probability of emergence of drug-resistant mutations is directly linked to the degree of viral replication. Incomplete virus suppression results from insufficient drug potency, noncompliance of the patients to the drug regimens, leading to reduced plasma levels of the drugs, "sanctuaries," which are inaccessible to the drugs, or drug resistance, either acquired under therapy or present a priori. In recent years, the application of powerful antiretroviral therapy in HIV-positive persons combined with the introduction of sensitive molecular techniques for virus quantification in the plasma led to the recognition that continuous massive viral production (about 10^{10} HIV particles per day) occurs, even in the early phase of infection related to clinical latency (14). Furthermore, the level of viremia early in infection was correlated to clinical disease progression (15). This new insight into mechanisms of viral pathogenesis resulted in the "hit hard and early" concept of modern antiretroviral therapy. The aim is to reduce viral load in the patients as early, as much, and as long as possible in order to prevent the emergence of resistant strains for as long as possible. This can potentially be achieved through the application of highly active antiretroviral therapy (HAART), which consists of the simultaneous administration of at least three drugs, usually two RT inhibitors and one of the more potent protease inhibitors. First results showed that HAART can indeed decrease viral load in the plasma to undetectable levels for quite a long time in a considerable proportion of treated patients and the concept of virus eradication seemed feasible (16,17). However, 2 to 3 years of experience with HAART and the introduction of ultrasensitive methods for viral load detection (limit of detection: 20 genome equivalents per milliliter plasma) revealed ongoing virus replication despite HAART. The reasons are addressed in this chapter.

It is difficult to generalize which combination of drugs is most appropriate for the "first shot" of HAART, which is the most important in terms of the aforementioned therapeutic goals. The presence of resistant viruses as a result of previous drug exposure, natural variation, or transmission, the complex interaction between resistance mutations, and the individual factors determining adherence of the patients to their drug regimens should be taken into account. The determination of individual resistance profiles, which can be determined phenotypically or genotypically, become extremely important in the prediction of resistance and the optimization of treatment decisions. Resistance data complement viral load data qualitatively and allow improved clinical management of HIV-positive persons. However, better standardization of the methods for resistance determination and better algorithms to interpret the results are still needed to transfer these methods into routine clinical practice.

Besides the primary therapeutic goal of efficient and sustained virus suppression, the management of viruses with increasing complexity of resistance in terms of number and type of accumulated resistance mutations in the infected population has to be considered in future drug development. The first compounds, which are specifically targeted against resistant viruses, are already in clinical trials (18). In addition, drugs with higher antiviral potency, better pharmacodynamics, and less toxicity are needed to minimize the development of drug resistance and hence the risk of increasing virus replication and disease progression.

II. RESISTANCE AS MAJOR CAUSE FOR TREATMENT FAILURE AND CLINICAL DETERIORATION

The development of resistant viruses is the major obstacle for sustained virus suppression and long-term clinical benefit of antiviral therapy against HIV infection. Several factors contribute to the development of resistance, for example, insufficient drug potency, suboptimal pharmacokinetics and drug activation, sanctuaries not accessible for the drugs, stage of disease, and patient compliance. In the early phase of HIV therapy, clearly, insufficient drug potency resulting from monotherapy or dual combination therapy with two nucleoside RT inhibitors (NRTIs) was the major reason for drug failure and the development of resistance. With more potent antiviral drugs, such as nonnucleoside reverse transcriptase inhibitors (NNRTIs) and protease inhibitors, being available for use in combination during HAART, insufficient drug potency is not the primary cause for the development of resistance. Rather, adherence of the patients to the very strict regimen (there are strict temporal and physiological conditions for taking pills as well as toxic side effects) has become a major factor for the development of resistance. Furthermore, the presence of drug-resistant HIV strains, caused by prior drug exposure or transmission of resistant virus strains, poses increasing problems for drug failure under HAART (19,20).

A. Identification of HIV Strains Resistant to Nucleoside RT Inhibitors

In the late 1980s, monotherapy with the nucleoside analogue AZT was the only treatment available for HIV-infected persons. Although initial clinical trials showed reduced mortality rates and clinical improvement accompanied by increasing CD4 cell counts (2), this clinical benefit was limited in time (21). Viruses with reduced susceptibility for AZT (i.e., increased IC_{50} values) as compared with pretreatment isolates were isolated from patients who received AZT for more than 6 months (3). Comparative nucleotide sequence analysis of the *pol* region coding for RT from pretreatment (sensitive) virus isolates and isolates under treatment (resistant) and subsequent in vitro studies led to the identification of defined amino acid substitutions in RT responsible for resistance (Fig. 1) (4). The major amino acid substitutions for AZT resistance are at positions 41, 67, 70, 215, and 219 of RT. Additional substitutions at positions 210 and 333 may contribute to resistance, if present, in combination with resistance mutations against other RT inhibitors

Amino acid position in RT

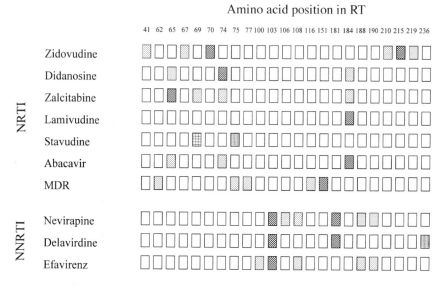

Figure 1   Known resistance mutations of reverse transcriptase (RT) inhibitors. For each drug, the position of mutated amino acids of drug-resistant HIV-1 isolates within RT is indicated with numbers. Primary resistance mutations are in dark gray; secondary resistance mutations are in pale gray; mutations known from *in vitro* studies, but rarely found in vivo, are hatched vertically; the grided amino acid shown for stavudine at position 69 corresponds to an insertion of three amino acids found *in vivo* and leading to multidrug resistance.

(22,23). Recently, a mechanism for AZT resistance was proposed that implied decreased binding of AZT triphosphate to the mutant enzyme in combination with increased pyrophosphorolytic cleavage of chain-terminated viral DNA resulting, overall, in decreased chain termination (24).

Resistance mutations accumulate gradually in the viral genomes, leading to increasing resistance under the selective pressure of the drugs (12,25). Although there seems to be a certain order in the acquisition of resistance mutations, individual differences are found, which are probably due to the sequence background in which these mutations occur (26). On the other hand, resistance mutations located at different sites of the viral genome can rapidly be linked through genetic recombination, as shown by in vitro studies (27–29).

Primary resistance mutations render the virus a selective advantage under therapy. However, in the absence of the drug, resistant viruses generally have reduced fitness as compared to the wild type (25,30). This was demonstrated by in vitro competition experiments between wild type and resistant virus strains. Similarly, secondary mutations outside the target for antiviral therapy can arise to compensate for the loss of fitness caused by primary resistance mutations. This is particularly the case for protease resistance mutations (31).

With the availability of additional antiviral substances against HIV, the era of combination therapy began. New RT inhibitors [didanosine (ddI), zalcitabine (ddC), and later lamivudine (3TC) and stavudine (d4T)] belonging to the same class of inhibitors as AZT (NRTIs) were used alone or in combination with AZT. Numerous clinical trials showed that combination therapy was superior to monotherapy in terms of delaying disease progression and prolonging survival (32–35). The introduction of sensitive tests for the quantitation of plasma viremia also clearly demonstrated improved efficacy of combination therapy in terms of the degree and the durability of viral load reduction (36). However, again drug-resistant strains emerged, although their appearance was delayed as compared with monotherapy (37).

As for AZT, defined amino acid exchanges within RT are associated with drug resistance for the other NRTIs (see Fig. 1). For ddI, the primary resistance mutation is at codon 74 of RT leading to a 10-fold resistance in vitro (5). Other codons involved in ddI resistance are at positions 65, 75, and 184 (38). Interestingly, ddI resistance can partially restore AZT sensitivity in patients with prior exposure to AZT (5). The ddI resistance mutation at position 74 seems to interact with the AZT resistance mutation at position 215, resulting in increased sensitivity toward AZT.

Resistance mutations for ddC are overlapping with those for ddI and, consequently, cross-resistance is observed between both substances (5,6,39). Mutations conferring ddC resistance are at positions 65, 69, 74, 75, and 184 of RT. An amino acid exchange at position 184 is also the primary mutation for resistance against 3TC, leading to about 1000-fold resistance in vitro (7,40). In patients given AZT and 3TC, the 184 mutation can counteract AZT resistance caused by mutations 215 and 41 (41). However, mutations at the carboxy-terminus of RT can result in dual resistance against AZT and 3TC (positions 333, 359, 371, and 395 of RT) (23).

Resistance against d4T seems to be more complicated from a virological point of view. Whereas an amino acid substitution at position 75 has been described for in vitro resistance, this mutation has rarely been observed in vivo (42). Rather, multiple genotypic changes associated with resistance mutations against other NRTIs are responsible for d4T resistance. These mutations include an insertion of two serines at position 69 and amino acid changes at positions 62, 69, 75, and 151 (see Fig. 1) (43). Particularly, the insertion at position 69 leads to cross-resistance against a variety of NRTIs. D4T resistance is higher if these mutations emerge in a background of AZT resistance mutations (44).

B. Multidrug Resistance to NRTIs

As shown for d4T, certain mutations within RT are associated with resistance against multiple drugs. Multidrug resistant (MDR) strains have been isolated from patients on prolonged combination therapy with NRTIs (45). The primary mutation conferring MDR is at position 151 ($Q \Rightarrow M$) (46). This mutation is associated with loss of fitness of the corresponding virus variants, which is compensated by additional mutations at positions 62, 75, 77, and 116. These viruses are resistant to AZT, ddI, ddC, d4T, and 3TC (46).

A second pathway involved in MDR is addressed earlier. An insertion of two serine amino acids at position 69, combined with mutations at position 62 and/or 75, leads to resistance to d4T, AZT, ddI, dC, 3TC, and the new carbocyclic NRTI, abacavir (1592) (43). The insertion alone results in a 3- to 10-fold reduction of virus susceptibility against these nucleotides (47).

For the NRTI abacavir, amino acid exchanges at positions 74 and 184 of RT have been linked to resistance based on in vitro studies (48). However, in vivo MDR pathways seem to play a major role in the development of resistance to abacavir. Patients with viruses carrying the 74 and 184 resistance mutations or AZT resistance mutations alone respond well to abacavir treatment. But, if multiple NRTI (41, 210, 215, 184, or 41, 215, insertion at 69) or the 151 MDR resistance mutations are present, abacavir response is attenuated or absent (48). Thus, abacavir treatment results in efficient virus suppression in a substantial proportion of NRTI-experienced patients.

C. Resistance to Nonnucleoside RT Inhibitors

The class of NNRTIs comprises a number of potent antiviral drugs, which inhibit RT directly by binding closely to the catalytic site in the hydrophobic pocket of the enzyme (49). NNRTIs inhibit HIV-1 strains of the main group M; generally, HIV-2 strains and HIV-1 viruses of group O are resistant to inhibition by NNRTIs (50,51). In monotherapy, the antiviral effect of NNRTIs is superior to NRTIs in terms of reduction of viral load in the plasma (52,53). However, drug-resistant HIV strains arise extremely rapidly within 4 weeks of drug administration in vitro and in vivo; a single amino acid exchange at position 181 (close to the active site of the enzyme) is sufficient to confer high level resistance (see Fig. 1) (9). Other mutations involved in NNRTI resistance are at positions 103, 106, 108, 188, and 190 (52,54). Resistance generally is not specific for the particular NNRTI administered, but leads to cross-resistance to other compounds in this class of inhibitors (55). Because of the drug potency of NNRTIs and the rapid emergence or resistance, compounds of this class of inhibitors are ideally suited for use in combination with other antiviral drugs during HAART. Clinical trials showed sustained virus suppression in triple combinations including one NNRTI, and no development of resistant viruses after 1 year of therapy in compliant patients was observed (56).

Nevirapine and delavirdine (BHAP) are approved antiretrovirals of the NNRTI class (57,58). Major resistance mutations include amino acid exchanges at positions 181 and 103 (see Fig. 1) (9). For delavirdine, an amino acid exchange at position 236 correlates with in vitro resistance. This mutation is rarely observed in vivo, probably because of reduced viral fitness (59).

Other very promising substances in terms of higher drug potency and altered resistance profiles are efavirenz (DMP266) and the quinoxaline HBY097, both of which are currently in clinical trials (52,60). The 181 resistance mutation, which is most frequently found with NNRTIs, is neither observed for efavirenz nor for HBY097. Rather, an amino acid exchange at position 103 seems to be the major resistance mutation for both substances in patients given these NNRTIs (52,60).

Additional substitutions at positions 100, 108, and 225 contribute to resistance for efavirenz (60). For HBY097, the major resistance mutations found in vitro (i.e., by cultivating wild type isolates in the presence of increasing drug concentrations) were at positions 171 and 190 (61). This is in contrast to the mutations observed in vivo and might be due to different viral or cellular backgrounds (laboratory strain/cell line versus primary strain/primary cells) or different effective drug concentrations in vitro and in vivo selecting for different virus mutants of the quasispecies. Like for d4T resistance already described, resistance mutations selected in vitro are not necessarily the ones selected for in vivo or, put in other words, resistance mutations found in vitro must not necessary predict the resistance mutations emerging in vivo.

D. Resistance to Protease Inhibitors

Besides RT, HIV protease is a second enzyme essential to the replication cycle of HIV (62). The enzyme catalyzes the cleavage of Gag-Pol and Gag precursor proteins into the mature components required for virus structure and replication, including protease itself, RT, and integrase (63). Therefore, this enzyme became a promising target for antiretroviral therapy. A number of peptidic substrate analogues have been identified, which specifically inhibit the HIV protease dimer (this volume, chapter by Redshaw). Four protease inhibitors (saquinavir, ritonavir, indinavir, and nelfinavir) are currently approved for antiretroviral therapy (see chapter on protease inhibitors), and others are in clinical trials. Protease inhibitors have been shown in numerous clinical trials to be potent inhibitors of HIV and, therefore, have become indispensable components of HAART (64–68). Combination therapies including at least one protease inhibitor result in more profound and prolonged virus suppression, which is reflected in delayed disease progression and substantial reduction in mortality rates (69). Also, at least partial immune reconstitution can be achieved in patients undergoing HAART, including protease inhibitors (70,71).

Like with RT inhibitors, however, the development of resistance is the major limitation of long-term efficacy of protease inhibitors. Resistance mutations have been identified for all protease inhibitors in therapeutic use (Fig. 2). These include primary resistance mutations at the sites of interaction between protease and inhibitors and secondary mutations, which usually compensate for loss in viral fitness induced by the primary mutations (30,31). Cross-resistance to the actual pro-

Amino acid position in protease

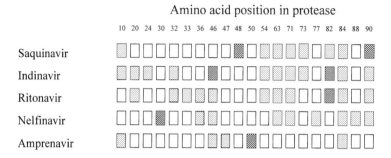

Figure 2 Known resistance mutations for protease inhibitors. For each drug, the position of mutated amino acids of drug-resistant HIV-1 isolates within protease is indicated with numbers. Primary resistance mutations are in dark gray, secondary mutations in pale gray.

tease inhibitors is particularly problematic and new drugs that specifically target resistant proteases are under development (72).

Saquinavir was the first protease inhibitor approved for HIV therapy in 1995 (64). Treatment with saquinavir resulted in a more profound reduction of plasma viral load than treatment with NRTIs (73). However, in patients given saquinavir for about 1 year, drug failure was observed because of the emergence of resistant HIV strains. Mutations associated with resistance to saquinavir are at positions 90 and 48 of the viral protease (10). Additional mutations at positions 10, 36, 46, 54, 63, 71, 82, and 84 arise later or under higher selective pressure (see Fig. 2). These mutations lead to cross-resistance to other protease inhibitors. Thus, switching therapy from saquinavir to indinavir, a second protease inhibitor, did not result in substantial clinical improvement (74,75).

Primary resistance mutations for indinavir are at positions 46 and 82, followed by mutations at positions 10, 20, 32, 54, 63, 71, 84, and 90 of the protease (see Fig. 2) (12). Viruses with both primary resistance mutations have reduced replication rates in vitro as compared with the wild type, which is compensated by additional mutations at protease cleavage sites in Gag (76). It seems that reduced protease activity caused by resistance mutations is compensated by altered protease cleavage sites, which restore protease functionality and, hence, viral replication capacity.

Also, for ritonavir, multiple mutations in the protease gene are associated with resistance, the major mutation being at position 82 (77). Further mutations commonly found in ritonavir-treated cases include positions 10, 20, 36, 54, 63, 71, 84, and 90 (see Fig. 2) (11). As expected from the overlapping patterns of resistance mutations observed for saquinavir, indinavir, and ritonavir, cross-resistance between these drugs is observed (78).

Nelfinavir, which is a nonpeptidic protease inhibitor, has a more complex pattern of resistance mutations. Whereas a mutation at position 30 is the primary mutation observed in patients receiving nelfinavir but no other protease inhibitors (13), this mutation is hardly observed in patients receiving nelfinavir after prior exposure to other protease inhibitors. In these patients, nelfinavir resistance is rather associated with common protease resistance mutations (36, 46, 63, 71, 77, 88, and 90) (see Fig 2) (79). Thus, viruses from patients taking nelfinavir as first protease inhibitor are still susceptible to the other protease inhibitors, whereas viruses from patients in whom nelfinavir is added to previous exposure to other protease inhibitors are resistant to nelfinavir.

A new protease inhibitor, amprenavir, which is currently being evaluated in clinical trials, has a different resistance profile compared with other protease inhibitors. Monotherapy with amprenavir results in mutations at positions 46, 47, and 50, all three mutations being necessary for high-level resistance (80). Therefore, amprenavir seems to be ideally suited for use in combination with other protease inhibitors or in protease-experienced patients. Interestingly, in vitro passage of amprenavir-resistance virus in the presence of saquinavir can restore susceptibility to amprenavir (81).

E. Cellular Resistance

Besides viral factors, cellular host factors may also play a role in drug failure. This effect has been described in vitro for cell lines under prolonged exposure to NRTIs (82,83). Resistance in this case is due to defects in thymidine kinase activity, which results in reduced levels of phosphorylated intermediates of NRTIs being the substrates of RT (84).

F. Resistance to Other Compounds Inhibiting the Retroviral Life Cycle

The development of resistance is not unique for RT or protease inhibitors. Recently, new inhibitors for virus entry have been identified in vitro; these inhibitors interfere with chemokine receptors acting as coreceptors for HIV entry (85,86). Bicyclams are substrate analogues for the chemokine receptor CXCR4 and consequently inhibit entry of HIV strains depending on this receptor (85). After extensive passaging of virus in the presence of AMD3100, a representative bicyclam, resistant viruses were isolated. They showed multiple single amino acid exchanges in gp120, suggesting that the overall conformation of the external viral glycoprotein plays a role in the development of resistance (87).

Similarly, RANTES-analogues have been identified as inhibitors of HIV isolates using the major coreceptor for HIV, CCR5, for entry (86). AOP-RANTES inhibits entry of CCR5-dependent HIV strains at nM concentrations. Resistant viruses have been selected after in vitro passage; however, resistance mutations have not yet been identified (88).

III. CORRELATION OF VIRUS REPLICATION, THE DEVELOPMENT OF RESISTANCE, AND CLINICAL DETERIORATION

In recent years, the application of powerful antiretroviral therapy in HIV-positive persons, combined with the introduction of sensitive molecular techniques for virus quantitation in the plasma, revolutionized modern understanding of viral pathogenesis (89,90). The recognition that a massive production of about 10^{10} HIV particles per day, accompanied by a rapid turnover of virus and acutely infected cells, is the driving force behind HIV pathogenesis, and that, furthermore, the level of viremia early in infection determines clinical progression (15), resulted in the "hit hard and early" concept of modern antiretroviral therapy (91). The goal is to achieve maximal virus suppression as early, as much, and as long as possible to prevent the development of resistant viruses for as long as possible through the early application of HAART.

The driving force behind evolution of the HIV quasispecies in the patient is the high error rate of RT (92), which misincorporates one "wrong" base pair per genome per replication cycle. However, this has to be considered in the background of the enormous amount of new viruses produced per day. Any mutation known to confer resistance to any antiviral drug will, thus, emerge by chance every day in every patient with unrestricted virus replication and contribute to resistance through further selection and evolution. The reason that drug-resistant HIV strains are not always found in untreated cases is because resistant viruses generally have reduced fitness as compared with wild type. Nevertheless, a considerable proportion of drug-naive patients harbor viruses with resistance mutations for RT, and even more so, for protease inhibitors (19,93,94). For example, the presence of AZT resistance mutations in AZT-naive patients is approximately 10% according to a number of studies (19,95). The protease gene is even more variable, and mutations conferring resistance for protease inhibitors are frequently present in untreated cases (20,94,96). Furthermore, the broad application of protease inhibitors in HIV therapy may lead to increased circulation and transmission of drug-resistant strains (20). As shown in Figure 3, protease resistance mutations increased over time in protease-naive HIV positive Germans since the introduction of protease inhibitors into standard combination therapy (20).

Other retrospective studies showed that the presence of baseline resistance mutations is indeed predictive for drug failure and is much more predictive than, and independent of, clinical and drug history predictors (97). Thus, therapy response to the protease inhibitor nelfinavir strongly depended on the presence of re-

	with 63	without 63
1997	22/26 (84.6%)	16/26 (61.5%)
1996	13/18 (72.2%)	9/18 (50.0%)
1995	20/30 (66.7%)	12/30 (40.0%)
1994	14/21 (66.7%)	6/21 (28.6%)

(a)

	with 63	without 63
1997	36/22 (1.64)	23/16 (1.44)
1996	23/13 (1.77)	9/9 (1.00)
1995	26/20 (1.30)	12/12 (1.00)
1994	20/14 (1.43)	7/6 (1.17)

(b)

Figure 3   (a) Increase of protease resistance mutations in protease-inhibitor–naive HIV-1 positive Germans since the introduction of protease inhibitors into standard combination therapy in 1995. Protease resistance mutations were determined by direct sequencing of polymerase chain reaction fragments derived from the protease gene after reverse transcription of viral RNA in plasma. The frequency of mutated samples was analyzed according to the year of sampling. Because the amino acid at position 63 is mutated frequently in untreated cases, the analysis was also done without considering mutations at this position (second column). (b) Also, the number of protease resistance mutations per sample increased over time. The mutated samples shown in Fig. 3a were analyzed with regard to the number of resistance mutations present per sample, again with or without considering the amino acid at position 63.

sistance mutations at positions 48, 82, 84, and 90 in protease-experienced patients. Eighty-four percent of the patients with no or one mutation at these positions were responders, whereas only 33% of the patients with two or more mutations responded to nelfinavir treatment (97). Similarly, in the same study, baseline phenotypic resistance was shown to be a strong predictor for therapeutic response. Seventy-four percent of the patients harboring viruses with less than four-fold resistance responded to nelfinavir, whereas only 20% of responders were found among patients with viruses with more than 10-fold resistance. Furthermore, a recent prospective study, Viradapt, comparing current standard of care triple therapy drug selection practices with drug selection based on genotypic resistance analyses, showed higher viral load reductions and a higher percentage of patients with undetectable viral load in the group of patients in which therapy was guided by genotypic resistance testing (97a).

Because of the strong predictive value of resistance determinations for drug response and clinical failure, resistance determinations should enter into routine clinical practice in order to optimize antiviral therapy individually (98). In particular, resistance determinations should be performed before start of therapy in order to attack the virus with the most effective combination of drugs (as predicted by the resistance profiles) from the beginning. This is important because many resistance mutations are present a priori as a result of natural variation, transmission, or previous drug exposure, and the "first shot" is the most effective in terms of viral load suppression and therapeutic benefit (99). Furthermore, resistance determinations at the time points of therapy failure, as indicated by increasing viral load in the plasma, would help to analyze qualitatively the causes for this increase and to choose the next drug combination appropriately.

IV. METHODS TO MONITOR DRUG RESISTANCE

Principally, drug resistance can be determined phenotypically or genotypically. Phenotypic assays for drug resistance determination are performed in vitro and are based on the direct determination of drug susceptibility of patient viruses, either as isolated or as recombinant viruses bearing the target enzyme for the drug (RT or protease) of the patient's viruses. Genotypic assays are based on the determination of resistance point mutations of the patient's viruses, either by direct sequencing or by hybridization techniques. Because of the complexity of the assays for resistance determination concerning performance or interpretation of results, so far these analyses have largely been restricted to the research setting or large clinical trials. However, more practical tests for routine applications are being developed and companies start to offer resistance determinations as a service to physicians or drug companies.

Usually, for the sake of simplicity, the starting material is the patient's plasma or peripheral blood mononuclear cells (PBMCs). However, this is just one compartment of the body and other compartments may harbor other virus variants with different resistance profiles (100). In fact, divergent resistance profiles have been described for virus sequences derived from cerebrospinal fluid (CSF) (101), lymph nodes (16,102), and semen (103) as compared with the respective plasma samples. Thus, the absence of resistant viruses from plasma does not necessarily imply the absence of resistant viruses in the body.

A. Phenotypic Assays for Resistance Determination

Assays to detect phenotypic resistance of HIV are designed to determine the (altered) growth parameters of HIV in vitro in the presence of therapeutic drugs as compared with drug-susceptible strains of HIV (ideally pretherapy isolates from the same patient). Various methods are employed to determine the phenotypic resistance of HIV isolates to antiretroviral drugs. Common to all methods is the determination of the concentration of antiretroviral drug required to inhibit virus specific growth parameters by 50% (IC_{50}). Usually, this is achieved by infection of suitable indicator cells with the HIV isolate in question. The infected cells are cultivated in the presence of increasing concentrations of the drug. After an appropriate period of cultivation, the replication of the virus is determined quantitatively. Subsequently, the IC_{50} is calculated according to standard algorithms. It is not yet clear, however, which IC_{50} values are clinically relevant for each component of a multidrug regimen (98).

The *direct (biological) approach* (104,105) (Fig. 4) involves isolation of the patient's PBMCs by density gradient centrifugation. Subsequently, the HIV-infected cells are cocultivated with mitogen-stimulated donor PBMCs isolated from regular blood donations. In this way, sufficient quantities of the patient's virus are obtained for subsequent IC_{50}- determination.

In a next step, the patient's virus is titrated on susceptible indicator cells to determine the titer of infectious virus particles (expressed as $TCID_{50}$, tissue culture infectious dose). Once the $TCID_{50}$ is determined, indicator cells are infected at a defined multiplicity of infection (m.o.i.), that is, infectious particles per susceptible target cell. The infected indicator cells are then cultivated in the presence of increasing concentrations of the antiretroviral drugs. Finally, the replication of the virus is determined by suitable assay endpoints, for example, concentration of viral proteins in the cell culture supernatant or virus-specific cytopathic effects of the virus toward the indicator cells. Figure 5 shows an example of determination of zidovudine resistance in serial patient isolates.

The *molecular approach* (Fig. 6) comprises amplification by polymerase chain reaction (PCR) of the RT gene and the protease gene, respectively, from the patient's virus in plasma. After cloning into HIV vectors deficient for the RT or protease gene, the recombinant viruses are biologically amplified in suitable target cells. Subsequently, the recombinant viruses are titrated and subjected to IC_{50} determination as described previously (106,107)

An alternative molecular approach comprises the determination of resistance by directly measuring the specific catalytic activity of RT and protease in the presence of various concentrations of the antiretroviral drugs (108,109). Half maximal inhibitory concentrations of the drugs tested are then defined. The system is based on expression cloning of the viral enzymes after amplication by PCR from the patient's virus or on direct measurements of enzymatic activity in pelleted virions.

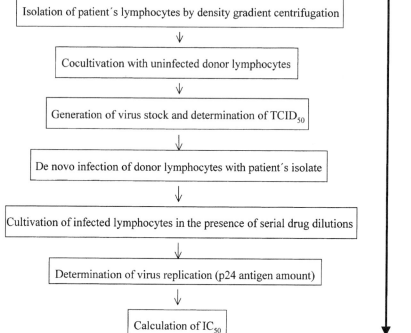

Figure 4   Schematic overview on the methodological steps involved in phenotypic drug resistance determination.

B.   Genotypic Assays for Resistance Determination (Genotypic Resistance Profile)

Genotypic assays for resistance determinations ask for the presence of resistance mutations in the viral genomes of treated patients. Resistance is implied from previous identification of these resistance mutations in vitro, where HIV is grown in the presence of increasing concentrations of the drugs.

Point mutation assays for the specific detection of resistance mutations are based on oligonucleotide probes specific for wild type or mutant codons, which interrogate for the presence of these codons in the patient sample (110). In the case of the line probe assay (LIPA) (111), the target sequence is amplified by PCR from the patient sample and biotinylated PCR-products are hybridized to the respective oligonucleotide probes. Hybrids can be detected by a colorimetric assay after biotinstreptavidin coupling. The assay is rapid and easy to perform, and it allows detection of mixtures of wild type and mutant codons in the sample. However, the assay requires the knowledge of all possible mutations leading to resistance and the introduction of all these mutations into oligonucleotide probes.

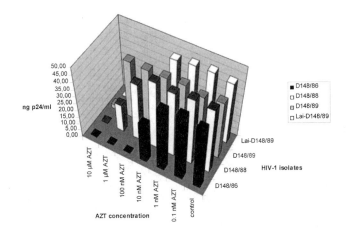

	10 µM AZT	1 µM AZT	100 nM AZT	10 nM AZT	1 nM AZT	0.1 nM AZT	control
86	0,00	0,00	0,00	27,90	44,00	46,20	44,10
88	0,00	19,90	40,30	47,30	45,40	46,90	46,10
89	3,30	40,80	40,40	40,60	41,10	38,50	40,20
48/89	0,00	0,00	15,60	43,20	44,80	45,30	43,30

Figure 5 Phenotypic resistance for zidovudine (AZT) of consecutive HIV-1 isolates from patient D148 under AZT treatment. Patient isolates were grown in the presence of the indicated concentrations of AZT and p24 antigen amount was determined. D148/86 (black) is an isolate derived before therapy, D148/88 (vertical stripes) and D148/89 (gray) are derived from the same patient 25 months and 32 months, respectively, after start of AZT therapy. Lai-D148/89 (horizontal stripes) is a recombinant virus bearing the RT of D148/89 in the background of HIV-1Lai. As shown in the diagram and the table, half-maximal virus inhibition (IC_{50}) is shifted toward higher AZT concentrations in resistant isolates. Note that the same RT-sequence in a different viral background may influence the IC_{50} as shown for Lai-D148/89 and D148/89 by a factor of about 50. This should be considered when using the molecular approach for phenotypic resistance determination (see Fig. 6).

For hybridization assays, different subtypes of HIV-1 can differ in the resistance codons yet result in the same amino acid substitutions. For example, subtype E viruses usually differ from subtype B by having ACC instead of ACT encoding threonine at position 69 of RT, but ACT instead of ACC encoding this amino acid at position 215 of RT (own unpublished data). The use of hybridization assays for resistance determinations requires continuous actualization as more and newer drugs are being introduced into HAART and consequently new resistance mutations arise.

In contrast, direct sequencing of PCR products from the drug target genes from patients' viruses (112,113) (Fig. 7) allows detection of all kinds of mutations deviating from master sequences derived from sensitive viruses. Potentially, every codon altered with respect to the pretreatment sequence from the same patient may

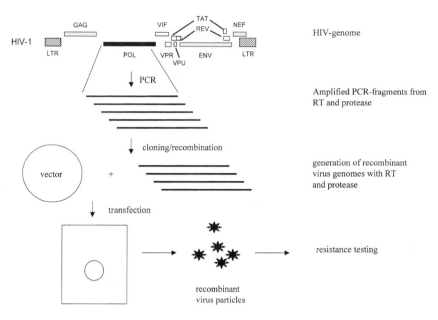

Figure 6 Schematic representation of the molecular approach for phenotypic resistance determination. The *pol*-region coding for RT and protease (black) is amplified by polymerase chain reaction (PCR) and either cloned or recombined into an HIV genetic vector deficient for this region of the viral genome. After transfection into susceptible cells, recombinant virus particles are produced bearing the RT and protease of the patient's viruses. These viruses are then grown in the presence of increasing concentrations of antiviral drugs, and the IC_{50} values are determined as previously described.

represent resistance mutations to the drugs used for therapy. Thus, if sequences from different patients receiving the same therapy have common changes in the target genes, these altered codons are candidates for resistance mutations emerging under the given drug combination. This is important because resistance mutations emerging in vivo are not necessarily the ones observed in vitro when growing viruses under increasing concentrations of the drugs. Viral fitness and immune selection play an important role in vivo in defining the virus variants replicating in the patients. Thus, the optimal combination of mutations conferring drug resistance, increased viral fitness, and immune evasion are overrepresented in vivo as compared with in vitro conditions.

Direct sequencing is a rapid and sensitive method to detect resistance mutations. Depending on sequencing techniques and devices, resistance mutations are detectable at levels as low as 5% to 10%.

The number of resistance mutations increases with the number of drugs used during combination therapy and synergistic or antagonistic interactions between

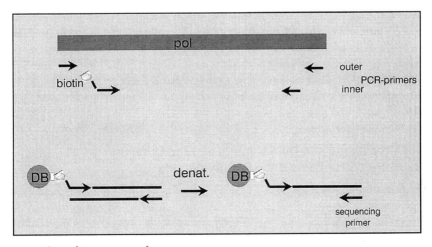

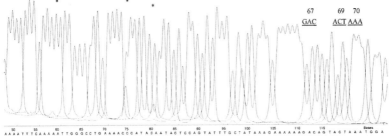

Figure 7 Determination of genotypic resistance profile by direct sequencing. The *pol* region containing RT or protease from the patient's isolate is amplified by PCR. One of the inner PCR primers is biotinylated to purify PCR fragments by streptavidin-coated magnetic beads (dynabeads, DB). After denaturation, the single DNA strand is sequenced directly. The lower panel shows part of a fluorogram of a sequence derived from RT around positions 67, 69, and 70, where amino acid substitutions may lead to resistance for AZT and ddC (see Fig. 1). Asterisks mark the presence of more than one nucleotide in the sequence that are due to variants being present in the quasispecies of the patient.

resistance mutations are becoming more complex. Therefore, certain genetic resistance profiles have to be interpreted in correlation with the corresponding phenotypic resistance profiles. Algorithms can then be used to deduce the actual degree of resistance from sequence data. A software product that links resistance genotype to phenotype is currently under development (114). A preliminary evaluation has shown that the accuracy of such software for predicting protease inhibitor phenotypic resistance from genotype is 98%.

The gene chip technology introduced recently combines hybridization techniques with sequencing data (115). Each nucleotide of the target sequence is interrogated by a panel of oligonucleotides, which are arranged on a high-density array (approximately 10.000 oligos per chip). Fluorescein-labeled fragmented target RNA is hybridized to the oligonucleotide array and sequence-specific hybridization is subsequently detected on the chip using an epifluorescence confocal microscope. Gene chip technology is available for RT and protease sequencing, and concordance with conventional sequencing techniques is greater than 98% (116).

C. Advantages and Disadvantages of the Different Methods for Resistance Determinations

All methods described have particular advantages and disadvantages. Compared with genotypic assays for detection of viral resistance, the phenotypic assays reflect the biological properties of the viral quasispecies isolated from the HIV-infected patient more appropriately. In addition, the phenotypic approach offers the opportunity to monitor the response of the viruses to all combinations of various drugs in vitro.

Clearly, disadvantageous is the great effort required to perform phenotypic resistance assays: All tests have to be performed in a Biosafety Level III containment by highly skilled and trained staff. In addition, the use of recombinant viruses necessitates particular requirements be adhered to with respect to national gene technology laws. In addition, assays that involve cell culture techniques are expensive.

Furthermore, phenotypic assays are time consuming. Results usually are obtained after 5 to 8 weeks. The biological approach involves a period of virus cultivation in vitro, by which the selective amplification of a viral subpopulation might be accomplished. The recombinant viruses made up from a genetic "background" of a laboratory virus strain and viral genes from the patient's viral quasispecies might behave biologically different than virus isolates that are not genetically manipulated. For instance, an RT gene derived from a patient isolate with 100-fold resistance for zidovudine, which carries the zidovudine resistance mutations at positions 41, 67, 70, and 215, after cloning into an HIV-vector deleted for RT, led to recombinant viruses with only about 10-fold resistance for zidovudine (own unpublished data). This means that the genetic backbone can influence phenotypic resistance determinations, in that viral fitness and replication parameters influence the readout of the system.

Finally, the phenotypic approaches require a minimum number of input viral particles for the subsequent amplification, be it by cultivation or cloning. Genetic methods for resistance determinations are faster and, consequently, less expensive than phenotypic assays. A clear disadvantage is that resistance mutations have to be known a priori and that interpretation of genetic resistance profiles becomes more difficult as more and more drugs are added to the therapeutic regimen of a patient. Resistance mutations for different drugs can influence each other positively or negatively, and all this knowledge should be considered when interpreting the genetic resistance profiles. Computer algorithms are being developed to link genetic resistance data to phenotypic resistance data. Once these algorithms are optimized, genetic resistance determinations should be broadly applicable in the routine clinical setting, and phenotypic resistance assays will be reserved for more special applications.

D. Quality Control and Standardization

Several different methods are used for resistance testing by various laboratories and companies. Standardization is urgently needed in order to compare results between different performers. Once consensus protocols for genotypic assays that involve direct sequencing of HIV nucleic acid are established, the issue of quality control should be manageable. Participating laboratories should be provided with standardized source material, for example, negative plasma spiked with defined quantities of plasmids containing mutations at various positions and in various proportions. These blinded samples are then subjected to the entire procedure of the genotyping assay, such as extraction of nucleic acid (reverse transcription), amplification of DNA, sequencing reactions, and evaluation of the sequence data.

Like for all routine testing in the setting of a clinical laboratory, "Ringversuche" have to be organized. Depending on the performance in the Ringversuch, permission might be granted to each participating laboratory to further offer and perform genotypic resistance assays.

Still in its infancy, clearly, is the standardization of assays that involve cell culture techniques. As for the genotyping assay, detailed consensus protocols must be developed to establish, for example, the procedures of virus isolation, type of target cell used for virus propagation, endpoint in the IC_{50} determination, and reagents used for IC_{50} determination.

No obvious approach is available to provide a range of participating laboratories with sufficient quantities of standardized biological material reflecting the diversity of the drug-resistant quasispecies of HIV.

V. CONCLUSIONS: MANAGEMENT OF RESISTANCE IN CLINICAL PRACTICE

The emergence of drug-resistant viruses under therapy or the presence of drug-resistant strains resulting from prior drug exposure, natural variation, or transmission is the major cause for failure of antiretroviral therapy. Whereas viral load measurements are able to indicate drug failure during therapy through an increase in viral load, viral load measurements do not indicate the presence of resistant viruses before start of therapy. Furthermore, an increase in viral load during therapy results from incomplete virus suppression, but it cannot be deduced from the viral load data per se which drugs of the combination were the ones that failed. This more qualitative aspect of drug failure can be determined by genotypic or phenotypic resistance assays.

Resistance determinations were shown in a number of studies to have high predictive value for therapeutic response. Therefore, it is important to monitor the presence or the emergence of drug-resistant HIV strains in the patients in order to choose appropriately the optimal drug combinations for therapeutic use in the individual patients. The introduction of resistance determinations into clinical practice would allow the monitoring of patients' resistance profiles individually and, consequently, the treatment of patients rationally according to these data. The costs of routine resistance determinations are lower than the expenses caused by ineffective therapy, which is predestinated to fail and to eventually lead to much higher additional costs resulting from hospitalizations caused by drug failure.

Clearly, resistance determinations have to be optimized in order to enter regular clinical use. Easy-to-use algorithms must be found to help predict phenotypic resistance from viral genotype and clinical failure from phenotypic resistance. Nevertheless, the identification of resistant viruses in the patients clearly is an indication for therapy switch, regardless of the degree of resistance.

REFERENCES

1. Barré-Sinoussi F, Chermann JC, Rey F, Nugeyre MT, Chamaret S, Gruest J, Dauguet C, Axler-Blin C, Brun-Vezinet F, Rouzioux C, Rozenbaum W, Montagnier L. Isolation of a T-lymphotropic retrovirus from a patient at risk for acquired immune deficiency syndrome (AIDS). Science 1983; 220:868–871.
2. Fischl MA, Richman DD, Grieco MH, Gottlieb MS, Volberding PA, Laskin OL, Leedom JM, Groopman JE, Mildvan D, Schooley RT, Jackson GG, Durack DT, King D, The AZT Collaborative Working Group. The efficacy of azidothymidine (AZT) in the treatment of patients with AIDS and AIDS-related complex: a double-blind placebo-controlled trial. N Engl J Med 1987; 317:185–191.
3. Larder BA, Darby G, Richman DD. HIV with reduced sensitivity to zidovudine (AZT) isolated during prolonged therapy. Science 1989; 243:1731–1734.
4. Larder BA, Kemp SD. Multiple mutations in HIV-1 reverse transcriptase confer high-level resistance to zidovudine. Science 1989; 246:1155–1158.
5. St Clair MH, Martin JL, Tudor-Williams G, Bach MC, Vavro CL, King DM, Kellam P, Kemp SD, Larder BA. Resistance to ddI and sensitivity to AZT induced by a mutation in HIV-1 reverse transcriptase. Science 1991; 253:1557–1559.
6. Craig C, Moyle G. The development of resistance of HIV-1 to zalcitabine. AIDS 1997; 11:271–279.
7. Tisdale M, Kemp SD, Parry NR, Larder BA. Rapid in vitro selection of human immunodeficiency virus type 1 resistant to 3′-thiacytidine inhibitors due to a mutation

in the YMDD region of reverse transcriptase. Proc Natl Acad Sci U S A 1993; 90: 5653–5656.

8. Lacy SF, Larder BA. Novel mutation (V75T) in human immunodeficiency virus type 1 reverse transcriptase confers resistance to 2´,3-didehydro-2´,3´- dideoxythymidine in cell culture. Antimicrob Agents Chemother 1994; 38:1428–1432.

9. Richman DD, Havlir D, Corbeil J, Looney D, Ignacio C, Spector SA, Sullivan J, Cheeseman S, Barringer K, Pauletti D, Shih CK, Myers M, Griffin J. Nevirapine resistance mutations of human immunodeficiency virus type 1 selected during therapy. J Virol 1994; 68:1660–1666.

10. Jacobsen H, Haenggi M, Ott M, Duncan IB, Andreoni M, Vella S, Mous J. Reduced sensitivity to saquinavir: an update on genotyping from phase I/II trials. Antiviral Res 1996; 29:95–97.

11. Molla A, Korneyeva M, Gao Q, Vasavanonda S, Schipper PJ, Mo HM, Markowitz M, Chernyavskiy T, Niu P, Lyons N, Hsu A, Granneman GR, Ho DD, Boucher CA, Leonard JM, Norbeck DW, Kempf DJ. Ordered accumulation of mutations in protease confers resistance to ritonavir. Nat Med 1996; 2:760–766.

12. Condra JH, Holder DJ, Schleif WA, Blahy OM, Danovich RM, Gabryelski LJ, Graham DJ, Laird D, Quintero JC, Rhodes A, Robbins HL, Roth E, Shivaprakesh M, Yang T, Chodakewitz JA, Deutsch PJ, Leavitt RY, Massari FE, Mellors JW, Squires KE, Steigbigel RT, Teppler H, Emini EA. Genetic correlates of in vivo viral resistance to indinavir, a human immunodeficiency virus type 1 protease inhibitor. J Virol 1997; 70:8270–8276.

13. Patick AK, Duran M, Cao Y, Ho T, Zhou P, Keller MR, Chapman S, Anderson R, Kuritzkes D, Shugarts D, Ho D, Markowitz M. Genotypic analysis of HIV-1 variants isolated from patients treated with the protease inhibitor nelfinavir, alone or in combination with d4T or AZT and 3TC. 4th Conference on Retroviruses and Opportunistic Infections, Washington, DC, Jan 22–26, 1997.

14. Coffin JM. HIV population dynamics in vivo: implications for genetic variation, pathogenesis, and therapy. Science 1995; 267:483–489.

15. Mellors JW, Rinaldo CR Jr, Gupta P, White RM, Todd JA, Kingsley LA. Prognosis in HIV-1 infection predicted by the quantity of virus in plasma. Science 1996; 272:1167–1170.

16. Wong JK, Gunthard H, Havlir DV, Zhang ZQ, Haase AT, Ignacio CC, Kwok S, Emini E, Richman DD. Reduction of HIV-1 in blood and lymph nodes following potent antiretroviral therapy and the virological correlates of treatment failure. Proc Natl Acad Sci U S A 1997; 94:12574–12579.

17. Pantaleo G, Perrin L. Can HIV be eradicated? AIDS 1998; 12(suppl A):S175–S180.

18. Palmer S, Shafer R, Merigan TC. New drug combinations against highly drug-resistant HIV isolates in vitro. 2nd International Workshop on HIV Drug Resistance and Treatment Strategies, Lake Maggiore, Italy, Jun 24–27, 1998.

19. Nájera I, Holguín A, Quiñones-Mateu M, Muñoz-Fernández MA, Nájera R, López-Galíndez C. Pol gene quasispecies of HIV: mutations associated with drug resistance in virus from patients undergoing no drug therapy. J Virol 1995; 69:23–31.

20. Dietrich U, Knechten H, Jäger H, Husak R, Ruppach H, von Briesen H. High prevalence of protease resistance mutations in therapy-naive HIV-1 positive German seroconvertors irrespective of viral subtype. 12th World AIDS Conference, Geneva, Switzerland, Jun 28–Jul 3, 1998.

21. Volberding PA, Lagakos SW, Grimes JM, Mitsuyasu RT, Fischl MA, Soiero R, for the AIDS Clinical Trials Group. The duration of zidovudine benefit in persons with asymptomatic HIV infection. Prolonged evaluation of protocol 019 of the AIDS Clinical Trials Group. JAMA 1994; 272:437–442.
22. Hooker DJ, Tachedjian G, Solomon AE, Gurusinghe AD, Land S, Birch C, Anderson JL, Roy BM, Arnold E, Deacon NJ. An in vivo mutation from leucine to tryptophan at position 210 in human immunodeficiency virus type 1 reverse transcriptase contributes to high-level resistance to 3′-azido-3′-deoxythymidine. J Virol 1996; 70: 8010–8018.
23. Miller V, Stazewski S, Rottmann K, Pauwels R, De Bethune MP, Hertogs K, van den Eynde C, Schel P, van Cauwenberge A, Larder BA, Harrigan PR, Tisdale M, Kemp SD, Bloor S, Stone C, Kohli A, Myers R, Mellors J, Shi C. Dual resistance to AZT and AZT/3TC- treated patients. 4th Conference on Retroviruses and Opportunistic Infections, Washington, DC, Jan 22–26, 1997.
24. Arion D, Kaushik N, McCormick S, Borkow G, Parniak MA. Phenotypic mechanism of HIV-1 resistance to 3′-azido- 3′-deoxythymidine (zidovudine). 2nd International Workshop on HIV Drug Resistance and Treatment Strategies, Lake Maggiore, Italy, Jun 24–27, 1998.
25. Keulen W, de Graaf L, Berkhout B, Boucher C. Evolution of zidovudine resistance mutations in vivo can be explained by differences in viral fitness. 2nd International Workshop on HIV Drug Resistance and Treatment Strategies, Lake Maggiore, Italy, Jun 24–27, 1998.
26. Leigh-Brown AJ, Richman DD. HIV-1: gambling on the evolution of drug resistance? Nat Med 1997; 3:268–271.
27. Kellam P, Larder BA. Retroviral recombination can lead to linkage of reverse transcriptase mutations that confer increased zidovudine resistance. J Virol 1995; 69: 669–674.
28. Moutouh L, Corbeil J, Richman DD. Recombination leads to the rapid emergence of HIV-1 dually resistant mutants under selective drug pressure. Proc Natl Acad Sci USA 1996; 93:6106–6111.
29. Yusa K, Kavlick MF, Mitsuya H. HIV-1 acquires resistance to multiple classes of antiviral drugs through recombination. 4th Conference on Retroviruses and Opportunistic Infections, Washington, DC, Jan 22–26, 1997.
30. Croteau G, Doyon L, Thibeault D, McKercher G, Pilote L, Lamarre D. Impaired fitness of human immunodeficiency virus type 1 variants with high-level resistance to protease inhibitors. J Virol 1997; 71:1089–1096.
31. Nijhuis M, Schuurman R, Schipper P, de Jong D, van Bommel T, de Groot T, Molla A, Borleffs J, Danner S, Boucher C. Reduced replication potential of HIV-1 variants initially selected during ritonavir therapy is restored upon selection of additional substitutions. 4th Conference on Retroviruses and Opportunistic Infections, Washington, DC, Jan 22–26, 1997.
32. Delta Coordinating Committee. Delta: a randomized double-blind controlled trial comparing combinations of zidovudine plus didanosine or zalcitabine with zidovudine. Lancet 1996; 348:283–291.
33. Hammer SM, Katzenstein DA, Hughes MD, Gundacker H, Jackson JB, Fiscus S, Rasheed S, Elbeik T, Reichman R, Japour A, Merigan TC, Hirsch MS, for the AIDS

Clinical Trials Group 175 Study Team. A trial comparing nucleoside monotherapy with combination therapy in HIV-infected adults with CD4 cell counts from 200 to 500 per cubic millimeter. N Engl J Med 1996; 335:1081–1090.

34. Schooley RT, Ramirez-Ronda C, Lange JMA, Cooper DA, Lavelle J, Lefkowitz L, Moore M, Larder BA, St. Clair M, Mulder JW, McKinnis R, Pennington KN, Harrigan PR, Kinghorn I, Steel H, Rooney JF, and the Wellcome Resistance Study Collaborative Group. Virological and immunological benefits of initial combination therapy with zidovudine and zalcizabine or didanosine compared with zidovudine monotherapy. J Infect Dis 1996; 173:1354–1366.

35. Katlama C, on behalf of the CAESAR Coordinating Committee. Clinical and survival benefit of 3TC in combination with zidovudine containing regimens in HIV-1 infection: interim results of the CAESAR study. AIDS 1996; 10:S9.

36. Montaner JSG, Reiss P, Cooper D, Vella S, Harris M, Conway B, Wainberg MA, Smith D, Robinson P, Hall D, Myers M, Lange JM. A randomized, double-blind trial comparing combinations of nevirapine, didanosine, and zidovudine for HIV-infected patients. The INCAS trial. JAMA 1998; 279:930–937.

37. Prichard MN, Shipman C Jr. Analysis of combination of antiviral drugs and design of effective multidrug therapies. Antiviral Ther 1996; 1:9–20.

38. Gu Z, Gao H, Li X, Parniak MA, Wainberg MA. Novel mutation in the human immunodeficiency virus type 1 reverse transcriptase gene that encodes cross-resistance to 2′,3′-dideoxyinosine and 2′,3′- dideoxycytidine. J Virol 1992; 66:7128–7135.

39. Shirasaka T, Yarchoan R, O'Brien MC, Husson RN, Anderson BD, Kojima E, Shimada T, Broder S, Mitsuya H. Changes in drug sensitivity of human immunodeficiency virus type 1 during therapy with azidothymidine, dideoxycytidine and dideoxyinosine: an in vitro comparative study. Proc Natl Acad Sci U S A 1993; 90:5 62–566.

40. Schuurman R, Nijhuis M, van Leeuwen R, Schipper P, de Jong D, Collis P, Danner SA, Mulder J, Loveday C, Christopherson C. Rapid changes in human immunodeficiency virus type 1 RNA load and appearance of drug-resistant virus populations in persons treated with lamivudine (3TC). J Infect Dis 1995; 171:1411–1419.

41. Larder BA, Kemp SD, Harrigan PR, Potential mechanism for sustained antiretroviral efficacy of AZT-3TC combination therapy. Science 1995; 269:696–699.

42. Soriano V, Dietrich U, Villalba N, Immelmann A, Gil- Aguado A, Echevarría S, Clotet B, Ocaña I, Santamaría JM, Bouza E, Borona V, Gatell JM, González-Lahóz J. Lack of emergence of genotypic resistance to stavudine (D4T) after 2 years of monotherapy. AIDS 1997; 11:696–697.

43. Whitcomb JM, Limoli K, Wrin T, Smith D, Tian H, Parkin N, Lie YS, Petropoulos CJ. Phenotypic and genotypic analysis of stavudine-resistant isolates of HIV-1. 2nd International Workshop on HIV Drug Resistance and Treatment Strategies, Lake Maggiore, Italy, Jun 24–27, 1998.

44. Bloor S, Hertogs K, Desmet RL, Pauwels R, Larder BA. Virological basis for HIV-1 resistance to stavudine investigated by analysis of clinical samples. 2nd International Workshop on HIV Drug Resistance and Treatment Strategies, Lake Maggiore, Italy, Jun 24–27, 1998.

45. Shirasaka T, Kavlick MF, Ueno T, Gao WY, Kojima E, Alcaide ML, Chokekijchai S, Roy BM, Arnold E, Yarchoan R, Mitsuya H. Emergence of human immunodeficiency

virus type 1 variants with resistance to multiple dideoxynucleosides in patients receiving therapy with dideoxynucleosides. Proc Natl Acad Sci U S A 1995; 92: 2398–2402.

46. Iversen AK, Shafer RW, Wehrly K, Winters MA, Mullins JI, Chesebro B, Merigan TC. Multidrug-resistant human immunodeficiency virus type 1 strains resulting from combination antiretroviral therapy. J Virol 1996; 70:1086–1090.

47. Winters MA, Coolley KL, Girard YA, Levee DJ, Hamdan H, Katzenstein DA, Shafer RW, Merigan TC. Phenotypic and molecular analysis of HIV-1 isolates possessing 6 bp inserts in the reverse transcriptase gene that confer resistance to nucleoside analogues. 2nd International Workshop on HIV Drug Resistance and Treatment Strategies, Lake Maggiore, Italy, Jun 24–27, 1998.

48. Lanier R, Danehower S, Daluge S, Cutrell A, Tisdale M, Pearce G, Spreen B, Lafon S, Kemp SD, Bloor S, Larder BA. Genotypic and phenotypic correlates of response to abacavir (ABC,1592). 2nd International Workshop on HIV Drug Resistance and Treatment Strategies, Lake Maggiore, Italy, Jun 24–27, 1998.

49. De Clerq E. HIV-1 specific RT inhibitors: highly selective inhibitors of human immunodeficiency virus type 1 that are specifically targeted at the viral reverse transcriptase. Med Res Rev 1993; 13:229–258.

50. Romero DL, Busso M, Tan CK, Reusser F, Palmer JR, Poppe SM, Aristoff PA, Downey KM, So AG, Resnick L, Tarpley WG. Nonnucleoside reverse transcriptase inhibitors that potently and specifically block human immunodeficiency virus type 1 replication. Proc Natl Acad Sci U S A 1991; 88:8806–8810.

51. Descamps D, Collin G, Loussert-Ajaka I, Saragosti S, Simon F, Brun-Vézinet F. HIV-1 group O sensitivity to antiretroviral drugs. AIDS 1995; 9:977–978.

52. Rübsamen-Waigmann H, Huguenel E, Paessens A, Kleim JP, Wainberg MA, Shah A. Second generation non-nucleosidic reverse transcriptase inhibitor HBY097 and HIV-1 viral load. Lancet 1997; 349:1517.

53. Saag MS, Emini EA, Laskin OL, Douglas J, Lapidus WI, Schleif WA, Whitley RJ, Hildebrand C, Byrnes VW, Kappes JC. A short-term clinical evaluation of L-697,661, a non-nucleoside inhibitor of HIV-1 reverse transcriptase. N Engl J Med 1993; 329: 1065–1072.

54. Havlir D, McLaughlin MM, Richman DD. A pilot-study to evaluate the development of resistance to nevirapine in asymptomatic human immunodeficiency virus-infected patients with CD4 cell counts greater than 55/mm^3. J Infect Dis 1995; 5:1379–1383.

55. Tantillo C, Ding J, Jacobo-Molina A, Nanni RG, Boyer PL, Hughes SH, Pauwels R, Andries K, Janssen PAJ, Arnold E. Location of anti-AIDS drug binding sites and resistance mutations in the three-dimensional structure of HIV-1 reverse transcriptase. Implications for mechanisms of drug inhibition and resistance. J Mol Biol 1994; 243: 369–387.

56. Wainberg MA, Birch C. Phenotypic and genotypic resistance emergence in naive HIV-1 patients treated with combinations of reverse transcriptase inhibitors. AIDS 1996; 10(suppl 2).

57. Havlir D, Cheeseman SH, Mc Laughlin M, Murphy R, Erice A, Spector SA, Greenough TC, Sullivan JL, Hall D, Myers M, et al. High-dose nevirapine: safety, pharmacokinetics, and antiviral effect in patients with human immunodeficiency virus infection. J Infect Dis 1995; 171:537–545.

58. Davey RT, Chaitt DG, Reed GF, Freimuth WW, Herpin BR, Metcalf JA, Eastman PS, Falloon J, Kovacs JA, Polis MA, Walker RE, Masur H, Boyle J, Coleman S, Cox SR, Wathen L, Daenzer CL, Lane HC. Randomised, controlled phase I/II trial of combination therapy with delavirdine (U-90152S) and conventional nucleosides in human immunodeficiency virus type 1-infected patients. Antimicrob Agents Chemother 1996; 40:1657–1664.

59. Demeter LM, Gerondelis P, Archer RH, Palaniappan C, Reichman RC, Bambara R. Impact of the P236L delavirdine resistance mutation on HIV-1 replication and reverse transcriptase function. International Workshop on HIV Drug Resistance, Treatment Strategies and Eradication, St. Petersburg, FL, Jun 25–28, 1997.

60. Bacheler LT, Anton E, Jeffrey S, George H, Hollis G, Abremski K, and the Sustiva Resistance Study Team. RT gene mutations associated with resistance to efavirenz. 2nd International Workshop on HIV Drug Resistance and Treatment Strategies, Lake Maggiore, Italy, Jun 24–27, 1998.

61. Kleim JP, Bender R, Kirsch R, Meichsner C, Paessens A, Rosner M, Rübsamen-Waigmann H, Kaiser R, Wichers M, Schneweis KE, et al. Preclinical evaluation of HBY097, a new nonnucleoside reverse transcriptase inhibitor of human immunodeficiency virus type 1 replication. Antimicrob Agents Chemother 1995; 39:2253–2257.

62. Kohl NE, Emini EA, Schlief WA, Davis LJ, Hermbach MC, Dixon RAF, Scolnick EM, Sigel IS. Active human immunodeficiency virus protease is required for viral infectivity. Proc Natl Acad Sci U S A 1988: 85:4686–4690.

63. Peng C, Ho BK, Chang TW, Chang NT. Role of human immunodeficiency virus type 1-specific protease in core protein maturation and infectivity. J Virol 1989; 63: 2550–2556.

64. Kitchen VS, Skinner C, Ariyoshi K, Lane EA, Duncan IB, Burckhardt J, Burger HU, Bragman K, Pinching AJ, Weber JN. Safety and activity of saquinavir in HIV infection. Lancet 1995; 345:952–955.

65. Danner SA, Carr A, Leonard JM. A short-term study of the safety, pharmacokinetics, and efficacy of ritonavir, an inhibitor of HIV-1 protease. N Engl J Med 1995; 333:1528–1533.

66. Mellors J, Steigbigl R, Gulick R, Frank I, Berry P, McMahon D, Fuhrer J, Farthing C, Hildebrand C, Schleif W, Condra J, Nessly M, Calandra G, Emini E, Chodakewitz J. Antiretroviral activity of the oral protease inhibitor MK-639 in p24 antigenemic, HIV-1 infected patients with <500 CD4/mm^3. 35th Interscience Conference on Antimicrobial Agents and Chemotherapy, San Francisco, Sept 17–30, 1995.

67. Moyle G, Youle M, Chapman S, Peterkin J, Monaghan J, Parnell A, Higgs C, Prince W, Carey W, Lant A, Nelson MA. Phase I/II dose escalating study of the novel protease inhibitor AG1343. 5th European Conference on Clinical Aspects and Treatment of HIV Infection, Copenhagen, Denmark, Sept 26–29, 1995.

68. Wang Y, Freimuth WW, Daenzer CL, Borin MT, Tutton CM, Piergies AA, Wurtz RM, Li HI, Davis JW, Crampton DJ, and the PNU-140690 Team. Safety and efficacy of PNU-140690, a new non-peptidic HIV protease inhibitor, and HIV genotypic changes in patients in a phase II study. 2nd International Workshop on HIV Drug Resistance and Treatment Strategies, Lake Maggiore, Italy, Jun 24–27, 1998.

69. Pallela F, Moorman A, Delaney K, Loveless M, Fuhrer J, Aschman D, Holmby S.

Dramatically declining morbidity and mortality in an ambulatory HIV-infected population. 5th Conference on Retroviruses and Opportunistic Infections, Feb 1–5, 1998.

70. Autran B, Carcelain G, Li TS, Blanc C, Mathez D, Tubiana R, Katlama C, Debre P, Leibowitch J. Positive effects of combined antiretroviral therapy on CD4+ T cell homeostasis and function in advanced HIV disease. Science 1997; 277:112–116.

71. Pantaleo G, Soudeyns H, Demarest JF, Vaccarezza M, Graziosi C, Paolucci S, Daucher M, Cohen OJ, Denis F, Biddison WE, Sekaly RP, Fauci AS. Evidence for rapid disappearance of initially expanded HIV-specific CD8+ T cell clones during primary infection. Proc Natl Acad Sci U S A 1997; 94:9848–9853.

72. Tisdale M. HIV protease inhibitors–resistance issues. Int Antiviral News 1996; 4:41–43.

73. Schapiro JM, Winters MA, Stewart F, Efron B, Norris J, Kozal MJ, Merigan TC. The effect of high-dose saquinavir on viral load and CD4+ T-cell counts in HIV-infected patients. Ann Intern Med 1996; 124:1039–1050.

74. Ermolieff J, Hong L, Lin X, Foundling S, Hartsuck JA, Tang J. Kinetic and structural basis of saquinavir resistance of HIV-1 protease mutants. International Workshop on HIV Drug Resistance, Treatment Strategies and Eradication, St. Petersburg, FL, Jun 25–28, 1997.

75. Dulioust A, Paulous S, Guillemot L, Boue F, Galanaud P, Clavel F. Selection of saquinavir-resistant mutants by indinavir following a switch from saquinavir. International Workshop on HIV Drug Resistance, Treatment Strategies and Eradication, St. Petersburg, FL, Jun 25–28, 1997.

76. Zhang YM, Imamichi H, Imamichi T, Lane HC, Fallon J, Vasudevachari MB, Salzman NP. Drug resistance during indinavir therapy is caused by mutations in the protease gene and in the Gag substrate cleavage sites. International Workshop on HIV Drug Resistance, Treatment Strategies and Eradication, St. Petersburg, FL, Jun 25–28, 1997.

77. Schmit JC, Ruiz L, Clotet B, Raventos A, Tor J, Leonard J, Dasmyter J, De Clerq E, Vandamme AM. Resistance-related mutations in the HIV-1 protease gene of patients treated for 1 year with the protease inhibitor ritonavir. 4th Conference on Retroviruses and Opportunistic Infections, Washington, DC, Jan 22–26, 1997.

78. Chen C, Niu P, Kati W, Norbeck D, Sham H, Kempf D, Kohlbrenner W, Plattner J, Leonard J, Molla A. Activity of ABT-378 against HIV protease containing mutations conferring resistance to ritonavir. 4th Conference on Retroviruses and Opportunistic Infections, Washington, DC, Jan 22–26, 1997.

79. Lawrence J, Schapiro J, Pesano R, Winters M, Cain P, Winslow D, Merigan TC. Clinical response and genotypic resistance patterns of sequential therapy with nelfinavir followed by indinavir plus nevirapine in saquinavir/reverse transcriptase inhibitor-experienced patients. 4th Conference on Retroviruses and Opportunistic Infections, Washington, DC, Jan 22–26, 1997.

80. Myers RE, Snowden W, Randall S, Tisdale M. Unique resistance profile of the protease inhibitor amprenavir (141W94) observed in vitro and in the clinic. 2nd International Workshop on HIV Drug Resistance and Treatment Strategies, Lake Maggiore, Italy, Jun 24–27, 1998.

81. Markland W, Zuchowski L, Black J, Rao BG, Parsons JD, Pazhanisamy S, Fulgham J, Griffith JP, Tisdale M, Tung R. Kinetic and structural analysis of HIV-1 protease mutations: amprenavir resistance, cross-resistance and resensitization. 2nd Interna-

tional Workshop on HIV Drug Resistance and Treatment Strategies, Lake Maggiore, Italy, Jun 24–27, 1998.

82. Dianzani F, Antonelli G, Turriziani O, Riva E, Simeoni E, Signoretti C, Strosselli S, Cianfriglia M. Zidovudine induces the expression of cellular resistance affecting its antiviral activity. AIDS Res Hum Retroviruses 1994; 10:1471–1478.

83. Magnani M, Brandi G, Casabianca A, Fraternale A, Schiavano GF, Rossi L, Chiarantini L, 2´-3´- Dideoxycytidine metabolism in a new drug-resistant cell line. Biochemical J 1995; 312:115–123.

84. Turriziani O, Antonelli G, Focher F, Bambacioni F, Dianzani F. Further study of the mechanism underlying the cellular resistance to AZT. Biochim Biophys Res Com 1996; 228:797–801.

85. Schols D, Este JA, Henson G, De Clerq E. Bicyclams, a class of potent anti-HIV agents, are targeted at the HIV coreceptor fusin/CXCR-4. Antiviral Res 1997; 35: 147–156.

86. Simmons G, Clapham PR, Picard L, Offord RE, Rosenkilde MM, Schwartz TW, Buser R, Wells TNC, Proudfoot AE. Potent inhibition of HIV-1 infectivity in macrophages and lymphocytes by a novel CCR5 antagonist. Science 1997; 272: 276–279.

87. De Vreese K, Kofler-Mongold V, Leutgeb C, Weber V, Vermeire K, Schacht S, Anne J, De Clerq E, Datema R, Werner G. The molecular target of bicyclams, potent inhibitors of human immunodeficiency virus replication. J Virol 1996; 70:689–696.

88. Arts EJ, Quiñones-Mateu ME, Albright JL, Lederman M, Offord RE. Intrinsic and selected resistance of primary NSI HIV-1 isolates to a chemokine analogue AOP-RANTES. 2nd International Workshop on HIV Drug Resistance and Treatment Strategies, Lake Maggiore, Italy, Jun 24–27, 1998.

89. Ho DD, Neumann AU, Perelson AS, Chen W, Leonard JM, Markowitz M. Rapid turnover of plasma virions and CD4 lymphocytes in HIV-1 infection. Nature 1995; 373:123–126.

90. Wei X, Gosh SK, Taylor ME, Johnson VA, Emini EA, Deutsch PP, Lifson JD, Bonhoeffer S, Nowak MA, Hahn BH, et al. Viral dynamics in human immunodeficiency virus type 1 infection. Nature 1995; 373:117–122.

91. Ho DD. Time to hit HIV, early and hard. N Engl J Med 1995; 333:450–451.

92. Roberts JD, Bebenek K, Kunkel TA. The accuracy of reverse transcriptase from HIV-1. Science 1988; 242:1171–1173.

93. Dietrich U, Ruppach H, Gehring S, Knechten H, Knickmann M, Jäger H, Wolf E, Husak R, Orfanos CE, Rübsamen-Waigmann H, Brede HD, von Briesen H. Large proportion of non-B HIV-1 subtypes and presence of AZT-resistance mutations among German Seroconvertors. AIDS 1997, 11:1532–1533.

94. Kozal M, Leahy N, Ross J, Swack N, Tapleton J. Prevalence of protease inhibitors (PRI) and reverse transcriptase inhibitor (RTI) drug-resistance mutations in rural Iowa HIV+ population: Implication for treatment. 4th Conference on Retroviruses and Opportunistic Infections, Washington, DC, Jan 22–26, 1997.

95. Gómez-Cano M, Rubio A, Puig T, Pérez- Olmeda M, Ruiz L, Soriano V, Pineda JA, Zamora L, Xaus N, Clotet B, Leal M. Prevalence of genotypic resistance to nucleoside analogues in antiretroviral-naive and antiretroviral-experienced HIV-infected patients in Spain. AIDS 1998; 12:1015–1020.

96. Barrie KA, Perez EE, Lamers SL, Farmerie WG, Dunn BM, Sleasman JW, Goodenow MM. Natural variation in HIV-1 protease, Gag p7 and p6, and protease cleavage sites within gag/pol polyproteins: amino acid substitutions in the absence of protease inhibitors in mothers and children infected by human immunodeficiency virus type 1. Virology 1996; 219:407–416.

97. Patick AK, Zhang M, Hertogs K, Griffiths L, Mazabel E, Pauwels R, Becker M. Correlation of virological response with genotype and phenotype of plasma HIV-1 variants in patients treated with nelfinavir in the US expanded access program. 2nd International Workshop on HIV Drug Resistance and Treatment Strategies, Lake Maggiore, Italy, Jun 24–27, 1998.

97a. Durant J, Clevenbergh P, Halfon P, Delgindice P, Porsin S, Simonet P, Montagne N, Boucher CA, Schapiro JM, Dellamonica P. Drug-resistance genotyping in HIV-1 therapy: the VIRADAPT randomized controlled trial. Lancet 1999; 353:2195–2199.

98. Hirsch MS, Conway B, D'Aquila RT, Johnson VA, Brun-Vézinet F, Clotet B, Demeter LM, Hammer SM, Jacobsen DM, Kuritzkes DR, Loveday C, Mellors JW, Vella S, Richman DD, for the International AIDS Society—USA Panel. Antiretroviral drug resistance testing in adults with HIV infection: implications for clinical management. JAMA 1998; 279:1984–1991.

99. Lange J, Richman DD. The first blow is half the battle. Antiviral Ther 1997; 2:132–133.

100. Wong JK, Ignacio CC, Torriani F, Havlir D, Fitch NJ, Richman DD. In vivo compartmentalization of human immunodeficiency virus: evidence from the examination of pol sequences from autopsy tissues. J Virol 1997; 71:2059–2071.

101. Di Stefano M, Sabri F, Leitner T, Svennerholm B, Hagberg L, Norkrans G, Chiodi F. Reverse transcriptase sequence of paired isolates of cerebrospinal fluid and blood from patients infected with human immunodeficiency virus type 1 during zidovudine treatment. J Clin Microbiol 1995; 33:352–255.

102. Gunthard HF, Wong JK, Ignacio CC, Guatelli JC, Riggs NL, Havlir DV, Richman DD. Human immunodeficiency virus replication and genotypic resistance in blood and lymph nodes after a year of potent antiretroviral therapy. J Virol 1998; 72:2422–2428.

103. Eron JJ, Johnston D, Fiscus SA, Cohen MS, Alcorn T, Vernazza P. Emergence of HIV-1 resistance in seminal plasma of men on antiretroviral therapy. 5th Conference on Retroviruses and Opportunistic Infections, Feb 1–5, 1998.

104. Japour AJ, Mayers DL, Johnson VA, Kuritzkes DR, Beckett LA, Arduino JM, Lane J, Black RJ, Reichelderfer PS, D'Aquila RT, et al. Standardized peripheral blood mononuclear cell culture assay for the determination of drug-susceptibilities of clinical human immunodeficiency virus type 1 isolates. Antimicrob Agents Chemother 1993; 37:1095–1101.

105. Richman DD, Johnson VA, Shirasaka T, O'Brien MC, Mitsuya H. Measurement of susceptibility of HIV-1 to antiviral drugs. In: Strober W, Shevach E, eds. Current Protocols in Immunology. New York: Green Publishing Associates and Wiley-Interscience, 1993:12.9.1.

106. Kellam P, Larder BA. Recombinant virus assay: a rapid phenotypic assay for assessment of drug susceptibility of human immunodeficiency virus type 1 isolates. Antimicrob Agents Chemother 1994; 38:23–30.

107. Hertogs K, DeBethume MP, Miller V, Ivens T, Schel P, Van Cauwenberge A, Van Den Eynde C, van Gerwen V, Azijn H, Van Houtte M, Peeters F, Staszewski S, Conaut M,

Bloor S, Kemp S, Larder BA, Pauwels R. A rapid method for simultaneous detection of phenotypic resistance to inhibitors of protease and reverse transcriptase in recombinant human immunodeficiency virus type 1 isolates from patients treated with antiviral drugs. Antimicrob Agents Chemother 1998; 42:269–276.

108. García-Lerma JG, Weinstock H, Soriano V, Juodawlkis AS, Folks TM, Schinazi RF, Heneine W. Rapid phenotypic detection of HIV-1 resistance to lamivudine (3TC) by direct analysis of plasma reverse transcriptase (RT) activity. 5th Conference on Retroviruses and Opportunistic Infections, Washington, DC, Feb 1–5, 1998.

109. Zhang H, Dornadula G, Wu Y, Havlir D, Richman DD, Pomerantz RJ. Kinetic analysis of intravirion reverse transcription in the blood plasma of human immunodeficiency virus type 1-infected individuals: direct assessment of resistance to reverse transcriptase inhibitors in vivo. J Virol 1996; 70:628–634.

110. Boucher CA, Tersmette M, Lange JM, Kellam P, de Goede RE, Mulder JW, Darby G, Goudsmit J, Larder BA. Zidovudine sensitivity of human immunodeficiency viruses from high-risk, symptom-free individuals during therapy. Lancet 1990; 336: 585–593.

111. Stuyver L, Wyseur A, Rombout A, Louwagie J, Scarcez T, Verhofstede C, Rimland D, Schinazi RF, Rousseau R. Line probe assay for rapid detection of drug-selected mutations in the human immunodeficiency virus type 1 reverse transcriptase gene. Antimicrob Agents Chemother 1997; 41:284–291.

112. Wahlberg J, Albert J, Lundeberg J, Cox S, Wahren B, Uhlén M. Dynamic changes in HIV-1 quasispecies from azidothymidine (AZT) treated patients. FASEB J 1992; 6:2843–2847.

113. Larder BA, Kohli A, Kellam P, Kemp SD, Kronick M, Heufrey RD. Quantitative detection of HIV-1 drug resistance mutations by automated DANN sequencing. Nature 1993; 365:671–673.

114. Pauwels R, Hertogs K, Kemp S, Bloor S, Van Acker K, Hansen J, De Beukeleer W, Roelant C, Larder B, Stoffels P. Comprehensive HIV drug resistance monitoring using rapid, high-throughput phenotypic and genotypic assays with correlative data analysis. 2nd International Workshop on HIV Drug Resistance and Treatment Strategies, Lake Maggiore, Italy, Jun 24–27, 1998.

115. Kozal MJ, Shah N, Shen N, Yang R, Fucini R, Merigan TC, Richman DD, Morris D, Hubbell E, Chee M, Gingeras TR. Extensive polymorphisms observed in HIV-1 clade B protease gene using high-density oligonucleotide arrays. Nature Med 1996; 2:753–759.

116. Gingeras TR, Mamtora G, Shen N, Drenkow J, Winters M, Merigan T. Genetic analysis of HIV-1 in plasma using high-density oligonucleotide arrays and dideoxynucleotide sequencing. 5th International Workshop on HIV Drug Resistance, Whistler, Canada, Jul 3–6, 1996.

4
Reverse Transcriptase Inhibitors as Anti-HIV Drugs

Erik De Clercq
Rega Institute for Medical Research, Leuven, Belgium

I. INTRODUCTION

Of the 13 compounds that have been formally approved for the treatment of human immunodeficiency virus (HIV) infections, nine are targeted at the viral reverse transcriptase (RT), the other four (saquinavir, ritonavir, indinavir, and nelfinavir) being targeted as the viral protease. Of the nine RT inhibitors that have been licensed, six can be considered as nucleoside reverse transcriptase inhibitors (NRTIs), namely zidovudine, didanosine, zalcitabine, stavudine, lamivudine, and abacavir. The other three, namely nevirapine, delavirdine, and efavirenz, belong to the non-nucleoside reverse transcriptase inhibitors (NNRTIs). In addition to these six NRTIs and three NNRTIs, several other RT inhibitors of either the NRTI or NNRTI type have shown considerable potential as anti-HIV agents. Some of these compounds are still in the preclinical stage of development but others have already proceeded to phase I, II, or III clinical trials. Most advanced and/or most promising among the new RT inhibitors are (-)-FTC (emitricitabine), F-ddA (lodenosine), PMEA (adefovir) and its oral prodrug form bis(POM)-PMEA [adefovir dipivoxil (Preveon)], PMPA (tenofovir) and its oral prodrug form bis(POC)-PMPA (tenofovir disoproxil fumarate), which can all be considered as NRTIs (PMEA and PMPA being, in fact, nucleotide reverse transcriptase inhibitors); and α-APA R89439 (loviride), MKC-442 (emivirine), quinoxaline GW867, and thiocarboxanilide UC-781, which should be regarded as NNRTIs. Of this series, Preveon has already been made available under the expanded access program.

This review is limited to the description of the anti-HIV activity of the following categories of RT inhibitors: (a) $2',3'$-dideoxynucleoside (ddN) analogues

(Fig. 1); (b) acyclic nucleoside phosphonates (ANP) analogues (Fig. 2); and (c) nonnucleoside RT inhibitors (NNRTIs) (Fig. 3), the latter in contrast to the compounds from categories (a) and (b), which can both be considered as nucleoside (or nucleotide) type of RT inhibitors (NRTIs). The compounds are discussed from the following viewpoints: (a) activity, safety, and selectivity as anti-HIV agents, (b) intracellular metabolism to the active metabolite, (c) mechanism of interaction with the target enzyme (RT), (d) efficacy in animal models (when demonstrated), (e) clinical efficacy in HIV-infected individuals (with the RT inhibitors when used singly or in combination), and (f) development of HIV drug resistance and the implications thereof.

The description of the RT inhibitors as anti-HIV agents should be viewed in the broad scope of anti-HIV therapy (1) and therapeutic approaches for intervention with HIV infections (2), and strategies to overcome or prevent the problem of HIV resistance development to anti-HIV agents in general (3) and NNRTIs in particular (4). In previous reviews, we have addressed the issues that could be expected from NNRTIs (5) and acyclic nucleoside phosphonates (i.e., PMEA and PMPA) (6) in the treatment of HIV infections.

II. ACTIVITY, SAFETY, AND SELECTIVITY

The anti-HIV properties of the ddN analogues are well documented and have been the subject of several review articles [i.e., zidovudine (7), didanosine (8), zalcitabine (9,10), and stavudine (11,12)]. The anti-HIV effects of zidovudine (AZT), didanosine (ddI), and zalcitabine (ddC) were first described by Mitsuya et al. (13,14), whereas the anti-HIV activity of stavudine (d4T) was first described by Baba et al. (15) and that of lamivudine (3TC) by Soudeyns et al. (16). In fact, Soudeyns et al. (16) described the anti-HIV activity of the racemic 2´,3´-dideoxy-3´-thiacytidine (BCH-189). When the enantiomers of BCH-189 were resolved, they were found to be equipotent in anti-HIV activity (in MT-4 cells); yet, the (-)-enantiomer (i.e., 3TC) was considerably less cytotoxic than the (+)-enantiomer (17). In peripheral blood mononuclear cells (PBMCs), however, the (-)-enantiomer (3TC) was about 10-fold more potent than the (+)-enantiomer (18). In PBMC, 3TC was as potent as AZT [50% effective concentration (EC_{50}): 0.002 μM, respectively]; neither compound proved toxic to the host cells at a concentration of 100 μM (18).

In addition to AZT, ddI, ddC, d4T, and 3TC, several other ddN analogues have been described as potent and selective inhibitors of both HIV-1 and HIV-2 replication: the (-)-enantiomer of 2´,3´-dideoxy-5-fluoro-3´-thiacytidine [(-)- FTC] (19), which, akin to 3TC, has also proven to inhibit the replication of hepatitis B virus (HBV) (20,21); abacavir (1592U89), or (-)-4-[2-amino-6-cyclopropylamino)-pyrin-9-yl]-2-cyclopentene-1- methanol (22), which can be considered as

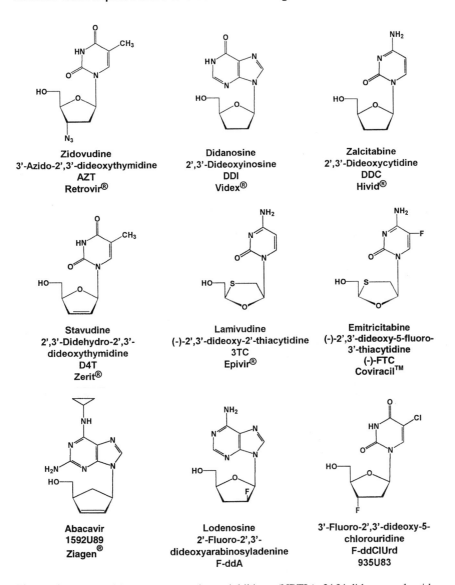

Figure 1   Nucleoside reverse transcriptase inhibitors (NRTIs): 2′,3′-dideoxynucleoside (ddN) analogues.

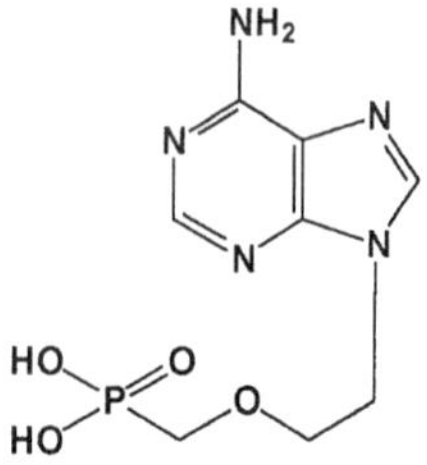

Adefovir
9-(2-Phosphonylmethoxyethyl)adenine
PMEA

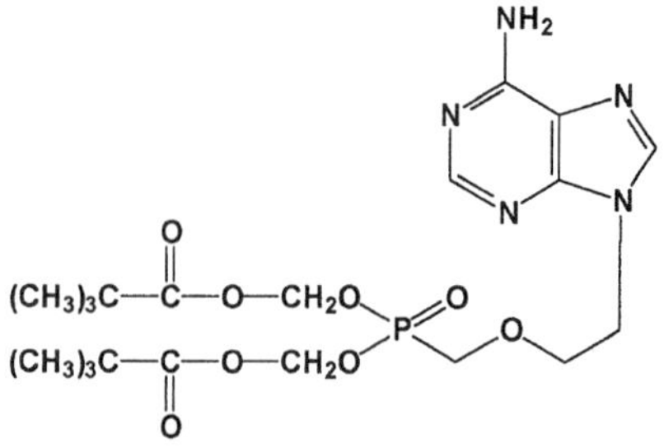

Adefovir dipivoxil
Bis(pivaloyloxymethyl) ester of
9-(2-phosphonylmethoxyethyl)adenine
Bis(POM)-PMEA
Preveon™

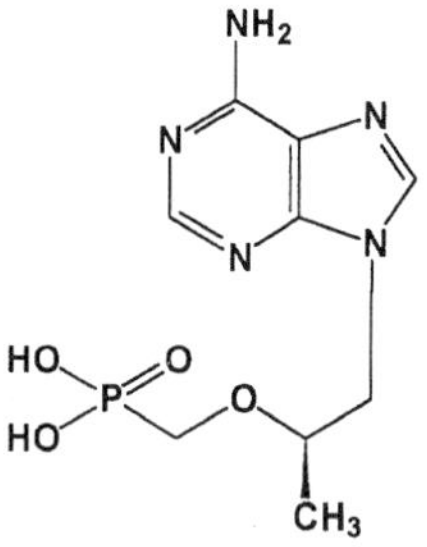

Tenofovir
(R)-9-(2-phosphonylmethoxypropyl)adenine
PMPA

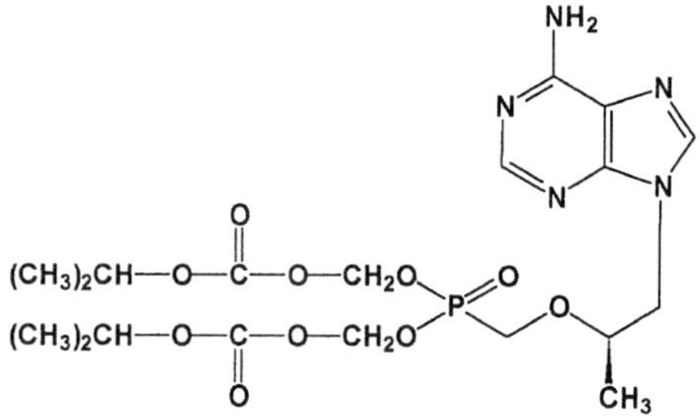

Tenofovir disoproxil fumarate
Bis(isopropyloxycarboxymethyl)ester of
(R)-9-(2-phosphonylmethoxypropyl)adenine
Bis(POC)-PMPA

Figure 2   Nucleotide reverse transcriptase inhibitors (NRTIs): acyclic nucleoside phosphonate (ANP) analogues.

the 6-cyclopropylamino derivative of carbovir (carbocyclic 2′,3′-didehydro- 2′,3′-dideoxyguanosine) (23); 2′-fluoro- 2′,3′-dideoxyarabinosyladenine (F-ddA), an acid-stable and metabolically stable analogue of ddI (24–26), which shows activity against AZT- and ddI resistant HIV strains (27); and 3′-fluoro-2′,3′-dideoxy-5-chlorouridine (F-ddClUrd, 935U83), which emerged as the most potent and selective anti-HIV agent among a series of 2′- and 3′-fluorinated -dideoxynucleoside analogues (28,29). Also, 935U83 retained activity against HIV strains that were resistant to AZT, ddI, or ddC, and showed a favorable pharmacokinetic and toxicological profile in animals (mice and monkeys) (30) and humans (31).

The acyclic nucleoside phosphonates (S)-9-(3-hydroxy-2-phosphonyl-methoxypropyl)-adenine (HPMPA) and 9-(2-phosphonylmethoxyethyl)adenine (PMEA) were first described by De Clercq et al. (32,33) as antiviral agents with a broad activity spectrum encompassing herpes-, adeno-, pox-, hepadna-, and retroviruses. Following PMEA (34), various other acyclic nucleoside phosphonates,

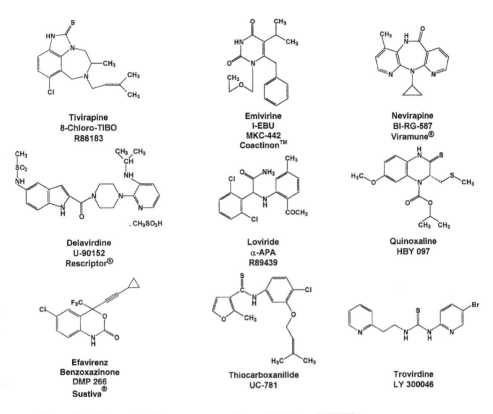

Figure 3 Nonnucleoside reverse transcriptase inhibitors (NNRTIs).

such as FPMPA [9-(3-fluoro-2-phosphonylmethoxypropyl)adenine] (35) and PMPA [9-(2-phosphonylmethoxypropyl)adenine] (36) and their 2,6-diaminopurine congeners FPMPDAP and PMPDAP were described as potent and selective anti-HIV agents. For all these compounds, the enantiomeric forms were synthesized [e.g., (R)- and (S)-FPMPA, (R)- and (S)-PMPA] and in all cases one enantiomeric form proved clearly more active than the other, thus (S)-FPMPA > (R)-FPMPA, (S)-FPMPDAP > (R)-FPMPDAP, (R)-PMPA > (S)-PMPA, and (R)-PMPDAP > (S)-PMPDAP. The most potent was (R)-PMPDAP with an EC$_{50}$ of 0.17 µM against HIV-1 in MT-4 cells and no cytotoxicity at 300 µM (36). Although PMEA and PMPA [viz (R)-PMPA] are not terribly potent anti-HIV agents in human T-cell lines (e.g., MT-4, CEM) that are routinely used for assessing anti-HIV activity, they are much more active in human monocytes and macrophages wherein they inhibit HIV replication at an EC$_{50}$ of 0.02 to 0.04 µM (37,38). From PMEA and PMPA, lipophilic ester forms, that is, bis(pivaloyloxymethyl) and bis(isopropyloxycarbonyloxymethyl) esters have been prepared in attempts to increase the oral bioavailability of the compounds, and these oral prodrugs of PMEA and PMPA, termed bis(POM)-PMEA (39) and bis(POC)-PMPA (40), respectively, have been further pursued in clinical studies.

Whereas the ddN analogues (e.g., AZT, ddI, ddC) and acylic nucleoside phosphonates (e.g., PMEA, PMPA) as substrate analogues (following their conversion to the triphosphate form) could reasonably be expected as RT inhibitors, it came as a surprise that compounds that were structurally unrelated to the natural substrates would also be able to block the reverse transcriptase reaction. The first compounds that were found to inhibit HIV replication through such an "unconventional" mechanism were the HEPT [1-(2-hydroxyethoxymethyl)-6-(phenylthio)thymine (41,42) and TIBO [tetrahydroimidazo(4,5,1-jk)(1,4)benzodiazepin-2(1H)-one] (43,44) derivatives. The unprecedented specificity of the TIBO derivatives (i.e., tivirapine), which were found to inhibit HIV-1 replication at concentrations that were 10,000- to 100,000-fold lower than the concentrations required to impair normal cell viability, was attributed to a specific interaction with the HIV-1 reverse transcriptase (43–45). For the HEPT derivatives, it became evident that they also interacted specifically with HIV-1 RT after a number of more active congeners (including MKC-442) had been synthesized (46–48). Following the HEPT and TIBO derivatives, various other, all structurally different, classes of compounds, including dipyridodiazepinones (i.e., nevirapine) (49,50), bis(heteroaryl)piperazine (BHAP) derivatives (i.e., delavirdine) (51,52), α-anilinophenylacetamide (α-APA) derivatives (i.e., loviride) (53), quinoxaline derivatives (i.e., HBY 097) (54,55,55a), quinazolinone/benzoxazinone derivatives (i.e., efavirenz) (56,57), phenethylthiazolethiourea (PETT) derivatives (i.e., trovirdine) (58,59), thiocarboxanilide derivatives (i.e., UC-781) (60,61), and several other classes of compounds (4,5) have been reported to act as specific HIV-1 RT inhibitors. All these compounds are collectively referred to as NNRTIs. What they all have in common, and this is inherent to the definition of NNRTIs, is that they must interact with a specific non–substrate-binding site of HIV-1 RT, which is present only in the reverse transcriptase of HIV-1 but not that of HIV-2 or any other retrovirus (4).

Synergistic anti-HIV activity may be expected if the RT inhibitors are used in combination: for example, when AZT is combined with ddI (62,63), even against AZT-resistant HIV strains (64). Strong synergistic anti-HIV activity has also been noted for PMEA in combination with AZT (65,66) and for PMPA in combination with AZT (66). Similarly, synergistic anti-HIV activity has been described for combinations of AZT with any of the NNRTIs, such as tivirapine (67), nevirapine (68), delavirdine (69), and MKC-442 (70,71). Synergistic anti-HIV activity has also been reported for the combinations of AZT with phosphonoformate (foscarnet) (72), of AZT with protease inhibitors (i.e., saquinavir) (73), of delavirdine with interferon-α (74), and of HEPT with interferon- α (75). Thiocarboxanilides have an additive inhibitory effect on HIV-1 when combined with other antiretroviral drugs (reverse transcriptase inhibitors or protease inhibitors) (76).

When used at a sufficiently high concentration (i.e., 50 µM for ddA; 2 µM for ddC), these ddN analogues afford long-term suppression of HIV-1 replication (for 30 days in the presence of the compound, followed by 80 days in its absence) (77). Yet, AZT cannot prevent virus breakthrough, even in the continued presence of the drug (up to a concentration of 25 µM) (78). Under conditions in which AZT and ddI proved unable to protect the cells against the destruction by the virus, the NNRTIs TIBO, BHAP, and nevirapine were capable of completely suppressing HIV-1 infection when added to the cells at a sufficiently high concentration (1 to 10 µM, or 100 times their EC_{50}) (79). The infected cells could apparently be cleared from virus by the NNRTIs when used at these "knocking-out" concentrations, and the resultant healthy cell culture could be subsequently maintained without drug with no evidence of latent proviral DNA (79,80). The more potent quinoxaline (81) and thiocarboxanilide (82) derivatives achieved this "knocking-out" effect at even lower concentrations (0.1 to 1 µM), that is, at concentrations that should be readily attainable in the plasma following systemic administration to patients. Also DMP 266 (efavirenz) was found to completely suppress virus replication in PBMC at a concentration of 0.96 µM, and no regrowth occurred in the presence of compound after 10 weeks or in the absence of compound for 3 additional weeks (83). If, furthermore, the NNRTIs are used in combination with other RT inhibitors, such as delavirdine combined with AZT (84), MKC-442 combined with AZT (85), delavirdine combined with 3TC (86), MKC-442 combined with 3TC (86), or thiocarboxanilide combined with other NNRTIs, then virus breakthrough could be suppressed for a much longer time, and at much lower concentrations than if the compounds were used individually (87). Thus, drug combination regimens containing both nucleoside- and nonnucleoside-type RT inhibitors should be advocated for a number of reasons: They act synergistically against the virus (as explained in the preceding paragraph), they allow the individual compounds to be used at lower doses, and still to achieve complete virus suppression; and, in preventing virus breakthrough, they also prevent the virus from becoming resistant to the compounds. It must be well understood that the different compounds should be used in simultaneous combination regimens and not in sequential therapy, because the latter approach would enable the virus to rapidly acquire resistance mutations to the individual compounds (88).

III. INTRACELLULAR METABOLISM TO THE ACTIVE METABOLITE

All the ddN analogues, whether AZT, ddI, ddC, d4T, or 3TC, must be phosphorylated through three consecutive kinase reactions to the triphosphate form (ddNTP) before they can interact as competitive inhibitors with respect to the normal substrates (dNTPs) at the target enzyme (RT). As a rule, the relative ability of the dideoxynucleoside analogues to generate 5′-triphosphates intracellularly is of greater importance in determining the eventual capacity to block HIV replication than the relative abilities of the resultant ddNTPs to inhibit the viral reverse transcriptase (89). The intracellular metabolism of the ddN analogues appears to be highly varying from one cell species to another, AZT being readily phosphorylated to its 5′-triphosphate in murine cells, but poorly so in human cells, whereas ddC is more extensively phosphorylated to its 5′-triphosphate in human than in murine cells (90). Also, the anabolic state of the cells plays an important role: AZT and d4T are preferentially phosphorylated, yield higher ratios of ddNTP/dNTP, and exert more potent anti-HIV activity in activated PBMC than in resting cells, whereas other ddNs, such as ddI, ddA, ddC, 3TC, and F-ddA, produce higher ratios of ddNTP/dNTP and exert more potent anti-HIV activity in resting cells (91).

As originally demonstrated for AZT (92), three phosphorylation steps, catalyzed successively by a nucleoside kinase (i.e., thymidine kinase), a nucleoside monophosphate kinase (i.e., thymidylate kinase), and a nucleoside diphosphate (NDP) kinase [an enzyme that can use both purine and pyrimidine and ribo- or deoxy(ribo)nucleotides as substrates (93)] are required to convert the ddNs to their 5′-triphosphates. For most of the ddN analogues, the bottleneck in this anabolic pathway is the first phosphorylation step, which quite often determines why some ddNs (e.g., AZT) are active and others [e.g., 2′,3′- dideoxyuridine (ddU)] are not (94). For AZT, however, the bottleneck is the second phosphorylation step (95,96), because AZT 5′-monophosphate (AZT-MP) inhibits dTMP kinase, the enzyme that is needed to phosphorylate AZT-MP as well as dTMP. Consequently, AZT-MP accumulates (92,97,98). In contrast, d4T, which is less efficiently phosphorylated to its 5′-monophosphate than AZT, readily proceeds from its monophosphate onto its di- and triphosphate so that eventually equivalent levels of the active metabolites (AZT-TP and d4T-TP) are reached (97).

As for the pyrimidine ddN analogues, the purine ddN analogues [e.g., carbovir (99)], must be phosphorylated through three consecutive phosphorylation steps to proceed to the active metabolite (triphosphate), the first, and crucial, step in this phosphorylation process being ensured by the 5′-nucleotidase. This enzyme is using inosine 5′-monophosphate (IMP) as the phosphate donor, and hence, IMP dehydrogenase inhibitors (such as mycophenolic acid) that lead to an accumulation of IMP, significantly enhance the intracellular phosphorylation (and eventual anti-HIV activity) of carbovir (99,100) and other purine ddN analogues such as ddA and ddI (101). However, mycophenolic acid does not stimulate the intracellular anabolism of abacavir (1592U89), apparently because 1592U89 circumvents the 5′-nucleotidase step used by carbovir: 1592U89 is phosphorylated by adenosine phosphotransferase to 1592U89 monophosphate which is then converted by a cytosolic deaminase to carbovir monophosphate before being further processed to the di- and triphosphate of carbovir (100). This unique intracellular activation pathway enables 1592U89 to overcome the pharmacokinetic and toxicological deficiencies of carbovir while maintaining potent and selective anti-HIV activity.

Intervention with the intracellular metabolism of the ddN analogues may have a marked effect on their anti-HIV potency. As already mentioned, IMP dehydrogenase inhibitors such as mycophenolic acid, tiazofurin, and ribavirin (101) stimulate the intracellular phosphorylation of the purine ddN analogues to their triphosphates. The increased levels of the ddNTPs, together with the depletion of the corresponding dNTP pool levels, translate into a marked potentiating effect of the IMP dehydrogenase inhibitors on the anti-HIV activity of the purine ddN analogues (i.e., ddI) (101,102). Also, the pyrimidine ddN analogues (i.e., d4T) may be stimulated in their metabolism to the triphosphate form, that is, by thymidylate synthase inhibitors [such as methotrexate (103)] that shut off the synthesis of dTTP, an allosteric inhibitor of thymidine kinase. Because the latter is required for the initial phosphorylation of d4T and AZT, the decrease in dTTP levels may translate into increased metabolic activation and anti-HIV activity of AZT and d4T. Furthermore, the inhibitory effect of AZT-MP on dTMP kinase (a key enzyme in the biosynthesis of dTTP) may also be used as an argument for advocating the combination of AZT with d4T because the latter may be expected to undergo increased phosphorylation by thymidine kinase when feedback inhibition by dTTP is alleviated.

Because the first phosphorylation by nucleoside kinases is the rate-limiting step in the metabolic activation of most ddN analogues, several attempts have been made to circumvent or "bypass" this nucleoside kinase step. The problem cannot be overcome by supplying the preformed nucleotides because such compounds are unable to penetrate cells. Thus "masked" nucleotides (or pronucleotides) were created that can, as such, penetrate the cells, deliver the nucleoside 5′-monophosphate intracellularly, and "bypass" the nucleoside kinases: for example, bis(pivaloyloxymethyl)-ddUMP (104), S-acyl-2-thioethyl (SATE) derivatives of ddUMP, AZT-MP, and other ddN 5′-monophosphates (105–107); phosphoramidate triesters of AZT, d4T, and d4T analogues (108–111); and cyclic saligenyl phosphotriesters of d4T and ddA (112,113). In particular, So 324, a d4T-MP prodrug containing at the phosphate moiety a phenyl group, and the methylester of alanine linked to the phosphate through a phosphoramidate linkage showed anti-HIV activity that was superior to that of d4T, and, in contrast to d4T, proved also active against HIV in thymidine kinase–deficient cells (109). Following intracellular uptake, the d4T-MP triester So 324 gave rise to the formation of d4T-MP, d4T-DP, and d4T-TP and also a new metabolite, alaninyl d4T-MP, which could be considered as an intracellular depot form of d4T and/or d4T-MP (110). Recently, 5′-O-[(alkoxycarbonyl)phosphinyl]-3′-azido- 2′,3′-dideoxythymidines have been synthesized that could be considered as prodrugs of both azidothymidine (AZT) and phosphonoformate (PFA) (114); these PFA-AZT conjugates proved more potent than PFA, as well as AZT, against AZT-resistant HIV-1 strains.

In the acyclic nucleoside phosphonates (e.g., PMEA, PMPA), the phosphate has been built in as a phosphonate that can no longer be cleaved off by esterases, and, because these molecules can, as such, be taken by the cells, they also "bypass" the first phosphorylation step. Inside the cells, PMEA and PMPA need only two additional phosphorylations to be converted to the active, diphosphorylated forms PMEApp and PMPApp (Fig. 4). As has been shown specifically for PMEA and HPMPA, these acyclic nucleoside phosphonates can be converted to their diphosphate derivatives in either one step, through the aid of 5-phosphoribosyl-1-pyrophosphate (PRPP) synthetase with PRPP as the diphosphate donor (115,116), or two steps, through adenylate kinase with ATP as the phosphate donor (117,118). The diphosphate derivatives (e.g., HPMPApp, PMEApp, PMPApp) can be considered as analogous to the dNTPs, and, akin to the ddNTPs (e.g., AZT-TP, d4T-TP), PMEApp and its congeners may then be expected to interact as competitive inhibitors/alternate substrates at the HIV RT level.

Dideoxynucleoside analogues (i.e. ddC)

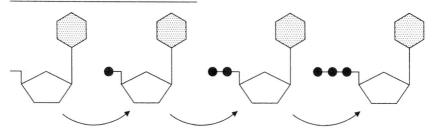

Acyclic nucleotide analogues (i.e. PMEA)

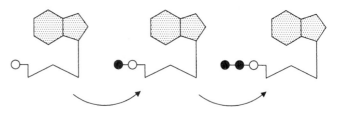

Figure 4   Intracellular metabolism of NRTIs: the 2′,3′-dideoxynucleoside (ddN) analogues [as exemplified for ddC (zalcitabine)] need three phosphorylation steps, whereas the acyclic nucleotide analogues [as exemplified for PMEA (adefovir)] only need two phosphorylation steps to be converted to their active metabolites [i.e., the 2′-deoxynucleoside 5′-triphosphate (dNTP) analogues].

In contrast to the ddN and ANP analogues, the NNRTIs do not need, or even want, any intracellular metabolism. They are able to interact directly with their target enzyme, the HIV-1 RT; and their eventual (in vitro) potency, as anti-HIV-1 agents, depends on their accessibility to, and their affinity for, the HIV-1 RT.

IV. MECHANISM OF INTERACTION WITH THE TARGET ENZYME

Whereas the ddN analogues are nonselectively phosphorylated, their triphosphate derivatives selectively interact with HIV RT, as exemplified for AZT-TP that has about 100-fold greater affinity for the HIV reverse transcriptase than for the cellular DNA polymerases α (92) and β (119). The ddNTP analogues, as again exemplified by AZT-TP, can serve as alternate substrates for HIV RT, and the resulting incorporation of ddNMP (e.g., AZT-MP) at the 3´-end causes chain termination (because of the unavailability of the 3´- hydroxylfunction required for further chain elongation) (119). Incorporation of ddNMP into the growing DNA chain, followed by chain termination, has also been demonstrated with various other ddNTPs, such as ddUTP (120) and 3TC-TP (121), and may well be regarded as the molecular basis for the anti-HIV activity of the ddN analogues (122).

The diphosphates of the acyclic nucleoside phosphonates (e.g., PMEApp, PMPApp), being alternative substrates to dATP, can also be incorporated at the 3´- end of the growing DNA chain, thus terminating further chain growth (35,36,115). Again, the incorporation of the chain-terminating acyclic nucleotides may be regarded as the molecular basis for their anti-HIV activity and selectivity. The acyclic nucleoside phosphonates can also be incorporated by cellular DNA polymerases α, β, γ, δ and ϵ (123,124), albeit at (much) lower efficiencies than by the HIV reverse transcriptase. Within the class of the ANP analogues, PMPApp is less efficiently incorporated by the cellular DNA polymerase than PMEApp (124), which is in agreement with the lower cytotoxicity of PMPA than of PMEA (36).

In contrast with the ddNAP analogues and ANP diphosphates, which interact with the substrate-binding site of HIV RT (see Fig. 4), the NNRTIs block the HIV-1 RT reaction through interaction with an allosterically located, non–substrate-binding site (4,5). This NNRTI-binding site ("pocket") is located at a close (about 10Å) distance from the substrate-binding site (125), and is not only spatially but also functionally (126) associated with the substrate-binding site. The cooperative interaction between these two sites (127) provides a means to increase the effectiveness of nucleoside and nonnucleoside RT inhibitors by using them in combination therapy.

Several studies have revealed a common mode of binding for the chemically diverse NNRTIs with their target site at the HIV-1 RT (128). The NNRTIs cause a repositioning of the three-stranded β-sheet in the p66 subunit (containing the catalytic aspartic acid residues 110, 185, and 186) (129). This suggests that the NNR-TIs inhibit HIV-1 RT by locking the active catalytic site in an inactive conformation, reminiscent of the conformation observed in the inactive p51 subunit (129). When bound into their pocket at the HIV-1 RT, the NNRTIs [i.e., α-APA (130), TIBO (131), 9-chloro-TIBO (132), and nevirapine (133)] maintain a very similar conformational "butterfly-like" shape. They roughly overlay each other in the binding pocket and appear to function as π-electron donors to aromatic side-chain residues surrounding the pocket (133). Side-chain residues of the pocket adapt to each bound inhibitor in a highly specific manner, closing down around the surface of the drug to make tight van der Waals contacts (133).

The binding of the thiocarboxanilide UC-781 in its HIV-1 RT pocket is shown in Figure 5 (134). The thiocarboxanilides bind to their pocket in a similar fashion as the other NNRTIs (134), that is, through hydrogen binding with the main chain oxygen of Lys-101 and hydrophobic interactions with Leu-100, Val-106, Val-179, Tyr-188, Phe-227, Leu-234, and His-235. The thiocarboxanilide UC-781 also makes important hydrophobic interactions with Trp-229. The BHAP U-90152 (delavirdine) occupies the same pocket as the other NNRTIs, but the complex is stabilized quite differently, in particular by hydrogen bonding to the main chain of

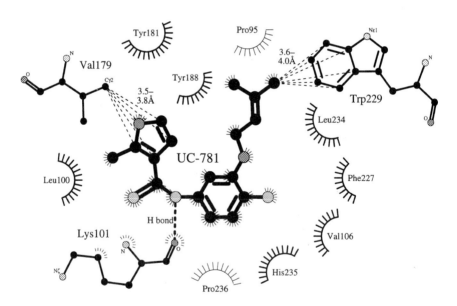

Figure 5 Schematic diagram of the interaction of UC-781 with HIV-1 reverse transcriptase. The hydrogen bond with Lys101 and the two methyl group-aromatic ring interactions are shown explicitly. Other major hydrophobic contacts are shown with bold lines, minor ones with faint lines. (From Ref. 134.)

Lys-103 and extensive hydrophobic contacts with Pro-236; when bound, part of U-90152 protrudes into the solvent creating a channel between Pro-236 and the polypeptide segments 225-226 and 105-106, thus providing evidence for the entry mode of NNRTIs (135).

Detailed evaluation of the mode of interaction of the different NNRTIs with their target site may provide important information on how to structurally modify or design NNRTIs so as to make their binding in the HIV-1 RT pocket more resilient to mutations.

V. ANTIRETROVIRUS ACTIVITY IN ANIMAL MODELS

Of all the HIV RT inhibitors that were shown to be effective against HIV replication in cell culture in vitro, the acyclic nucleoside phosphonates (i.e., PMEA and PMPA) have been most intensively pursued for their in vivo antiretrovirus activity. Whatever the animal model that was used to assess their in vivo potential, ANP analogues invariably proved more efficacious than ddN analogues such as AZT, that is, in the suppression of tumor formation and associated mortality in mice inoculated with Moloney murine sarcoma virus (MSV) (36,136). In this model, the antiretrovirus activity of PMEA increased when it was less frequently administered (137). In mice inoculated intracerebrally with MSV, PMEA effected a significant delay in tumor formation even at a dose as low as 1 mg/kg/day (138). In severe combined immune deficient (SCID) mice, oral bis(POM)-PMEA afforded anti-MSV efficacy that was equivalent to that of subcutaneous PMEA given at equimolar doses (39). The antiretroviral efficacy of PMEA has also been established in the murine AIDS (MAIDS) model [i.e., LP-BM5 virus-infected immunocompromised mice that are highly susceptible to opportunistic herpes simplex virus infections (139)], and in the hu-PBL-SCID mouse model [i.e., SCID mice reconstituted with human peripheral blood leukocytes (PBL) that are susceptible to infection with HIV (140)]. In the hu-PBL-SCID mouse model, F-ddA was tested in parallel with, and found more efficacious than, AZT in decreasing the HIV-1 infection rate [from 93% (control) to 31% (AZT) and 0% (F-ddA)] (141).

The acyclic nucleoside phosphonates were further evaluated in feline retrovirus models (6) [i.e., cats infected with feline immunodeficiency virus (FIV)]. In these studies, PMEA (at a daily dose of 5 to 10 mg/kg) was found to suppress the replication of HIV, as well as the symptoms of opportunistic infection (gingivitis, stomatitis, and diarrhea) (142). In a comparative study, (R)-PMPDAP proved to be superior to PMEA in terms of antiviral efficacy, as attested by a more significant reduction of FIV RNA titers in plasma (143). High therapeutic efficacy, without toxicity, has also been observed with (R)-PMPA and (S)-FPMPA in FIV-infected cats (6). Sheep infected with the neurotropic visna-maedi virus represent an attractive model for retrovirus infections of the central nervous system (CNS):

PMEA (injected subcutaneously at 10 mg/kg, three times a week) effected a marked suppression of visna virus replication in the CNS, and associated brain lesions, in lambs inoculated intracerebrally with the virus (144).

PMEA, and more recently, PMPA have also been investigated in the simian immunodeficiency virus (SIV) model, which is generally accepted as the most representative model for HIV infections in humans. In SIV-infected rhesus macaques, PMEA (at a dose of 10 or 20 mg/kg/day, starting 1 day before SIV infection, and continued for 29 days) clearly reduced SIV p26 antigenemia and delayed the onset of antibody production (145). An even higher efficacy with PMEA was observed in another study (146), in which PMEA (at a dose of 20 mg/kg/day, starting 2 days before SIV inoculation, and continued for 28 days) completely blocked virus replication in 83% of the animals (macaques). PMEA proved clearly superior to AZT, which was protective against SIV infection in only 6% of the animals (147). Moreover, in contrast to the severe anemia seen with AZT, no hematological toxicity was observed in the PMEA-treated monkeys.

When PMPA was administered (at 30 mg/kg/day) for 4 weeks, beginning either 48 hours before, 4 hours after, or 24 hours after virus inoculation, it completely protected all macaques against SIV infection without signs of toxicity (148). Under the same conditions, AZT failed to protect any animal, and, unlike AZT, PMPA was devoid of any hematological toxicity. PMPA appears to have excellent potential as an effective and nontoxic agent for the postexposure prophylaxis of HIV infections (i.e., in persons who have been accidentally exposed to HIV) and for the prevention of maternal transmission of HIV. In addition, PMPA may also be useful in preventing sexual HIV transmission (i.e., if applied topically as a vaginal microbicidal formulation). In rhesus macaques treated with a 10% PMPA vaginal gel at 1 day before, and then 0, 24, and 48 hours after intravaginal inoculation of SVI, 100% protection against vaginal SIV transmission was noted (6).

The long-term therapeutic and toxic effects of PMPA have also been evaluated in newborn rhesus macaques infected with SIV: PMPA (at 30 mg/kg/day, starting at 3 weeks after virus inoculation) provided a rapid, pronounced, and persistent reduction of viremia (in three of the four animals); all four PMPA-treated animals remained disease-free for more than 13 months, whereas three of the four untreated animals had died within 3 months (149). In another study, in which PMPA (at a dose of 30 mg/kg/day) was assessed for its efficacy in the treatment of an established SIV infection in macaques, it was found to reduce SIV levels by greater than 99% in the plasma or peripheral blood mononuclear cells (PBMC) within 2 weeks of treatment, again with no signs of toxicity (150).

In contrast to the ANP analogues that have proved to be highly efficacious, both prophylactically and therapeutically, in a variety of retrovirus models in mice, cats, sheep, and monkeys, the ddN analogues (other than AZT) have neither been extensively explored nor found significantly effective in animal retrovirus models. The poor efficacy of ddN analogues such as ddI, ddC, and 3TC in murine retrovirus infections has been generally attributed to the poor anabolism of the compounds to their triphosphate derivatives. Also, the NNRTIs have been very rarely studied in animal retrovirus models, essentially because their in vitro activity is limited to HIV-1. When evaluated in HIV-1 infected hu-PBL-SCID mice, NNR-TIs such as delavirdine (BHAP U-90152) and thiocarboxanilides protected the mice against HIV-1 infection (82). Similarly, nevirapine proved effective in preventing HIV-1 infection in chimpanzees (151).

VI. CLINICAL EFFICACY IN HIV-INFECTED INDIVIDUALS

As has been shown (1) with other ddN analogues (e.g., AZT, ddI, ddC) monotherapy with stavudine (d4T) has proven effective in delaying progression of HIV disease even if the patients had been previously given zidovudine (152). Monotherapy with adefovir dipivoxil (Preveon) has been shown to effect a significant increase in CD4$^+$ cell counts and significant decrease in HIV-1 RNA levels, as compared to placebo, over a 12-week treatment period (153). Also, NNRTIs have been the subject of short-term clinical studies (154–160). As a rule, the NNRTIs were very well tolerated [although rash developed in about half of the patients given nevirapine (158)]; they efficiently suppressed plasma viral load [up to $-1.38 \log_{10}$ (160)], but could not prevent the emergence of drug-resistant virus strains (156,158). Nevirapine-resistant virus was isolated from all subjects tested at 12 weeks (158), and by that time plasma HIV-1 RNA load had returned to baseline values (161). Although some patients given high-dose nevirapine (i.e., 400 mg daily) may experience sustained reduction in plasma HIV RNA despite the presence of resistant virus (162), this does not seem to hold true in previously untreated HIV-1-infected persons (161).

In one study (163), in patients with advanced HIV infection, combination therapy of AZT with either ddI or ddC did not prove superior to AZT therapy alone. In various other studies, however, combination therapy proved clearly superior to monotherapy. In AZT- naïve patients, combination of AZT with 3TC resulted in a more potent and sustained antiviral effect than AZT monotherapy (164); and in AZT-experienced patients, combination of AZT with 3TC provided a greater and more sustained increase in CD4$^+$ cell counts and decreases in viral load than continued AZT monotherapy (165). Also, combination of AZT with ddI (or ddC) resulted in a significant increase in CD4$^+$ cell counts through 72 weeks, as compared with AZT monotherapy, and a greater and more sustained decline in plasma HIV-1 RNA load (166); and for patients who began receiving AZT, changing to combination therapy (AZT with ddI or ddC) resulted in a significantly increased survival rate (167). Where different drug combination regimens were compared, the combination of AZT with ddI and the combination of AZT with 3TC seemed to be superior to the combination of AZT with ddC in terms of fewer clinical events (168) and greater immunological response (169), respectively. Another promising combination is that of d4T with 3TC: on short-term, this combination is well tolerated and associated with virological and immunological benefits, so that further evaluation of d4T and 3TC in combination is warranted (170).

Monotherapy with NNRTIs rapidly leads to the emergence of drug-resistant HIV strains (156,157); however, the rate of emergence of NNRTI-resistant virus is markedly reduced in subjects receiving AZT concomitantly with the NNRTI (i.e., pyridinone L-697,661) (171,172). NNRTIs, as demonstrated for nevirapine (173) and delavirdine (174), may be advantageously combined with ddN analogues such as AZT and thus achieve higher efficacy than when used alone. If this combination (AZT with nevirapine or delavirdine) is extended with another drug (i.e., ddI), the efficacy (in both immunological and virological terms) is further increased (174,175). Combined treatment of nevirapine with AZT and ddI has also proved effective in providing a sustained reduction of the plasma HIV-1 RNA load in infants (176). It was advocated (176) that such triple-drug combination therapy should be started as early as possible in infants with maternally acquired HIV-1 infection (probably within the first 2 to 4 weeks) to minimize the likelihood that antiretroviral resistance would emerge.

That triple-drug combinations are able to achieve a higher level of in vivo efficacy has also been demonstrated in a comparative study of AZT plus 3TC plus loviride versus AZT plus loviride (177). Addition of 3TC, or 3TC plus lovirid, to AZT-containing regimens added further incremental benefit in delaying disease progression over that seen with AZT (or AZT plus ddI or ddC) [CAESAR trial (178)]. Similarly, addition of an HIV protease inhibitor (such as saquinavir) to the combination of AZT with ddC provided a greater reduction in HIV-1 load and a greater increase in CD4$^+$ cell counts over those seen with the dual-drug combinations (AZT plus ddC, or AZT plus saquinavir) (179). Whereas treatment with AZT plus ddI (or ddC) is superior to treatment with AZT alone (180), three- drug combinations that include an HIV protease inhibitor (i.e., indinavir) and two ddN analogues (i.e., AZT and 3TC) are clearly more efficacious than dual drug combinations (AZT plus 3TC) (181). In fact, the combination of indinavir with AZT and 3TC has been found to reduce plasma HIV RNA levels to less than 500 copies per milliliter for as long as 1 year (182). The incremental reduction in viral load that is seen when switching from AZT monotherapy to AZT plus 3TC bitherapy and on to AZT plus 3TC plus indinavir tritherapy is virtually mirrored by an equivalent increase in the CD4$^+$ cell counts (Fig. 6) (183).

As a rule, triple-drug therapy can be considered as superior to dual-drug therapy, which, in turn, can be considered as superior to single-drug therapy, and it could a priori be expected that quadruple-drug therapy (184) may even be more effective than triple-, and quintuple-more so than quadruple-drug therapy. The drug combination regimens that have been most intensively pursued are depicted in Figure 7, but it is obvious that many more drug combinations could be envisaged, and, in fact, several additional combinations, involving nelfinavir, PMEA, efavirenz, and so on, are currently being evaluated for their clinical efficacy.

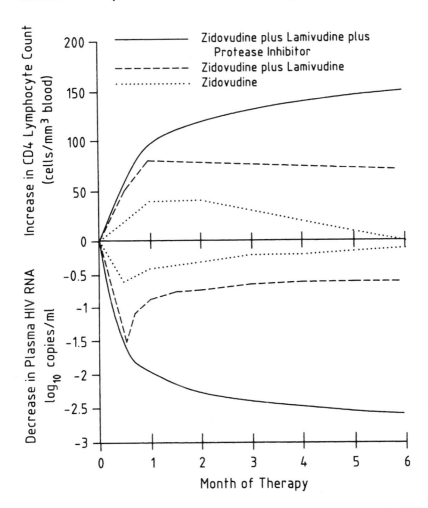

Figure 6 Idealized response of CD4 cell counts and HIV RNA plasma levels following initiation of therapy with one nucleoside analogue [i.e., AZT (zidovudine)] or two nucleoside analogues [i.e., AZT (zidovudine) plus 3TC [lamivudine]] or a protease inhibitor such as indinavir or ritonavir combined with the nucleoside analogues. (Modified from Ref. 183.)

VII. DRUG INTERACTIONS

As drug combinations are pursued at an increasing pace, they should be carefully monitored for drug interactions (185). It is unlikely that the protease inhibitors may interfere with the pharmacokinetics of the ddN analogues, because they follow different metabolic pathways. Protease inhibitors are metabolized by the cytochrome

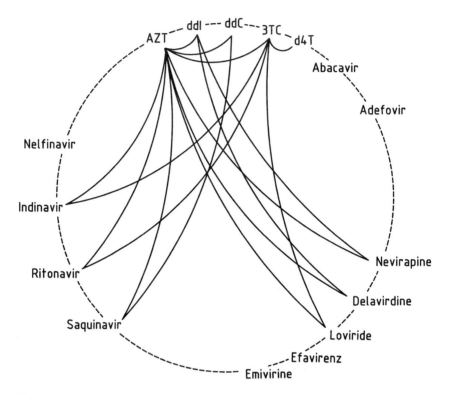

Figure 7   Combination drug therapy for HIV infections: those drug combinations that have been most intensively pursued (as indicated) could be readily extended to numerous other drug combinations (not indicated).

P450 (CYP) enzymes present in the liver and gut wall (186). Zidovudine (AZT) undergoes extensive hepatic glucuronidation, and didanosine (ddI) is catabolized by purine nucleoside phosphorylase to hypoxanthine and, finally, uric acid. Zalcitabine (ddC), stavudine (d4T), and lamivudine (3TC) are primarily eliminated by the kidney. Hence, no interference with the CYP enzymes responsible for the metabolism of the protease inhibitors would be anticipated. On the other hand, the ddN analogues require intracellular phosphorylation to their active triphosphate metabolites; the effect of the protease inhibitors on this phosphorylation process is unknown but should be determined.

    While possible interactions between protease inhibitors and ddN analogues are neither known nor anticipated, interactions between protease inhibitors and NNRTIs are likely to be expected because they are both hepatically metabolized (187). In addition to being metabolized by the P450 CYP enzymes (particularly

CYP 3A4), protease inhibitors have the potential to inhibit CYP 3A4 (in order of increasing inhibitory potency: saquinavir < indinavir < ritonavir). Ritonavir increases plasma saquinavir levels and may also be expected to increase the plasma levels of NNRTIs (such as delavirdine). Vice versa, delavirdine, being a CYP 3A4 inhibitor, may increase the plasma levels of saquinavir. Nevirapine, however, would rather act as a P450 enzyme inducer and thus reduce the plasma levels of hepatically metabolized drugs such as saquinavir (187).

VIII. HIV DRUG RESISTANCE

Drug resistance is the inevitable consequence of incomplete suppression of HIV replication. The rapid replication rate of HIV and its inherent genetic variation leads to the generation of a seemingly limitless number of viral variants that exhibit drug resistance (188). Mutations engendering HIV drug resistance can arise in any portion of the viral genome, including the viral RT gene. HIV drug resistance development was first recognized for AZT (189), and has since been documented for virtually all compounds that have been described as specific anti-HIV agents (188). For HIV to acquire high-level resistance to AZT, multiple mutations in the HIV-1 RT are required, that is, M41L, D67N, K70R, T215Y/F, and K219Q (190,191). In vivo, in patients given AZT, these mutations were shown to appear in an orderly fashion (192). Following the T215Y mutation, the L210W mutation may emerge and further contribute to high-level resistance to AZT (193).

Other mutations in HIV-1 RT are associated with resistance to ddI (i.e., L74V), ddC (i.e., K65R), d4T (i.e., V75T) (194), 3TC (i.e., M184V) (195,196), 1592U89 (i.e., K65R, L74V, M184V) (197), and FddA (i.e., P119S) (198) (Fig. 8). Whereas some of these mutations (e.g., M184V) may confer cross-resistance to different compounds (i.e, 3TC, ddI, ddC, and 1592U89), other mutations may actually suppress the drug-resistant phenotype and resensitize the virus to the drug. Thus, the ddI resistance mutation L74V has been found to increase the sensitivity of the virus to AZT (199) [although this resensitization does not occur in all genetic contexts (200)]; similarly, the 3TC resistance mutation M184V was found to counteract the AZT resistance phenotype based on the T215Y/F mutation (201). Even though just one amino acid substitution is sufficient for in vivo development of significant AZT resistance, multiple substitutions are required for the same level of AZT resistance in strains harboring the M184V mutation (202).

Multidrug-resistant HIV-1 strains containing the RT mutations A62V, V75I, F77L, F116Y, and Q151M (Fig. 9) have been reported in patients receiving combination therapy with AZT and ddI; together, these mutations confer resistance to AZT, ddI, ddC, and d4T (203,204). Accumulation of the HIV-1 RT mutations V75I, F77L, F116Y, Q151M, and M184V has also been found in a patient that was sequentially given AZT, ddI, ddC, d4T, and 3TC (205); the multidrug-resistant virus

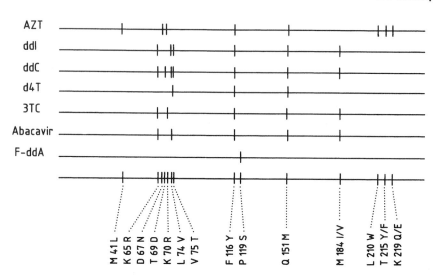

Figure 8 Mutations in the HIV reverse transcriptase that confer resistance to 2′,3′-dideoxynucleoside (ddN) analogues AZT, ddI, ddC, d4T, 3TC, abacavir, and F-ddA.

was resistant to all the ddN analogues but retained wild-type sensitivity to the ANPs (i.e., PMEA) and NNRTIs. Multidrug-resistant virus strains can acquire additional (i.e., NNRTI resistance) mutations (i.e., Y181C), without giving up their resistance to the ddN analogues (AZT, ddI) (206). The Q151M mutation may play a pivotal role in the multidrug resistance to ddN analogues. The Q151M mutation in SIV RT does not affect viral virulence. An AZT-resistant SIV mutant with the Q151M

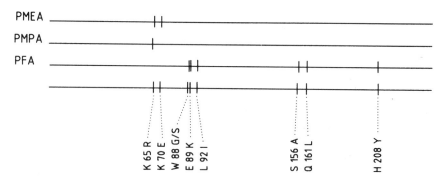

Figure 9 Mutations in the HIV reverse transcriptase that confer resistance to the acyclic nucleotide analogues (acyclic nucleoside phosphonates) PMEA and PMPA, and the pyrophosphate analogue foscarnet (PFA).

mutation was found to cause fatal immunodeficiency following inoculation into newborn rhesus macaques (207).

Resistance of HIV-1 to the pyrophosphate analogue foscarnet (phosphono-formic acid, PFA) is associated with RT mutations W99G/S, E89K, L92I, S156A, Q161L, and H208Y (208,209). PFA-resistant virus shows increased susceptibility to AZT, TIBO, and nevirapine (208). Furthermore, prolonged in vitro passage of wild-type or AZT-resistant HIV-1 strains with the combination AZT and PFA failed to generate coresistant virus. Strains selected by passage in the presence of PFA plus AZT were phenotypically susceptible to AZT despite multiple RT mutations known to confer AZT resistance. Thus, PFA resistance mutations can phenotypically reverse AZT resistance (209).

HIV can develop decreased sensitivity to acyclic nucleoside phosphonates (i.e., PMEA), but only after long-term in vitro exposure (i.e., 10 months), and this reduced sensitivity is associated with K65R, the same mutation that is associated with reduced sensitivity to ddI and ddC (210,211) (see Fig. 9). Again, the PMEA resistance mutation K65R was found to suppress phenotypic resistance to PMEA, which argues in favor of combined drug regimens containing both PMEA and AZT. The K70E mutation has also been associated with decreased susceptibility to PMEA as well as 3TC (212). If PMEA- and/or PMPA-resistant viruses do arise in vivo following prolonged treatment with the drugs [bis(POM)-PMEA and bis(POC)-PMPA], it will be interesting to determine whether they carry the K65R mutation, the K70E mutation, or any other mutations. From the clinical trials that are ongoing with bis(POM)-PMEA and bis(POC)-PMPA, it appears that they do not readily lead to the emergence of drug resistance mutations, and there is, at present, no evidence that antiviral drug resistance may compromise the clinical effectiveness of the acyclic nucleoside phosphonates.

The first RT mutations shown to be associated with, an to account for, HIV-1 resistance to NNRTIs were the K103N and Y181C mutations, engendering resistance to pyridinone (213), nevirapine (214), and TIBO 82150 (215). In fact, the mutations K103N and Y181C have been observed with virtually all NNRTIs (3,188) (Fig. 10), except for the quinoxalines (i.e., HBY 097). The latter preferentially induce mutations at RT position 190 (i.e., G190E) (216), particularly under high selective pressure (217) [whereas under low selective pressure, mutations L100I, K103N, V106A/I/L, Y181C, and G190A/T/V are induced (217)]. Concomitantly with the G109E mutation, HBY 097 induces the mutations L74V and V75I as well (218,219). However, in vivo the K103N mutation is preferentially induced (220). Other "specific" NNRTI mutations include L100I [TIBO 82150 (220a)], E138K [TSAO-T (221,222)], and P236L [BHAP (223)]. Resistance to the HEPT derivatives (i.e., MKC-442) can be associated with mutations at RT positions 103 (K103N), 108 (V108I), or 181 (Y181C) (224), or yet other sites (225), although MKC-442 (emivirine I-EBU) still retains sufficient activity against the Y181C mutant (IC_{50}: 0.22 μM), as compared to the wildtype (IC_{50}: 0.002 μM (226).

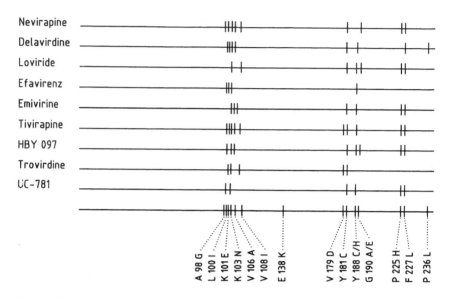

Figure 10   Mutations in the HIV-1 reverse transcriptase that confer resistance to the non-nucleoside reverse transcriptase inhibitors (NNRTIs).

The quinoxalines, and in particular HBY 097, retain pronounced activity against HIV-1 RT mutants containing the L100I, K103N, V106A, and Y181C mutation. Also, DMP 266 (efavirenz) is equally active against the V108I, V179D, Y181C mutant, and wild-type HIV-1 (57), and the thiocarboxanilides are only 10- to 20-fold less active against those HIV-1 mutants (i.e., L100I, V106A, E138K, and V179D) that they select for in vitro (82). More remarkably, the P236L mutation that confers resistance to BHAP U-90152 (delavirdine) causes hypersensitivity to other NNRTIs (e.g., nevirapine, TIBO, and pyridinone) (223). Recently, a novel mutation (P225H) was identified, that consistently appeared in a V106A mutant background and conferred additional resistance to all NNRTIs, except for delavirdine, which actually showed hypersensitivity toward the P225H mutant (227). Another novel mutation (F227L) that arose in a V106A mutant background was found to confer high-level resistance to virtually all NNRTIs that were examined (228).

The latter studies (227,228) confirm previous studies (57) that combinations of different mutations (i.e., L100I and K103N; K101D and K103N; K103N and Y181C) are needed for high-level resistance. It is not clear whether such double mutants may readily arise in vivo in patients under NNRTI treatment. With nevirapine, the most common mutation observed in vivo is Y181C, and this mutation is prevented from emerging by coadministration of AZT (229). Vice versa, the

Y181C or L100I mutation in an AZT resistance background significantly suppressed resistance to AZT (230,231), whereas the V106A mutation did not (230). Concomitant combination of the quinoxaline HBY 097 and 3TC prevented the emergence of virus resistance to HBY 097 (232). The mutually antagonistic effects of different resistance mutations (and the hypersensitivity that is seen under some conditions) further corroborated the conclusion repeatedly reached herein that different drugs should be used in concomitant combinations (i.e., AZT with 3TC with one or more NNRTIs). However, in one case an AZT resistance mutation appeared to potentiate the effect of the K103N mutation for HBY 097 (220a).

VIII. CONCLUSION

It has become increasingly clear that the best possible chemotherapy of HIV infections requires the combination of different anti-HIV drugs. While achieving synergism in their anti-HIV action, combination of different drugs may also reduce the risk of HIV drug resistance development and diminish the toxic side effects of the compounds (through reduction of the individual doses). Under no conditions should the compounds be used in sequential order, because such procedure (233) may allow the virus to acquire resistance mutations to all of the compounds (88). Instead, concomitant combination therapy, as demonstrated particularly with 3TC and NNRTIs (88), should be advocated. Of paramount importance is that these drug combination regimens should be started as soon as possible after HIV infection and that the individual compounds should be used at the highest possible doses so as to completely suppress virus replication and prevent drug-resistant virus strains from emerging. The latter recommendation is based on the virus "knocking-out" phenomenon (79–88) that has been observed in vitro with different NNRTIs when used at sufficiently high concentrations.

HIV-1 viremia, the hallmark of HIV infection, is sustained by a highly dynamic process involving continuous rounds of de novo virus replication and cell turnover (234,235). Productively infected cells have, on average, a life span of 2.2 days (half life = 1.6 days) and plasma virions have a mean life span of 0.3 days (half life = 0.24 days); the average total HIV-1 production is approximately 10^{10} virions per day, and the minimum duration of the HIV-1 life cycle in vivo is 1.2 days on average (236). Virus replication is the driving force in the progression to AIDS. Low viral load is associated with long-term nonprogression to AIDS (237,238), and even though both the plasma HIV RNA levels and CD4+ lymphocyte counts are both valid predictors of the clinical progression of HIV disease (239,240), plasma viral load is a more accurate predictor of progression to AIDS than the number of CD4+ T cells (241). Furthermore, the clinical course of HIV-1 infection may be already determined at the earliest phase of the disease, and this necessitates initiation of definitive treatment very early in HIV-1 infection (242).

Given that treatment of the HIV-1 infection should be initiated as early as possible (and that the treatment regimens should consist of the concomitant use of different anti-HIV agents at the highest possible doses), how long should this treatment be continued? An unequivocal answer to this question cannot be provided yet. Long-term treatment with the current combination drug regimens can effect a significant reduction in the plasma viral load (even to undetectable levels) and prevent the emergence of resistance. But, despite prolonged suppression of plasma viremia, replication-competent virus could still be recovered from resting CD4$^+$ T lymphocytes (243,244), even after 30 months of highly active antiretroviral therapy (HAART). These observations clearly indicate that, with the current drug treatment regimens available for the treatment of HIV disease, (a) virus replication can be suppressed, (b) resistance development can be prevented, (c) progression to AIDS can be arrested, but (d) latent virus cannot be eradicated from its reservoirs.

ACKNOWLEDGMENTS

I thank Christiane Callebaut for her proficient editorial assistance.

REFERENCES

1. De Clercq E. Antiviral therapy for human immunodeficiency virus infections. Clin Microbiol Rev 1995; 8:200–239.
2. De Clercq E. Toward improved anti-HIV chemotherapy: therapeutic strategies for intervention with HIV infections. J Med Chem 1995; 38:2491–2517.
3. De Clercq E. Development of resistance of human immunodeficiency virus (HIV) to anti-HIV agents: how to prevent the problem? Int J Antimicrob Agents 1997; 9:21–36.
4. De Clercq E. Non-nucleoside reverse transcriptase inhibitors (NNRTIs) for the treatment of human immunodeficiency virus type 1 (HIV-1) infections: strategies to overcome drug resistance development. Med Res Rev 1996; 16:125–157.
5. De Clercq E. What can be expected from non-nucleoside reverse transcriptase inhibitors (NNRTIs) in the treatment of human immunodeficiency virus type 1 (HIV-1) infections? Rev Med Virol 1996; 6:97–117.
6. Naesens L, Snoeck R, Andrei G, Balzarini J, Neyts J, De Clercq E, HPMPC (cidofovir), PMEA (adefovir) and related acyclic nucleoside phosphonate analogues: a review of their pharmacology and clinical potential in the treatment of viral infections. Antiviral Chem Chemother 1996; 8:1–23.
7. Langtry HD, Campoli-Richards DM. Zidovudine. A review of its pharmacodynamic and pharmacokinetic properties, and therapeutic efficacy. Drugs 1989; 37:408–450.
8. Faulds D, Brogden RN. Didanosine. A review of its antiviral activity, pharmacokinetic properties and therapeutic potential in human immunodeficiency virus infection. Drugs 1992; 44:94–116.

9. Whittington R, Brogden RN. Zalcitabine. A review of its pharmacology and clinical potential in acquired immunodeficiency syndrome (AIDS). Drugs 1992; 44:656–683.

10. Adkins JC, Peters DH, Faulds D. Zalcitabine. An update of its pharmacodynamic and pharmacokinetic properties and clinical efficacy in the management of HIV infection. Drugs 1997; 53:1054–1080.

11. Riddler SA, Anderson RE, Mellors JW. Antiretroviral activity of stavudine (2′,3′-didehydro-3′-deoxythymidine, D4T). Antiviral Res 1995; 27:189–203.

12. Moyle GJ. Stavudine: pharmacology, clinical use and future role. Exp Opin Invest Drugs 1997; 6:191–200.

13. Mitsuya H, Weinhold KJ, Furman PA, St. Clair MH, Nusinoff Lehrman S, Gallo RC, Bolognesi D, Barry DW, Broder S. 3′-Azido-3′-deoxythymidine (BW A509U): an antiviral agent that inhibits the infectivity and cytopathic effect of human T-lymphotropic virus type III/lymphadenopathy-associated virus in vitro. Proc Natl Acad Sci U S A 1985; 82:7096–7100.

14. Mitsuya H, Broder S. Inhibition of the in vitro infectivity and cytopathic effect of human T-lymphotrophic virus type III/lymphadenopathy-associated virus (HTLV-III/LAV) by 2′,3′-dideoxynucleosides. Proc Natl Acad Sci U S A 1986; 83:1911–1915.

15. Baba M, Pauwels R, Herdewijn P, De Clercq E, Desmyter J, Vandeputte M. Both 2′,3′-dideoxythymidine and its 2′,3′-unsaturated derivative (2′,3′-dideoxythymidinene) are potent and selective inhibitors of human immunodeficiency virus replication in vitro. Biochem Biophys Res Commun 1987; 142:128–134.

16. Soudeyns H, Yao X-J, Gao Q, Belleau B, Kraus J-L, Nguyen-Ba N, Spira B, Wainberg MA. Anti-human immunodeficiency virus type 1 activity and in vitro toxicity of 2′-deoxy- 3′-thiacytidine (BCH-189), a novel heterocyclic nucleoside analog. Antimicrob Agents Chemother 1991; 35:1386–1390.

17. Coates JAV, Cammack N, Jenkinson HJ, Mutton IM, Pearson BA, Storer R, Cameron JM, Penn CR. The separated enantiomers of 2′-deoxy-3′-thiacytidine (BCH 189) both inhibit human immunodeficiency virus replication in vitro. Antimicrob Agents Chemother 1992; 36:202–205.

18. Schinazi RF, Chu CK, Peck A, McMillan A, Mathis R, Cannon D, Jeong L-S, Beach JW, Choi W-B, Yeola S, Liotta DC. Activities of the four optical isomers of 2′,3′-dideoxy-3′-thiacytidine (BCH-189) against human immunodeficiency virus type 1 in human lymphocytes. Antimicrob Agents Chemother 1992; 36:672–676.

19. Schinazi RF, McMillan A, Cannon D, Mathis R, Lloyd RM, Peck A, Sommadossi J-P, St. Clair M, Wilson J, Furman PA, Painter G, Choi W-B, Liotta DC. Selective inhibition of human immunodeficiency viruses by racemates and enantiomers of cis-5-fluoro-1-[2-(hydroxymethyl)-1,3-oxathiolan-5-yl]cytosine. Antimicrob Agents Chemother 1992; 36:2423–2431.

20. Doong S-L, Tsai C-H, Schinazi RF, Liotta DC, Cheng Y-C. Inhibition of the replication of hepatitis B virus in vitro by 2′,3′-dideoxy-3-thiacytidine and related compounds. Proc Natl Acad Sci U S A 1991; 88:8495–8499.

21. Furman PA, Davis M, Liotta DC, Paff M, Frick LW, Nelson DJ, Dornsife RE, Wurster JA, Wilson LJ, Fyfe JA, Tuttle JV, Miller WH, Condreay L, Averett DR, Schinazi RF, Painter GR. The anti-hepatitis B virus activities, cytotoxicities, and anabolic profiles

of the (-) and (+) enantiomers of *cis*-5-fluoro-1-[2-(hydroxymethyl)- 1,3-oxathiolan-5-yl]cytosine. Antimicrob Agents Chemother 1992; 36:2686–2692.

22. Daluge SM, Good SS, Faletto MB, Miller WH, St. Clair MH, Boone LR, Tisdale M, Parry NR, Reardon JE, Dornsife RE, Averett DR, Krenitsky TA. 1592U89, A novel carbocyclic nucleoside analog with potent, selective anti-human immunodeficiency virus activity. Antimicrob Agents Chemother 1997; 41:1082–1093.

23. Vince R, Hua M, Brownell J, Daluge S, Lee F, Shannon WM, Lavelle GC, Qualls J, Weislow OS, Kiser R, Canonico PG, Schultz RH, Narayanan VL, Mayo JG, Shoemaker RH, Boyd MR. Potent and selective activity of a new carbocyclic nucleoside analog (carbovir: NSC 614846) against human immunodeficiency virus in vitro. Biochem Biophys Res Commun 1988; 156:1046–1053.

24. Herdewijn P, Pauwels R, Baba M, Balzarini J, De Clercq E. Synthesis and anti-HIV activity of various 2´- and 3´-substituted 2´,3´-dideoxyadenosines: a structure-activity analysis. J Med Chem 1987; 30:2131–2137.

25. Marquez VE, Tseng CK-H, Kelley JA, Mitsuya H, Broder S, Roth JS, Driscoll JS. 2´,3´-Dideoxy-2´-fluoro-ara-A: an acid-stable purine nucleoside active against human immunodeficiency virus (HIV). Biochem Pharmacol 1987; 36:2719–2722.

26. Masood R, Ahluwalia GS, Cooney DA, Fridland A, Marquez VE, Driscoll JS, Hao Z, Mitsuya H, Perno C-F, Broder S, Johns DG. 2´-Fluoro-2´,3´- dideoxyarabinosyladenine: a metabolically stable analogue of the antiretroviral agent 2´,3´-dideoxyadenosine. Mol Pharmacol 1989; 37:590–596.

27. Driscoll JS, Mayers DL, Bader JP, Weislow OS, Johns DG, Buckheit Jr RW. 2´-Fluoro-2´,3´- dideoxyarabinosyladenine (F-ddA): activity against drug-resistant human immunodeficiency virus strains and clades A-E. Antiviral Chem Chemother 1997; 8: 107–111.

28. Van Aerschot A, Herdewijn P, Balzarini J, Pauwels R, De Clercq E. 3´-Fluoro-2´,3´-dideoxy-5-chlorouridine: most selective anti-HIV-1 agent among a series of new 2´- and 3´-fluorinated 2´,3´- dideoxynucleoside analogues. J Med Chem 1989; 32:1743–1749.

29. Balzarini J, Van Aerschot A, Pauwels R, Baba M, Schols D, Herdewijn P, De Clercq E. 5-Halogeno-3´-fluoro- 2´,3´dideoxyuridines as inhibitors of human immunodeficiency virus (HIV): potent and selective anti-HIV activity of 3´-fluoro-2´,3´-dideoxy-5-chlorouridine. Mol Pharmacol 1989; 35:571–577.

30. Daluge SM, Purifoy DJM, Savina PM, St. Clair MH, Parry NR, Dev IK, Novak P, Ayers KM, Reardon JE, Roberts GB, Fyfe JA, Blum MR, Averett DR, Dornsife RE, Domin BA, Ferone R, Lewis DA, Krenitsky TA. 5-Chloro-2´,3´-dideoxy-3´-fluorouridine (935U83), a selective anti-human immunodeficiency virus agent with an improved metabolic and toxicological profile. Antimicrob Agents Chemother 1994; 38:1590–1603.

31. Riddler SA, Wang LH, Bartlett JA, Savina PM, Packard MV, McMahon KD, Blum MR, Dunn JA, Elkins MM, Mellors JW. Safety and pharmacokinetics of 5-chloro-2´,3´-dideoxy-3´- fluorouridine (935U83) following oral administration of escalating single doses in human immunodeficiency virus-infected adults. Antimicrob Agents Chemother 1996; 40:2842–2847.

32. De Clercq E, Holý A, Rosenberg I, Sakuma T, Balzarini J, Maudgal PC. A novel selective broad-spectrum anti-DNA virus agent. Nature 1986; 323:464–467.

33. De Clercq E, Sakuma T, Baba M, Pauwels R, Balzarini J, Rosenberg I, Holý. A. Antiviral activity of phosphonylmethoxyalkyl derivatives of purine and pyrimidines. Antiviral Res 1987; 8:261–272.

34. Pauwels R, Balzarini J, Schols D, Baba M, Desmyter J, Rosenberg I, Holý A, De Clercq E. Phosphonylmethoxyethyl purine derivatives, a new class of anti-human immunodeficiency virus agents. Antimicrob Agents Chemother 1988; 32:1025– 1030.

35. Balzarini J, Holý A, Jindrich J, Dvorakova H, Hao Z, Snoeck R, Herdewijn P, Johns DG, De Clercq E. 9-[(2RS)-3-fluoro-2-phosphonylmethoxypropyl] derivatives of purines: a class of highly selective antiretroviral agents in vitro and in vivo. Proc Natl Acad Sci U S A 1991; 88:4961–4965.

36. Balzarini J, Holý A, Jindrich J, Naesens L, Snoeck R, Schols D, De Clercq E. Differential antiherpesvirus and antiretrovirus effects of the (S and (R) enantiomers of acyclic nucleoside phosphonates: potent and selective in vitro and in vivo antiretrovirus activities of (R)-9-(2- phosphomethoxypropyl)-2,6-diaminopurine. Antimicrob Agents Chemother 1993; 37:332–338.

37. Balzarini J, Perno C-F, Schols D, De Clercq E. Activity of acyclic nucleoside phosphonate analogues against human immunodeficiency virus in monocyte/ macrophages and peripheral blood lymphocytes. Biochem Biophys Res Commun 1991; 178:329–335.

38. Balzarini J, Aquaro S, Perno C-F, Witvrouw M, Holý A, De Clercq E. Activity of the (R)-enantiomers of 9-(2-phosphonylmethoxypropyl)-adenine and 9-(2-phosphonyl-methoxypropyl)-2,6-diaminopurine against human immunodeficiency virus in different human cell systems. Biochem Biophys Res Commun 1996; 219:337–341.

39. Naesens L, Balzarini J, Bischofberger N, De Clercq E. Antiretroviral activity and pharmacokinetics in mice of oral bis(pivaloyloxymethyl)-9-(2-phosphonyl-methoxyethyl)adenine, the bis(pivaloyloxymethyl) ester prodrug of 9-(2-phospho-nylmethoxyethyl)adenine. Antimicrob Agents Chemother 1996; 40:22–28.

40. Naesens L, Bischofberger N, Augustijns P, Annaert P, Van den Mooter G, Arimilli MN, Kim CU, De Clercq E. Antiretroviral efficacy and pharmacokinetics of oral bis(isopropyloxycarbonyloxymethyl)-9-(2-phosphonylmethoxypropyl)adenine in mice. Antimicrob Agents Chemother 1998; 42:1568–1573.

41. Baba M, Tanaka H, De Clercq E, Pauwels R, Balzarini J, Schols D, Nakashima H, Perno C-F, Walker RT, Miyasaka T. Highly specific inhibition of human immunodeficiency virus type 1 by a novel 6-substituted acyclouridine derivative. Biochem Biophys Res Commun 1989; 165:1375–1381.

42. Miyasaka T, Tanaka H, Baba M, Hayakawa H, Walker RT, Balzarini J, De Clercq E. A novel lead for specific anti-HIV-1 agents: 1-[(2-hydroxyethoxy)methyl]-6-(phenylthio)thymine. J Med Chem 1989; 32:2507–2509.

43. Pauwels R, Andries K, Desmyter J, Schols D, Kukla M- J, Breslin HJ, Raeymaeckers A, Van Gelder J, Woestenborghs R, Heykants J, Schellekens H, Janssen MAC, De Clercq E, Janssen PAJ. Potent and selective inhibition of HIV-1 replication in vitro by a novel series of TIBO derivatives. Nature 1990; 343:470–474.

44. Debyser Z, Pauwels R, Andries K, Desmyter J, Kukla M, Janssen PAJ, De Clercq E. An antiviral target on reverse transcriptase of human immunodeficiency virus type 1 revealed by tetrahydroimidazo[4,5,1-jk][1,4]benzodiazepin-2(1H)- one and -thione derivatives. Proc Natl Acad Sci U S A 1991; 88:1451–1455.

45. Pauwels R, Andries K, Debyser Z, Kukla M-J, Schols D, Breslin HJ, Woestenborghs R, Desmyter J, Janssen MAC, De Clercq E, Janssen PAJ. New tetrahydroimidazo[4,5,1-jk][1,4]-benzodiazepin-2(1H)-one and -thione derivatives are potent inhibitors of human immunodeficiency virus type 1 replication and are synergistic with 2′,3′-dideoxynucleoside analogs. Antimicrob Agents Chemother 1994; 38:2863–2870.

46. Baba M, De Clercq E, Tanaka H, Ubasawa M, Takashima H, Sekiya K, Nitta I, Umezu K, Nakashima H, Mori S, Shigeta S, Walker RT, Miyasaka T. Potent and selective inhibition of human immunodeficiency virus type 1 (HIV-1) by 5-ethyl-6-phenyltiouracil derivatives through their interaction with the HIV-1 reverse transcriptase. Proc Natl Acad Sci U S A 1991; 88:2356–2360.

47. Baba M, De Clercq E, Tanaka H, Ubasawa M, Takashima H, Sekiya K, Nitta I, Umezu K, Walker RT, Mori S, Ito M, Shigeta S, Miyasaka T. Highly potent and selective inhibition of human immunodeficiency virus type 1 by a novel series of 6-substituted acyclouridine derivatives. Mol Pharmacol 1991; 39:805–810.

48. Baba M, Shigeta S, Yuasa S, Takashima H, Sekiya K, Ubasawa M, Tanaka H, Miyasaka T, Walker RT, De Clercq E. Preclinical evaluation of MKC-442, a highly potent and specific inhibitor of human immunodeficiency virus type 1 in vitro. Antimicrob Agents Chemother 1994; 38:688–692.

49. Merluzzi VJ, Hargrave KD, Labadia M, Grozinger K, Skoog M, Wu JC, Shih C-K, Eckner K, Hattox S, Adams J, Rosenthal AS, Faanes R, Eckner RJ, Koup RA, Sullivan JL. Inhibition of HIV-1 replication by a non-nucleoside reverse transcriptase inhibitor. Science 1990; 250:1411–1413.

50. Koup RA, Merluzzi VJ, Hargrave KD, Adams J, Grozinger K, Eckner RJ, Sullivan JL. Inhibition of human immunodeficiency virus type 1 (HIV-1) replication by the dipyridodiazepinone BI-RG-587. J Infect Dis 1991; 163:966–970.

51. Romero DL, Busso M, Tan C-K, Reusser F, Palmer JR, Poppe SM, Aristoff PA, Downey KM, So AG, Resnick L, Tarpley WG. Nonnucleoside reverse transcriptase inhibitors that potently and specifically block human immunodeficiency virus type 1 replication. Proc Natl Acad Sci U S A 1991; 88:8806–8810.

52. Romero DL, Morge RA, Genin MJ, Biles C, Busso M, Resnick L, Althaus IW, Reusser F, Thomas RC, Tarpley WG. Bis(heteroaryl)piperazine (BHAP) reverse transcriptase inhibitors: structure-activity relationships of novel substituted indole analogues and the identification of 1-[(5-methanesulfonamido-1H-indol-2-yl)carbonyl]-4-[3-[(1-methyl-ethyl)amino]pyridinyl] piperazine monomethanesulfonate (U-90152S), a second-generation clinical candidate. J Med Chem 1993; 36:1505–1508.

53. Pauwels R, Andries K, Debyser Z, Van Daele P, Schols D, Stoffels P, De Vreese K, Woestenborghs R, Vandamme A-M, Janssen CGM, Anné J, Cauwenbergh G, Desmyter J, Heykants J, Janssen MAC, De Clercq E, Janssen PAJ. Potent and highly selective human immunodeficiency virus type 1 (HIV-1) inhibition by a series of α-anilinophenylacetamide derivatives targeted at HIV-1 reverse transcriptase. Proc Natl Acad Sci U S A 1993; 90:1711–1715.

54. Kleim J-P, Bender R, Billhardt U-M, Meichsner C, Riess G, Rösner M, Winkler I, Paessens A. Activity of a novel quinoxaline derivative against human immunodeficiency virus type 1 reverse transcriptase and viral replication. Antimicrob Agents Chemother 1993; 37:1659–1664.

55. Kleim J-P, Bender R, Kirsch R, Meichsner C, Paessens A, Rösner M, Rübsamen-Waigmann H, Kaiser R, Wichers M, Schneweis KE, Winkler I, Riess G. Preclinical evaluation of HBY 097, a new nonnucleoside reverse transcriptase inhibitor of human immunodeficiency virus type 1 replication. Antimicrob Agents Chemother 1995; 39: 2253–2257.

55a. Rübsamen-Waigmann H, Huguenel E, Paessens A, Kleim J-P, Wainberg A, Shah A. Second-generation non-nucleosidic reverse transcriptase inhibitor HBY 097 and HIV-1 viral load. Lancet 1997; 394:1517.

56. Tucker TJ, Lyle TA, Wiscount CM, Britcher SF, Young SD, Sanders WM, Lumma WC, Goldman ME, O'Brien JA, Ball RG, Homnick CF, Schleif WA, Emini EA, Huff JR, Anderson PS. Synthesis of a series of 4-(arylethynyl)-6-chloro-4-cyclopropyl-3,4-dihydroquinazolin-2(1H)-ones as novel non-nucleoside HIV-1 reverse transcriptase inhibitors. J Med Chem 1994; 37:2437–2444.

57. Young SD, Britcher SF, Tran LO, Payne LS, Lumma WC, Lyle TA, Huff JR, Anderson PS, Olsen DB, Carroll SS, Pettibone DJ, O'Brien JA, Ball RG, Balani SK, Lin JH, Chen I-W, Schleif WA, Sardana VV, Long WJ, Byrnes VW, Emini EA. L-743,726 (DMP-266): a novel, highly potent nonnucleoside inhibitor of the human immunodeficiency virus type 1 reverse transcriptase. Antimicrob Agents Chemother 1995; 39:2602–2605.

58. Ahgren C, Backro K, Bell FW, Cantrell AS, Clemens M, Colacino JM, Deeter JB, Engelhardt JA, Högberg M, Jaskunas SR, Johansson NG, Jordan CL, Kasher JS, Kinnick MD, Lind P, Lopez C, Morin Jr JM, Meusing MA, Noreen R, Öberg B, Paget CJ, Palkowitz JA, Parrish CA, Pranc P, Sahlberg C, Ternansky RJ, Vasileff RT, Vrang L, West SJ, Zhang H, Zhou X-X. The PETT series, a new class of potent nonnucleoside inhibitors of human immunodeficiency virus type 1 reverse transcriptase. Antimicrob Agents Chemother 1995; 39:1329–1335

59. Bell FW, Cantrell AS, Högberg M, Jaskunas SR, Johansson NG, Jordan CL, Kinnick MD, Lind P, Morin Jr JM, Noreen R, Öberg B, Palkowitz JA, Parrish CA, Pranc P, Sahlberg C, Ternansky RJ, Vasileff RT, Vrang L, West SJ, Zang H, Zhou X-X. Phenethylthiazolethiourea (PETT) compounds, a new class of HIV-1 reverse transcriptase inhibitors. 1. Synthesis and basis structure-activity relationship studies of PETT analogs. J Med Chem 1995; 38:4929–4936.

60. Balzarini J, Brouwer WG, Felauer EE, De Clercq E, Karlsson A. Activity of various thiocarboxanilide derivatives against wild-type and several mutant human immunodeficiency virus type 1 strains. Antiviral Res 1995; 27:219–236.

61. Balzarini J, Brouwer WG, Dao DC, Osika EM, De Clercq E. Identification of novel thiocarboxanilide derivatives that suppress a variety of drug-resistant mutant human immunodeficiency virus type 1 strains at a potency similar to that for wild-type virus. Antimicrob Agents Chemother 1996; 40:1454–1466.

62. Dornsife RE, St. Clair MH, Huang AT, Panella TJ, Koszalka GW, Burns CL, Averett DR. Anti-human immunodeficiency virus synergism by zidovudine (3′-azidothymidine) and didanosine (dideoxyinosine) contrasts with their additive inhibition of normal human marrow progenitor cells. Antimicrob Agents Chemother 1991; 35:322–328.

63. Antonelli G, Dianzani F, Bellarosa D, Turriziani O, Riva E, Gentile A. Drug combination of AZT and ddI: synergism of action and prevention of appearance of AZT-resistance. Antiviral Chem Chemother 1994; 5:51–55.

64. Johnson VA, Merrill DP, Videler JA, Chou T-C, Byington RE, Eron JJ, D'Aquila RT, Hirsch MS. Two-drug combinations of zidovudine, didanosine, and recombinant interferon-α inhibit replication of zidovudine-resistant human immunodeficiency virus type 1 synergistically in vitro. J Infect Dis 1991; 164:646–655.

65. Smith MS, Brian EL, De Clercq E, Pagano JS. Susceptibility of human immunodeficiency virus type 1 replication in vitro to acyclic adenosine analogs and synergy of the analogs with 3′-azido-3′-deoxythymidine. Antimicrob Agents Chemother 1989; 33:1482–1486.

66. Mulato AS, Cherrington JM. Anti-HIV activity of adefovir (PMEA) and PMPA in combination with antiretroviral compounds: in vitro analyses. Antiviral Res 1997; 36:91–97.

67. Buckheit Jr RW, White EL, Germany-Decker J, Allen LB, Ros LJ, Shannon WM, Janssen PAJ, Chirigos MA. Cell-based and biochemical analysis of the anti-HIV activity of combinations of 3′-azido-3′-deoxythymidine and analogues of TIBO. Antiviral Chem Chemother 1994; 5:35–42.

68. Richman D, Rosenthal AS, Skoog M, Eckner RJ, Chou T- C, Sabo JP, Merluzzi VJ. BI-RG-587 is active against zidovudine-resistant human immunodeficiency virus type 1 and synergistic with zidovudine. Antimicrob Agents Chemother 1991; 35:305–308.

69. Chong K-T, Pagano PJ, Hinshaw RR. Bisheteroarylpiperazine reverse transcriptase inhibitor in combination with 3′-azido-3′-deoxythymidine or 2′,3′-dideoxycytidine synergistically inhibits human immunodeficiency virus type 1 replication in vitro. Antimicrob Agents Chemother 1994; 38:288–293.

70. Brennan TM, Taylor DL, Bridges CG, Leyda JP, Tyms AS. The inhibition of human immunodeficiency virus type 1 in vitro by a non-nucleoside reverse transcriptase inhibitor MKC-442, alone and in combination with other anti-HIV compounds. Antiviral Res 1995; 26:173–187.

71. Yuasa S, Sadakata Y, Takashima H, Sekiya K, Inouye N, Ubasawa M, Baba M. Selective and synergistic inhibition of human immunodeficiency virus type 1 reverse transcriptase by a non-nucleoside inhibitor, MKC-442. Mol Pharmacol 1993; 44: 895–900.

72. Kong X-B, Zhu Q-Y, Ruprecht RM, Watanabe KA, Zeidler JM, Gold JWM, Polsky B, Armstrong D, Chou T-C. Synergistic inhibition of human immunodeficiency virus type 1 replication in vitro by two-drug and three-drug combinations of 3′-azido- 3′-deoxythymidine, phosphonoformate, and 2′,3′- dideoxythymidine. Antimicrob Agents Chemother 1991; 35:2003–2011.

73. Craig JC, Duncan IB, Whittaker L, Roberts NA. Antiviral synergy between inhibitors of HIV proteinase and reverse transcriptase. Antiviral Chem Chemother 1990; 4: 161–166.

74. Pagano PJ, Chong K-T. In vitro inhibition of human immunodeficiency virus type 1 by a combination of delavirdine (U- 90152) with protease inhibitor U-75875 or interferon-α. J Infect Dis 1995; 171:61–67.

75. Ito M, Baba M, Shigeta S, De Clercq E, Walker RT, Tanaka H, Miyasaka T. Synergistic inhibition of human immunodeficiency virus type 1 (HIV-1) replication in vitro by 1-[(2-hydroxyethoxy)methyl]-6-phenylthiothymine (HEPT) and recombinant alpha interferon. Antiviral Res 1991; 15:323–330.

76. Balzarini J, De Clercq E. The thiocarboxanilides UC- 10 and UC-781 have an additive inhibitory effect against human immunodeficiency virus type 1 reverse transcriptase and replication in cell culture when combined with other antiretroviral drugs. Antiviral Chem Chemother 1997; 8:197–204.

77. Mitsuya H, Jarrett RF, Matsukura M, Di Marzo Veronese F, DeVico AL, Sarngadharan MG, Johns DG, Reitz MS, Broder S. Long-term inhibition of human T-lymphotropic virus type III/lymphadenopathy-associated virus (human immunodeficiency virus) DNA synthesis and RNA expression in T cells protected by 2′,3′-dideoxynucleosides in vitro. Proc Natl Acad Sci U S A 1987; 84:2033–2037.

78. Smith MS, Brian EL, Pagano JS. Resumption of virus production after human immunodeficiency virus infection of T lymphocytes in the presence of azidothymidine. J Virol 1987; 61:3769–3773.

79. Balzarini J, Karlsson A, Pérez-Pérez M- J, Camarasa M-J, De Clercq E. Knocking-out concentrations of HIV-1- specific inhibitors completely suppress HIV-1 infection and prevent the emergence of drug-resistant virus. Virology 1993; 196:576–585.

80. Vasudevachari MB, Battista C, Lane HC, Psallidopoulos MC, Zhao B, Cook J, Palmer JR, Romero DL, Tarpley WG, Salzman NP. Prevention of the spread of HIV-1 infection with nonnucleoside reverse transcriptase inhibitors. Virology 1992; 190: 269–277.

81. Balzarini J, Karlsson A, Meichsner C, Paessens A, Riess G, De Clercq E, Kleim J-P. Resistance pattern of human immunodeficiency virus type 1 reverse transcriptase to quinoxaline S-2720. J Virol 1994; 68:7986–7992.

82. Balzarini J, Pelemans H, Aquaro S, Perno C-F, Witvrouw M, Schols D, De Clercq E, Karlsson A. Highly favorable antiviral activity and resistance profile of the novel thiocarboxanilide pentenyloxy ether derivatives UC-781 and UC-82 as inhibitors of human immunodeficiency virus type 1 replication. Mol Pharmacol 1996; 50:394–401.

83. Winslow DL, Garber S, Reid C, Scarnati H, Baker D, Rayner MM, Anton ED. Selection conditions affect the evolution of specific mutations in the reverse transcriptase gene associated with resistance to DMP 266. AIDS 1996; 10:1205–1209.

84. Dueweke TJ, Poppe SM, Romero DL, Swaney SM, So AG, Downey KM, Althaus IW, Reusser F, Busso M, Resnick L, Mayers DL, Lane J, Aristoff PA, Thomas RC, Tarpley WG. U-90152, a potent inhibitor of human immunodeficiency virus type 1 replication. Antimicrob Agents Chemother 1993; 37:1127–1131.

85. Okamoto M, Makino M, Yamada K, Nakade K, Yuasa S, Baba M. Complete inhibition of viral breakthrough by combination of MKC-442 with AZT during a long-term culture of HIV-1-infected cells. Antiviral Res 1996; 31:69–77.

86. Balzarini J, Pelemans H, Pérez-Pérez M- J, San-Félix A, Camarasa M-J, De Clercq E, Karlsson A. Marked inhibitory activity of non-nucleoside reverse transcriptase inhibitors against human immunodeficiency virus type 1 when combined with (-)2′,3′-dideoxy-3′-thiacytidine. Mol Pharmacol 1996; 49:882–890.

87. Balzarini J, Pérez-Pérez M-J, Vélazquez S, San-Félix A, Camarasa M-J, De Clercq E, Karlsson A. Suppression of the breakthrough of human immunodeficiency virus type 1 (HIV-1) in cell culture by thiocarboxanilide derivatives when used individually or in combination with other HIV-1-specific inhibitors (i.e., TSAO derivatives). Proc Natl Acad Sci U S A 1995; 92:5470–5474.

88. Balzarini J, Pelemans H, Karlsson A, De Clercq E, Kleim J-P. Concomitant combination therapy for HIV infection preferable over sequential therapy with 3TC and non-nucleoside reverse transcriptase inhibitors. Proc Natl Acad Sci U S A 1996; 93: 13152–13157.

89. Hao Z, Cooney DA, Hartman NR, Perno C-F, Fridland A, DeVico AL, Sarngadharan MG, Broder S, Johns DG. Factors determining the activity of 2′,3′-dideoxynucleosides in suppressing human immunodeficiency virus in vitro. Mol Pharmacol 1988; 34:431–435.

90. Balzarini J, Pauwels R, Baba M, Herdewijn P, De Clercq E, Broder S, Johns DG. The in vitro and in vivo anti-retrovirus activity, and intracellular metabolism of 3′-azido-2′,3′-dideoxythymidine and 2′,3′- dideoxycytidine are highly dependent on the cell species. Biochem Pharmacol 1988; 37:897–903.

91. Gao W-Y, Agbaria R, Driscoll JS, Mitsuya H. Divergent anti-human immunodeficiency virus activity and anabolic phosphorylation of 2′,3′-dideoxynucleoside analogs in resting and activated human cells. J Biol Chem 1994; 269:12633–12638.

92. Furman PA, Fyfe JA, St. Clair MH, Weinhold K, Rideout JL, Freeman GA, Nusinoff Lehrman S, Bolognesi D, Broder S, Mitsuya H, Barry DW. Phosphorylation of 3′-azido-3′-deoxythymidine and selective interaction of the 5′-triphosphate with human immunodeficiency virus reverse transcriptase. Proc Natl Acad Sci U S A 1986; 83: 8333–8337.

93. Bourdais J, Biondi R, Sarfati S, Guerreiro C, Lascu I, Janin J, Véron M. Cellular phosphorylation of anti-HIV nucleosides. J Biol Chem 1996; 271:7887–7890.

94. Hao Z, Cooney DA, Farquhar D, Perno C-F, Zhang K, Masood R, Wilson Y, Hartman NR, Balzarini J, Johns DG. Potent DNA chain termination activity and selective inhibition of human immunodeficiency virus reverse transcriptase by 2′,3′-dideoxyuridine-5′-triphosphate. Mol Pharmacol 1990; 37:157–163.

95. Lavie A, Schlichting I, Vetter IR, Konrad M, Reinstein J, Goody RS. The bottleneck in AZT activation. Nat Med 1997; 3:922–924.

96. Lavie A, Vetter IR, Konrad M, Goody RS, Reinstein J, Schlichting I. Structure of thymidylate kinase reveals the cause behind the limiting step in AZT activation. Nat Struct Biol 1997; 4:601–604.

97. Balzarini J, Herdewijn P, De Clercq E. Differential patterns of intracellular metabolism of 2′,3′- didehydro-2′,3′-dideoxythymidine and 3′-azido- 2′,3′-dideoxythymidine, two potent anti-human immunodeficiency virus compounds. J Biol Chem 1989; 264:6127–6133.

98. Ho H-T, Hitchcock MJM. Cellular pharmacology of 2′,3′-dideoxy-2′,3′-didehydrothymidine, a nucleoside analog active against human immunodeficiency virus. Antimicrob Agents Chemother 1989; 33:844–849.

99. Parker WB, Shaddix SC, Bowdon BJ, Rose LM, Vince R, Shannon WM, Bennett Jr LL. Metabolism of carbovir, a potent inhibitor of human immunodeficiency virus type 1, and its effects on cellular metabolism. Antimicrob Agents Chemother 1993; 37:1004–1009.

100. Faletto MB, Miller WH, Garvey EP, St. Clair MH, Daluge SM, Good SS. Unique intracellular activation of the potent anti-human immunodeficiency virus agent 1592U89. Antimicrob Agents Chemother 1997; 41:1099–1107.

101. Hartman NR, Ahluwalia GS, Cooney DA, Mitsuya H, Kageyama S, Fridland A, Broder S, Johns DG. Inhibitors of IMP dehydrogenase stimulate the phosphorylation of the anti-human immunodeficiency virus nucleosides 2′,3′-dideoxyadenosine and 2′,3′-dideoxyinosine. Mol Pharmacol 1991; 40:118–124.

102. Balzarini J, Lee C-K, Herdewijn P, De Clercq E. Mechanism of the potentiating effect of ribavirin on the activity of 2′,3′-dideoxyinosine against human immunodeficiency virus. J Biol Chem 1991; 266:21509–21514.

103. Ahluwalia GS, Gao W-Y, Mitsuya H, Johns DG. 2′,3′-Didehydro-3′-deoxythymidine: regulation of its metabolic activation by modulators of thymidine-5′-triphosphate biosynthesis. Mol Pharmacol 1996; 50:160–165.

104. Sastry JK, Nehete PN, Khan S, Nowak BJ, Plunkett W, Arlinghaus RB, Farquhar D. Membrane-permeable dideoxyuridine 5′-monophosphate analogue inhibits human immunodeficiency virus infection. Mol Pharmacol 1991; 41:441–445.

105. Puech F, Gosselin G, Lefebvre I, Pompon A, Aubertin A-M, Kirn A, Imbach J-L. Intracellular delivery of nucleoside monophosphates through a reductase-mediated activation process. Antiviral Res 1993; 22:155–174.

106. Lefebvre I, Périgaud C, Pompon A, Aubertin A-M, Girardet J-L, Kirn A, Gosselin G, Imbach J-L. Mononucleoside phosphotriester derivatives with S-acyl-2-thioethyl bioreversible phosphate-protecting groups: intracellular delivery of 3′-azido-2′,3′-dideoxythymidine 5′-monophosphate. J Med Chem 1995; 38:3941–3950.

107. Valette G, Pompon A, Girardet J-L, Cappellacci L, Franchetti P, Grifantini M, La Colla P, Loi AG, Périgaud C, Gosselin G, Imbach J-L. Decomposition pathways and in vitro HIV inhibitory effects of IsoddA pronucleotides: toward a rational approach for intracellular delivery of nucleoside 5′-monophosphates. J Med Chem 1996; 39: 1981–1990.

108. McGuigan C, Pathirana RN, Balzarini J, De Clercq E. Intracellular delivery of bioactive AZT nucleotides by aryl phosphate derivatives of AZT. J Med Chem 1993; 36: 1048–1052.

109. Balzarini J, Karlsson A, Aquaro S, Perno C-F, Cahard D, Naesens L, De Clercq E, McGuigan C. Mechanism of anti-HIV action of masked alaninyl d4T-MP derivatives. Proc Natl Acad Sci U S A 1996; 93:7295–7299.

110. Balzarini J, Egberink H, Hartmann K, Cahard D, Vahlenkamp T, Thormar H, De Clercq E, McGuigan C. Antiretrovirus specificity and intracellular metabolism of 2′,3′-didehydro-2′,3′-dideoxythymidine (stavudine) and its 5′-monophosphate triester prodrug So324. Mol Pharmacol 1996; 50:1207–1213.

111. McGuigan C, Vélazquez S, De Clercq E, Balzarini J. Synthesis and evaluation of 5-halo 2′,3′-didehydro-2′,3′-dideoxynucleosides and their blocked phosphoramidates as potential anti-human immunodeficiency virus agents: an example of "kinase bypass." Antiviral Chem Chemother 1997; 8:519–527.

112. Meier C, Lorey M, De Clercq E, Balzarini J. Cyclic saligenyl phosphtriesters of 2′,3′-dideoxy-2′,3′-didehydrothymidine (d4T)—a new pro-nucleotide approach. Bioorg Med Chem Lett 1997; 7:99–104.

113. Meier C, Knispel T, De Clercq E, Balzarini J. ADA-bypass by lipophilic cycloSal-ddAMP pro-nucleotides. A second example of the efficiency of the cycloSal-concept. Bioorg Med Chem Lett 1997; 7:1577–1582.

114. Rosowsky A, Fu H, Pai N, Mellors J, Richman DD, Hostetler KY. Synthesis and in vitro activity of long-chain 5′-O-[(alkoxycarbonyl)phosphinyl]-3′-azido-3′-deoxythymidines against wild-type and AZT-and foscarnet-resistant strains of HIV-1. J Med Chem 1997; 40:2482–2490.

115. Balzarini J, Hao Z, Herdewijn P, Johns DG, De Clercq E. Intracellular metabolism and mechanism of anti-retrovirus action of 9-(2-phosphonylmethoxyethyl)adenine, a potent anti-human immunodeficiency virus compound. Proc Natl Acad Sci U S A 1991; 88:1499–1503.

116. Balzarini J, De Clercq E. 5-Phosphoribosyl 1-pyrophosphate synthetase converts the acyclic nucleoside phosphonates 9-(3-hydroxy-2-phosphonylmethoxypropyl)adenine and 9-(2-phosphonylmethoxyethyl)adenine directly to their antivirally active diphosphate derivatives. J Biol Chem 1991; 266:8686–8689.

117. Merta A, Votruba I, Jindrich J. Holý A, Cihlar T, Rosenberg I, Otmar M, Herve TY. Phosphorylation of 9-(2-phosphonomethoxyethyl)adenine and 9-(S)-(3-hydroxy-2-phosphonomethoxypropyl)adenine by AMP(dAMP) kinase from L1210 cells. Biochem Pharmacol 1992; 44:2067–2077.

118. Robbins BL, Greenhaw J, Connelly MC, Fridland A. Metabolic pathways for activation of the antiviral agent 9-(2-phosphonylmethoxyethyl)adenine in human lymphoid cells. Antimicrob Agents Chemother 1995; 39:2304–2308.

119. St. Clair MH, Richards CA, Spector T, Weinhold KJ, Miller WH, Langlois AJ, Furman PA. 3′-Azido-3′-deoxythymidine triphosphate as an inhibitor and substrate of purified human immunodeficiency virus reverse transcriptase. Antimicrob Agents Chemother 1987; 31:1972–1977.

120. Hao Z, Cooney DA, Farquhar D, Perno C-F, Zhang K, Masood R, Wilson Y, Hartman NR, Balzarini J, Johns DG. Potent DNA chain termination activity and selective inhibition of human immunodeficiency virus reverse transcriptase by 2′,3′-dideoxyuridine-5′-triphosphate. Mol Pharmacol 1989; 37:157–163.

121. Gray NM, Marr CLP, Penn CR, Cameron JM, Bethell RC. The intracellular phosphorylation of (-)-2′-deoxy-3′-thiacytidine (3TC) and the incorporation of 3TC 5′-monophosphate into DNA by HIV-1 reverse transcriptase and human DNA polymerase gamma. Biochem Pharmacol 1995; 50:1043–1051.

122. Huang P, Farquhar D, Plunkett W. Selective action of 3′-azido-3′-deoxythymidine 5′-triphosphate on viral reverse transcriptases and human DNA polymerases. J Biol Chem 1990; 265:11914–11918.

123. Kramata P, Votruba I, Otova B, Holý A. Different inhibitory potencies of acyclic phosphonomethoxyalkyl nucleotide analogs toward DNA polymerases α, δ, ε. Mol Pharmacol 1996; 49:1005–1011.

124. Cihlar T, Chen MS. Incorporation of selected nucleoside phosphonates and anti-human immunodeficiency virus nucleotide analogues into DNA by human DNA polymerases α, β and gamma. Antiviral Chem Chemother 1997; 8:187–195.

125. Tantillo C, Ding J, Jacobo-Molina A, Nanni RG, Boyer PL, Hughes SH, Pauwels R, Andries K, Janssen PAJ, Arnold E. Locations of anti-AIDS drug binding sites and resistance mutations in the three-dimensional structure of HIV-1 reverse transcriptase. Implications for mechanisms of drug inhibition and resistance. J Mol Biol 1994; 243:369–387.

126. Dueweke TJ, Kézdy FJ, Waszak GA, Deibel Jr MR, Tarpley WG. The binding of a novel bisheteroarylpiperazine mediates inhibition of human immunodeficiency virus type 1 reverse transcriptase. J Biol Chem 1992; 267:27–30.

127. Spence RA, Kati WM, Anderson KS, Johnson KA. Mechanism of inhibition of HIV-1 reverse transcriptase by nonnucleoside inhibitors. Science 1995; 267:988–993.

128. Ren J, Esnouf R, Garman E, Somers D, Ross C, Kirby I, Keeling J, Darby G, Jones Y, Stuart D, Stammers D. High resolution structures of HIV-1 RT from four RT-inhibitor complexes. Nat Struct Biol 1995; 2:293–302.

129. Esnouf R, Ren J, Ross C, Jones Y, Stammers D, Stuart D. Mechanism of inhibition of HIV-1 reverse transcriptase by non-nucleoside inhibitors. Nat Struct Biol 1995; 2:303–308.

130. Ding J, Das K, Tantillo C, Zhang W, Clark Jr AD, Jessen S, Lu X, Hsiou Y, Jacobo-Molina A, Andries K, Pauwels R, Moereels H, Koymans L, Janssen PAJ, Smith Jr RH, Kroeger Koepke M, Michejda CJ, Hughes SH, Arnold E. Structure of HIV-1 reverse transcriptase in a complex with the non-nucleoside inhibitor α-APA R 95845 at 2.8 A resolution. Structure 1995; 3:365–379.

131. Ding J, Das K, Moereels H, Koymans L, Andries K, Janssen PAJ, Hughes SH, Arnold E. Structure of HIV-1 RT/TIBO R 86183 complex reveals similarity in the binding of diverse nonnucleoside inhibitors. Nat Struct Biol 1995; 2:407–415.

132. Ren J, Esnouf R, Hopkins A, Ross C, Jones Y, Stammers D, Stuart D. The structure of HIV-1 reverse transcriptase complexed with 9-chloro-TIBO: lessons for inhibitor design. Structure 1995; 3:915–926.

133. Kroeger Smith MB, Rouzer CA, Taneyhill LA, Smith NA, Hughes SH, Boyer PL, Janssen PAJ, Moereels H, Koymans L, Arnold E, Ding J, Das K, Zhang W, Michejda CJ, Smith Jr RH. Molecular modeling studies of HIV-1 reverse transcriptase nonnucleoside inhibitors: total energy of complexation as a predictor of drug placement and activity. Protein Sci 1995; 4:2203–2222.

134. Esnouf RM, Stuart DI, De Clercq E, Schwartz E, Balzarini J. Models which explain the inhibition of reverse transcriptase by HIV-1-specific (thio)carboxanilide derivatives. Biochem Biophys Res Commun 1997; 234:458–464.

135. Esnouf RM, Ren J, Hopkins AL, Ross CK, Jones EY, Stammers DK, Stuart DI. Unique features in the structure of the complex between HIV-1 reverse transcriptase and the bis(heteroaryl)piperazine (BHAP) U-90152 explain resistance mutations for this nonnucleoside inhibitor. Proc Natl Acad Sci U S A 1997; 94:3984–3989.

136. Balzarini J, Naesens L, Herdewijn P, Rosenberg I, Holý A, Pauwels R, Baba M, Johns DG, De Clercq E. Marked in vivo antiretrovirus activity of 9-(2-phosphonylmethoxyethyl)adenine, a selective anti-human immunodeficiency virus agent. Proc Natl Acad Sci U S A 1989; 86:332–336.

137. Balzarini J, Naesens L, De Clercq E. Anti-retrovirus activity of (9-(2-phosphonylmethoxyethyl)adenine (PMEA) in vivo increases when it is less frequently administered. Int J Cancer 1990; 46:337–340.

138. Balzarini J, Sobis H, Naesens L, Vandeputte M, De Clercq E. Inhibitory effects of 9-(2-phosphonylmethoxyethyl)adenine and 3′-azido-2′,3′-dideoxythymidine on tumor development in mice inoculated intracerebrally with moloney murine sarcoma virus. Int J Cancer 1990; 45:486–489.

139. Gangemi JD, Cozens RM, De Clercq E, Balzarini J, Hochkeppel H-K. 9-(2-Phosphonylmethoxyethyl)adenine in the treatment of murine acquired immunodeficiency disease and opportunistic herpes simplex virus infections. Antimicrob Agents Chemother 1989; 33:1864–1868.

140. Bridges CG, Taylor DL, Ahmed PS, Brennan TM, Hornsperger J-M, Navé J-F, Casara P, Tyms AS. MDL 74,968, a new acyclonucleotide analog: activity against human immunodeficiency virus in vitro and in the hu-PBL-SCID.beige mouse model of infection. Antimicrob Agents Chemother 1996; 40:1072–1077.

141. Ruxrungtham K, Boone E, Ford Jr H, Driscoll JS, Davey Jr RT, Lane HC. Potent activity of 2′-β-fluoro-2′,3′-dideoxyadenosine against human immunodeficiency virus type 1 infection in hu-PBL-SCID mice. Antimicrob Agents Chemother 1996; 40: 2369–2374.

142. Egberink H, Borst M, Niphuis H, Balzarini J, Neu H, Schellekens H, De Clercq E, Horzinek M, Koolen M. Suppression of feline immunodeficiency virus infection in vivo by 9-(2-phosphonomethoxyethyl)adenine. Proc Natl Acad Sci U S A 1990; 87: 3087–3091.

143. Vahlenkamp TW, De Ronde A, Balzarini J, Naesens L, De Clercq E, van Eijk MJT, Horzinek MC, Egberink HF. (R)-9-(2-phosphonylmethoxypropyl)-2,6-diaminopurine is a potent inhibitor of feline immunodeficiency virus infection. Antimicrob Agents Chemother 1995; 39:746–749.

144. Thormar H, Georgsson G, Palsson PA, Balzarini J, Naesens L, Torsteinsdottir S, De Clercq E. Inhibitory effect of 9-(2-phosphonylmethoxyethyl)adenine on visna virus infection in lambs: a model for in vivo testing of candidate anti-human immunodeficiency virus drugs. Proc Natl Acad Sci U S A 1995; 92:3283–3287.

145. Balzarini J, Naesens L, Slachmuylders J, Niphuis H, Rosenberg I, Holý A, Schellekens H, De Clercq E. 9-(2-Phosphonylmethoxyethyl)adenine (PMEA) effectively inhibits retrovirus replication in vitro and simian immunodeficiency virus infection in rhesus monkeys. AIDS 1991; 5:21–28.

146. Tsai C-C, Follis KE, Sabo A, Grant RF, Bartz C, Nolte RE, Benveniste RE, Bischofberger N. Preexposure prophylaxis with 9-(2-phosphonylmethoxyethyl)adenine against simian immunodeficiency virus infection in macaques. J Infect Dis 1994; 169:260–266.

147. Tsai C-C, Follis KE, Grant R, Sabo A, Nolte R, Bartz C, Bischofberger N, Benveniste R. Comparison of the efficacy of AZT and PMEA treatment against acute SIV$_{mne}$ infection in macaques. J Med Primatol 1994; 23:175–183.

148. Tsai C-C, Follis KE, Sabo A, Beck TW, Grant RF, Bischofberger N, Benveniste RE, Black R. Prevention of SIV infection in macaques by (R)-9-(2-phosphonylmethoxypropyl)adenine. Science 1995; 270:1197–1199.

149. Van Rompay KKA, Cherrington JM, Marthas ML, Berardi CJ, Mulato AS, Spinner A, Tarara RP, Canfield DR, Telm S, Bischofberger N, Pedersen NC, 9-[2-(Phosphonomethoxy)propyl]adenine therapy of established simian immunodeficiency virus infection in infant rhesus macaques. Antimicrob Agents Chemother 1996; 40:2586–2591.

150. Tsai C-C, Follis KE, Beck TW, Sabo A, Bischofberger N, Dailey PJ. Effects of (R)-9-(2-phosphonylmethoxypropyl)adenine monotherapy on chronic SIV infection in macaques. AIDS Res Hum Retroviruses 1997; 13:707–712.

151. Grob PM, Cao Y, Muchmore E, Ho DD, Norris S, Pav JW, Shih C-K, Adams J. Prophylaxis against HIV-1 infection in chimpanzees by nevirapine, a nonnucleoside inhibitor of reverse transcriptase. Nat Med 1997; 3:665–670.

152. Spruance SL, Pavia AT, Mellors JW, Murphy R, Gathe Jr J, Stool E, Jemsek JG, Dellamonica P, Cross A, Dunkle L. Clinical efficacy of monotherapy with stavudine compared with zidovudine in HIV-infected, zidovudine-experienced patients. A randomized, double-blind, controlled trial. Ann Intern Med 1997; 126:355–363.

153. Deeks SG, Collier A, Lalezari J, Pavia A, Rodrigue D, Drew WL, Toole J, Jaffe HS, Mulato AS, Lamy PD, Li W, Cherrington JM, Hellmann N, Kahn J. The safety and efficacy of adefovir dipivoxil, a novel anti-human immunodeficiency virus (HIV) therapy, in HIV-infected adults: a randomized, double-blind, placebo-controlled trial. J Infect Dis 1997; 176:1517–1523.

154. Pialoux G, Youle M, Dupont B, Gazzard B, Cauwenbergh GFMJ, Stoffels PAM, Davies S, De Saint Martin J, Janssen PAJ. Pharmacokinetics of R 82913 in patients with AIDS or AIDS-related complex. Lancet 1991; 338:140–143.

155. De Wit S, Hermans P, Sommereijns B, O'Doherty E, Westenborghs R, Van De Velde V, Cauwenbergh GFMJ, Clumeck N. Pharmacokinetics of R 82913 in AIDS patients: a phase I dose-finding study of oral administration compared with intravenous infusion. Antimicrob Agents Chemother 1992; 36:2661–2663.

156. Davey Jr RT, Dewar RL, Reed GF, Vasudevachari MB, Polis MA, Kovacs JA, Falloon J, Walker RT, Masur H, Haneiwich SE, O'Neill DG, Decker MR, Metcalf JA, Deloria MA, Laskin OL, Salzman N, Lane HC. Plasma viremia as a sensitive indicator of the antiretroviral activity of L-697,661. Proc Natl Acad Sci U S A 1993; 90: 5608–5612.

157. Saag MS, Emini EA, Laskin OL, Douglas J, Lapidus WI, Schleif WA, Whitley RJ, Hildebrand C, Byrnes VW, Kappes JC, Anderson KW, Massari FE, Shaw GM, the L-697-661 Working Group. A short-term clinical evaluation of L-697,661, a non-nucleoside inhibitor of HIV-1 reverse transcriptase. N Engl J Med 1993; 329:1065–1072.

158. Havlir D, Cheeseman SH, McLaughlin M, Murphy R, Erice A, Spector SA, Greenough TC, Sullivan JL, Hall D, Myers M, Lamson M, Richman DD. High-dose nevirapine: safety, pharmacokinetics, and antiviral effect in patients with human immunodeficiency virus infection. J Infect Dis 1995; 171:537–545.

159. Staszewski S, Miller V, Kober A, Colebunders R, Vandercam B, Delescluse J, Clumeck N, Van Wanzeele F, De Brabander M, De Creé J, Moeremans M, Andries K, Boucher C, Stoffels P, Janssen PAJ, members of the Loviride Collaborative Study Group. Evaluation of the efficacy and tolerance of R 018893, R 089439 (loviride) and placebo in asymptomatic HIV-1-infected patients. Antiviral Therapy 1996; 1:42–50.

160. Rübsamen-Waigmann H, Huguenel E, Paessens A, Kleim J-P, Wainberg MA, Shah E. Second-generation non-nucleosidic reverse transcriptase inhibitor HBY097 and HIV-1 viral load. Lancet 1997; 349:1517.

161. de Jong MD, Vella S, Carr A, Boucher CAB, Imrie A, French M, Hoy J, Sorice S, Pauluzzi S, Chiodo F, Weverling GJ, van der Ende ME, Frissen PJ, Weigel HM, Kauffmann RH, Lange JMA, Yoon R, Moroni M, Hoenderdos E, Leitz G, Cooper DA, Hall D, Reiss P. High-dose nevirapine in previously untreated human immunodeficiency virus type 1-infected persons does not result in sustained suppression of viral replication. J Infect Dis 1997; 175:966–970.

162. Havlir D, McLaughlin MM, Richman DD. A pilot study to evaluate the development of resistance to nevirapine in asymptomatic human immunodeficiency virus-infected patients with CD4 cell counts of >500 mm^3: AIDS clinical trials group protocol 208. J Infect Dis 1995; 172:1379–1383.

163. Saravolatz LD, Winslow DL, Collins G, Hodges JS, Pettinelli C, Stein DS, Markowitz N, Reves R, Loveless MO, Crane L, Thompson M, Abrams D, investigators for the Terry Beirn Community Programs for Clinical Research on AIDS. Zidovudine alone or in combination with didanosine or zalcitabine in HIV-infected patients with the acquired immunodeficiency syndrome or fewer than 200 CD4 cells per cubic millimeter. N Engl J Med 1996; 335:1099–1106.

164. Katlama C, Ingrand D, Loveday C, Clumeck N, Mallolas J, Staszewski S, Johnson M, Hill AM, Pearce G, McDade H. Safety and efficacy of lamivudine-zidovudine combination therapy in antiretroviral-naive patients. A randomized controlled comparison with zidovudine monotherapy. JAMA 1996; 276:118–125.

165. Staszewski S, Loveday C, Picazo JJ, Dellamonica P, Skinhoj P, Johnson MA, Danner SA, Harrigan PR, Hill AM, Verity L, McDade H. Safety and efficacy of lamivudine-zidovudine combination therapy in zidovudine-experienced patients. A randomized controlled comparison with zidovudine monotherapy. JAMA 1996; 276:111–117.

166. Schooley RT, Ramirez-Ronda C, Lange JMA, Cooper DA, Lavelle J, Lefkowitz L, Moore M, Larder BA, St. Clair M, Mulder JW, McKinnis R, Pennington KN, Harrigan PR, Kinghorn I, Steel H, Rooney JF, the Wellcome Resistance Study Collaborative Group. Virologic and immunologic benefits of initial combination therapy with zidovudine and zalcitabine or didanosine compared with zidovudine monotherapy. J Infect Dis 1996; 173:1354–1366.

167. Graham NMH, Hoover DR, Park LP, Stein DS, Phair JP, Mellors JW, Detels R, Saah AJ. Survival in HIV-infected patients who have received zidovudine: comparison of combination therapy with sequential monotherapy and continued zidovudine monotherapy. Ann Intern Med 1996; 124:1031–1038.

168. Mauss S, Adams O, Willers R, Jablonowski H. Combination therapy with ZDV + DDI versus ZDV + DDC in patients with progression of HIV-infection under treatment with ZDV. J Acquir Immune Defic Syndr Hum Retrovirol 1996; 11:469–477.

169. Bartlett JA, Benoit SL, Johnson VA, Quinn JB, Sepulveda GE, Ehmann WC, Tsoukas C, Fallon MA, Self PL, Rubin M, Lamivudine plus zidovudine compared with zalcitabine plus zidovudine in patients with HIV infection. A randomized, double-blind, placebo-controlled trial. Ann Intern Med 1996; 125:161–172.

170. Rouleau D, Conway B, Raboud J, Rae S, Fransen S, Shillington A, Zala C, O'Shaughnessy MV, Montaner JSG. Stavudine plus lamivudine in advanced human immunodeficiency virus disease: a short-term pilot study. J Infect Dis 1997; 176:1156–1160.

171. Staszewski S, Massari FE, Kober A, Gohler R, Durr S, Anderson KW, Schneider CL, Waterbury JA, Bakshi KK, Taylor VI, Hildebrand CS, Kreisl C, Hoffstedt B, Schleif WA, von Briesen H, Rübsamen-Waigmann H, Calandra GB, Ryan JL, Stille W, Emini EA, Byrnes VW. Combination therapy with zidovudine prevents selection of human immunodeficiency virus type 1 variants expressing high level resistance to L-697,661, a non-nucleoside reverse transcriptase inhibitor. J Infect Dis 1995; 171: 159–165.

172. Schooley RT, Campbell TB, Kuritzkes DR, Blaschke T, Stein DS, Rosandich ME, Phair J, Pottage JC, Messari F, Collier A, Kahn J, the ACTG 184 Protocol Team.

Phase 1 study of combination therapy with L-697,661 and zidovudine. J Acquir Immune Defic Syndr Hum Retrovirol 1996; 12:363–370.

173. Carr A, Vella S, de Jong MD, Sorice F, Imrie A, Boucher CA, Cooper DA. A controlled trial of nevirapine plus zidovudine versus zidovudine alone in P24 antigenaemic HIV-infected patients. AIDS 1996; 10:635–641.

174. Davey RT Jr, Chaitt DG, Reed GF, Freimuth WW, Herpin BR, Metcalf JA, Eastman PS, Falloon J, Kovacs JA, Polis MA, Walker RE, Masur H, Boyle J, Coleman S, Cox SR, Wathen L, Daenzer CL, Lane HC. Randomized, controlled phase I/II trial of combination therapy with delavirdine (U-90152S) and conventional nucleosides in human immunodeficiency virus type 1-infected patients. Antimicrob Agents Chemother 1996; 40:1657–1664.

175. D'Aquila RT, Hughes MD, Johnson VA, Fischl MA, Sommadossi J-P, Liou S-H, Timpone J, Myers M, Basgoz N, Niu M, Hirsch MS, the National Institute of Allergy and Infectious Diseases AIDS Clinical Trials Group Protocol 241 Investigators. Nevirapine, zidovudine, and didanosine compared with zidovudine and didanosine in patients with HIV-1 infection. A randomized, double-blind, placebo-controlled trial. Ann Intern Med 1996; 124:1019–1030.

176. Luzuriaga K, Bryson Y, Krogstad P, Robinson J, Stechenberg B, Lamson M, Cort S, Sullivan JL. Combination treatment with zidovudine, didanosine, and nevirapine in infants with human immunodeficiency virus type 1 infection. N Engl J Med 1997; 336:1343–1349.

177. Staszewski S, Miller V, Rehmet S, Stark T, De Creé J, De Brabander M, Peeters M, Andries K, Moeremans M, De Raeymaeker M, Pearce G, Van Den Broeck R, Verbiest W, Stoffels P. Virological and immunological analysis of a triple combination pilot study with loviride, lamivudine and zidovudine in HIV-1 infected patients. AIDS 1996; 10:F1–F7.

178. CAESAR Coordinating Committee. Randomised trial of addition of lamivudine or lamivudine plus loviride to zidovudine-containing regimens for patients with HIV-1 infection: the CAESAR trial. Lancet 1997; 349:1413–1421.

179. Collier AC, Coombs RW, Schoenfeld DA, Basset RL, Timpone J, Baruch A, Jones M, Facey K, Whitacre C, McAuliffe VJ, Friedman HM, Merigan TC, Reichman RC, Hooper C, Corey L. Treatment of human immunodeficiency virus infection with saquinavir, zidovudine and zalcitabine. N Engl J Med 1996; 334:1011–1017.

180. Hammer SM, Katzenstein DA, Hughes MD, Gundacker H, Schooley RT, Haubrich RH, Henry WK, Lederman MM, Phair JP, Niu M, Hirsch MS, Merigan TC. A trial comparing nucleoside monotherapy with combination therapy in HIV-infected adults with CD4 cell counts from 200 to 500 per cubic millimeter. N Engl J Med 1996; 335: 1081–1090.

181. Hammer SM, Squires KE, Hughes MD, Grimes JM, Demeter LM, Currier JS, Eron JJ Jr, Feinberg JE, Balfour HH Jr, Deyton LR, Chodakewitz JA, Fischl MA. A controlled trial of two nucleoside analogues plus indinavir in persons with human immunodeficiency virus infection and CD4 cell counts of 200 per cubic millimeter or less. N Engl J Med 1997; 337:725–735.

182. Gulick RM, Mellors JW, Havlir D, Eron JJ, Gonzalez C, McMahon D, Richman DD, Valentine FT, Jonas L, Meibohm A, Emini EA, Chodakewitz JA. Treatment with indinavir, zidovudine, and lamivudine in adults with human immunodeficiency virus infection and prior antiretroviral therapy. N Engl J Med 1997; 337:734–739.

183. Havlir DV, Richman DD. Viral dynamics of HIV: implications for drug development and therapeutic strategies. Ann Intern Med 1996; 124:984–994.

184. Tamalet C, Lafeuillade A, Fantini J, Poggi C, Yahi N. Quantification of HIV-1 viral load in lymphoid and blood cells: assessment during four-drug combination therapy. AIDS 1997; 11:895–901.

185. Taburet A-M, Singlas E. Drug interactions with antiviral drugs. Clin Pharmacokinet 1996; 30:385–401.

186. Barry M, Gibbons S, Back D, Mulcahy F. Protease inhibitors in patients with HIV disease. Clin Pharmacokinet 1997; 32:194–209.

187. Sahai J. Risks and synergies from drug interactions. AIDS 1996; 10(suppl 1):S21–S25.

188. Schinazi RF, Larder BA, Mellors JW. Mutations in retroviral genes associated with drug resistance. Int Antiviral News 1997; 5:129–142.

189. Larder BA, Darby G, Richman DD. HIV with reduced sensitivity to zidovudine (AZT) isolated during prolonged therapy. Science 1989; 243:1731–1734.

190. Larder BA, Kemp SD. Multiple mutations in HIV-1 reverse transcriptase confer high-level resistance to zidovudine (AZT). Science 1989; 246:1155–1158.

191. Kellam P, Boucher CAB, Larder BA. Fifth mutation in human immunodeficiency virus type 1 reverse transcriptase contributes to the development of high-level resistance to zidovudine. Proc Natl Acad Sci U S A 1992; 89:1934–1938.

192. Boucher CAB, O'Sullivan E, Mulder JW, Ramautarsing C, Kellam P, Darby G, Lange JMA, Goudsmit J, Larder BA. Ordered appearance of zidovudine resistance mutations during treatment of 18 human immunodeficiency virus-positive subjects. J Infect Dis 1992; 165:105–110.

193. Hooker DJ, Tachedjian G, Solomon AE, Gurusinghe AD, Land S, Birch C, Anderson JL, Roy BM, Arnold E, Deacon NJ. An in vivo mutation from leucine to tryptophan at position 210 in human immunodeficiency virus type 1 reverse transcriptase contributes to high-level resistance to 3′-azido-3′-deoxythymidine. J Virol 1996; 70: 8010–8018.

194. Lacey SF, Larder BA. Novel mutation (V75T) in human immunodeficiency virus type 1 reverse transcriptase confers resistance to 2′,3′-didehydro-2′,3′-dideoxythymidine in cell culture. Antimicrob Agents Chemother 1994; 38;1428–1432.

195. Tisdale M, Kemp SD, Parry NR, Larder BA. Rapid in vitro selection of human immunodeficiency virus type 1 resistant to 3′-thiacytidine inhibitors due to a mutation in the YMDD region of reverse transcriptase. Proc Natl Acad Sci U S A 1993; 90: 5653–5656.

196. Kavlick MF, Shirasaka T, Kojima E, Pluda JM, Hui F Jr, Yarchoan R, Mitsuya H. Genotypic and phenotypic characterization of HIV-1 isolated from patients receiving (-)-2′,3′-dideoxy-3′-thiacytidine. Antiviral Res 1995; 28:133–146.

197. Tisdale M, Alnadaf T, Cousens D. Combination of mutations in human immunodeficiency virus type 1 reverse transcriptase required for resistance to the carbocyclic nucleoside 1592U89. Antimicrob Agents Chemother 1997; 41:1094–1098.

198. Tanaka M, Srinivas RV, Ueno T, Kavlick MF, Hui FK, Fridland A, Driscoll JS, Mitsuya H. In vitro induction of human immunodeficiency virus type 1 variants resistant to 2′-β-fluoro-2′,3′-dideoxyadenosine. Antimicrob Agents Chemother 1997; 41: 1313–1318.

199. St. Clair MH, Martin JL, Tudor-Williams G, Bach MC, Vavro CL, King DM, Kellam P, Kemp SD, Larder BA. Resistance to ddI and sensitivity to AZT induced by a mutation in HIV-1 reverse transcriptase. Science 1991; 253:1557–1559.

200. Eron JJ, Chow Y-K, Caliendo AM, Videler J, Devore KM, Cooley TP, Liebman HA, Kaplan JC, Hirsch MS, D'Aquila RT. *pol* Mutations conferring zidovudine and didanosine resistance with different effect in vitro yield multiply resistant human immunodeficiency virus type 1 isolates in vivo. Antimicrob Agents Chemother 1993; 37:1480–1487.

201. Larder BA, Kemp SD, Harrigan PR. Potential mechanism for sustained antiretroviral efficacy of AZT-3TC combination therapy. Science 1995; 269:696–699.

202. Nijhuis M, Schuurman R, de Jong D, van Leeuwen R, Lange J, Danner S, Keulen W, de Groot T, Boucher CAB. Lamivudine-resistant human immunodeficiency virus type 1 variants (184V) require multiple amino acid changes to become co-resistant to zidovudine in vivo. J Infect Dis 1997; 176:398–405.

203. Shirasaka T, Kavlick MF, Ueno T, Gao W-Y, Kojima E, Alcaide ML, Chokekijchai S, Roy BM, Arnold E, Yarchoan R, Mitsuya H. Emergence of human immunodeficiency virus type 1 variants with resistance to multiple dideoxynucleosides in patients receiving therapy with dideoxynucleosides. Proc Natl Acad Sci U S A 1995; 92:2398–2402.

204. Iversen AKN, Shafer RW, Wehrly K, Winters MA, Mullins JI, Chesebro B, Merigan TC. Multidrug-resistant human immunodeficiency virus type 1 strains resulting from combination antiretroviral therapy. J Virol 1996; 70:1086–1090.

205. Schmit J-C, Cogniaux J, Hermans P, Van Vaeck C, Sprecher S, Van Remoortel B, Witvrouw M, Balzarini J, Desmyter J, De Clercq E, Vandamme A-M. Multiple drug resistance to nucleoside analogues and nonnucleoside reverse transcriptase inhibitors in an efficiently replicating human immunodeficiency virus type 1 patient strain. J Infect Dis 1996; 174:962–968.

206. Shafer RW, Winters MA, Iversen AKN, Merigan TC. Genotypic and phenotypic changes during culture of a multinucleoside-resistant human immunodeficiency virus type 1 strain in the presence and absence of additional reverse transcriptase inhibitors. Antimicrob Agents Chemother 1996; 40:2887–2890.

207. Van Rompay KKA, Greenier JL, Marthas ML, Otsyula MG, Tarara RP, Miller CJ, Pedersen NC. A zidovudine-resistant simian immunodeficiency virus mutant with a Q151M mutation in reverse transcriptase causes AIDS in newborn macaques. Antimicrob Agents Chemother 1997; 41:278–283.

208. Mellors JW, Bazmi HZ, Schinazi RF, Roy BM, Hsiou Y, Arnold E, Weir J, Mayers DL. Novel mutations in reverse transcriptase of human immunodeficiency virus type 1 reduce susceptibility to foscarnet in laboratory and clinical isolates. Antimicrob Agents Chemother 1995; 39:1087–1092.

209. Tachedjian G, Mellors J, Bazmi H, Birch C, Mills J. Zidovudine resistance is suppressed by mutations conferring resistance of human immunodeficiency virus type 1 to foscarnet. J Virol 1996; 70:7171–7181.

210. Gu Z, Salomon H, Cherrington JM, Mulato AS, Chen MS, Yarchoan R, Foli A, Sogocio KM, Wainberg MA. K65R mutation of human immunodeficiency virus type 1 reverse transcriptase encodes cross-resistance to 9-(2-phosphonylmethoxyethyl)adenine. Antimicrob Agents Chemother 1995; 39:1888–1891.

211. Foli A, Sogocio KM, Anderson B, Kavlick MF, Saville MW, Wainberg MA, Gu Z, Cherrington JM, Mitsuya H, Yarchoan R. In vitro selection and molecular characterization of human immunodeficiency virus type 1 with reduced sensitivity to 9-[2-(phosphonomethoxy)ethyl]adenine (PMEA). Antiviral Res 1996; 32:91–98.

212. Cherrington JM, Mulato AS, Fuller MD, Chen MS. Novel mutation (K70E) in human immunodeficiency virus type 1 reverse transcriptase confers decreased susceptibility to 9-[2-(phosphonomethoxy)ethyl]adenine in vitro. Antimicrob Agents Chemother 1996; 40:2212–2216.

213. Nunberg JH, Schleif WA, Boots EJ, O'Brien JA, Quintero JC, Hoffman JM, Emini EA, Goldman ME. Viral resistance to human immunodeficiency virus type 1-specific pyridinone reverse transcriptase inhibitors. J Virol 1991; 65:4887–4892.

214. Richman D, Shih C-K, Lowy I, Rose J, Prodanovich P, Goff S, Griffin J. Human immunodeficiency virus type 1 mutants resistant to nonnucleoside inhibitors of reverse transcriptase arise in tissue culture. Proc Natl Acad Sci U S A 1991; 88:11241–11245.

215. Mellors JW, Dutschman GE, Im G-J, Tramontano E, Winkler SR, Cheng Y-C. In vitro selection and molecular characterization of human immunodeficiency virus-1 resistant to non-nucleoside inhibitors of reverse transcriptase. Mol Pharmacol 1991; 41:446–451.

216. Kleim J-P, Bender R, Kirsch R, Meichsner C, Paessens A, Riess G. Mutational analysis of residue 190 of human immunodeficiency virus type 1 reverse transcriptase. Virology 1994; 200:696–701.

217. Kleim J-P, Winkler I, Rösner M, Kirsch R, Rübsmen-Waigmann H, Paessens A, Riess G. In vitro selection for different mutational patterns in the HIV-1 reverse transcriptase using high and low selective pressure of the nonnucleoside reverse transcriptase inhibitor HBY 097. Virology 1997; 231:112–118.

218. Kleim J-P, Rösner M, Winkler I, Paessens A, Kirsch R, Hsiou Y, Arnold E, Riess G. Selective pressure of a quinoxaline nonnucleoside inhibitor of human immunodeficiency virus type 1 (HIV-1) reverse transcriptase (RT) on HIV-1 replication results in the emergence of nucleoside RT-inhibitor-specific (RT Leu-74 → Val or Ile and Val-75 → Leu or Ile) HIV-1 mutants. Proc Natl Acad Sci U S A 1996; 93:34–38.

219. Boyer PL, Gao H-Q, Hughes SH. A mutation at position 190 of human immunodeficiency virus type 1 reverse transcriptase interacts with mutations at positions 74 and 75 via the template primer. Antimicrob Agents Chemother 1998; 42:447–452.

220. Mellors JW, Im G-J, Tramontano E, Winkler SR, Medina DJ, Dutschman GE, Bazmi HZ, Piras G, Gonzalez CJ, Cheng Y-C. A single conservative amino acid substitution in the reverse transcriptase of human immunodeficiency virus-1 confers resistance to (+)-(5S)-4,5,6,7-tetrahydro-5-methyl-6-(3-methyl-2-butenyl)imidazo[4,5,1-jk][1,4]benzo diazepin-2(1H)-thione (TIBO R82150). Mol Pharmacol 1993; 43: 11–16.

220a. Rübsamen-Waigmann H, Huguenel E, Shah A, Ruoff H-J, von Briesen H, Immelmann A, Wainberg MA, Dietrich U. Resistance mutations selected in vivo under therapy with anti-HIV drug HBY 097 differ from resistance pattern selected in vitro. Antiviral Research 1999; 42:15–24.

221. Jonckheere H, Taymans J-M, Balzarini J, Velazquez S, Camarasa M-J, Desmyter J, De Clercq E, Anné J. Resistance of HIV-1 reverse transcriptase against [2′,5′-bis-O-(tert-butyldimethylsilyl)-3′-spiro-5″-(4″-amino-1″,2″-oxathiole-2″,2″-dioxide)]

(TSAO) derivatives is determined by the mutation Glu^{138} → Lys on the p51 subunit. J Biol Chem 1994; 269:25255–25258.

222. Boyer PL, Ding J, Arnold E, Hughes SH. Subunit specificity of mutations that confer resistance to nonnucleoside inhibitors in human immunodeficiency virus type 1 reverse transcriptase. Antimicrob Agents Chemother 1994; 38:1909–1914.

223. Dueweke TJ, Pushkarskaya T, Poppe SM, Swaney SM, Zhao JQ, Chen ISY, Stevenson M, Tarpley WG. A mutation in reverse transcriptase of bis(heteroaryl)piperazine-resistant human immunodeficiency virus type 1 that confers increased sensitivity to other nonnucleoside inhibitors. Proc Natl Acad Sci U S A 1993; 90:4713–4717.

224. Seki M, Sadakata Y, Yuasa S, Baba M. Isolation and characterization of human immunodeficiency virus type 1 mutants resistant to the non-nucleotide reverse transcriptase inhibitor MKC-442. Antiviral Chem Chemother 1995; 6:73–79.

225. Buckheit RW Jr, Fliakas-Boltz V, Yeagy-Bargo S, Weislow O, Mayers DL, Boyer PL, Hughes SH, Pan B-C, Chu S-H, Bader JP. Resistance to 1-[(2-hydroxyethoxy) methyl]-6-(phenylthio)thymine derivatives is generated by mutations at multiple sites in the HIV-1 reverse transcriptase. Virology 1995; 210:186–193.

226. Balzarini J, Baba M, De Clercq E. Differential activities of 1-[(2-hydroxyethoxy) methyl]-6-(phenylthio)thymine derivatives against different human immunodeficiency virus type 1 mutant strains. Antimicrob Agents Chemother 1995; 39:998–1002.

227. Pelemans H, Esnouf R, Dunkler A, Parniak MA, Vandamme A-M, Karlsson A, De Clercq E. Kleim J-P, Balzarini J. Characteristics of the Pro225His mutation in human immunodeficiency virus type 1 (HIV-1) reverse transcriptase that appears under selective pressure of dose-escalating quinoxaline treatment of HIV-1. J Virol 1997; 71: 8195–8203.

228. Balzarini J, Pelemans H, Esnouf R, De Clercq E. A novel mutation (F227L) arises in the reverse transcriptase of human immunodeficiency virus type 1 on dose-escalating treatment of HIV type 1-infected cell cultures with the nonnucleoside reverse transcriptase inhibitor thiocarboxanilide UC-781. AIDS Res Hum Retroviruses 1998; 14:255–260.

229. Richman DD, Havlir D, Corbeil J, Looney D, Ignacio C, Spector SA, Sullivan J, Cheeseman S, Barringer K, Pauletti D, Shih C-K, Myers M, Griffin J. Nevirapine resistance mutations of human immunodeficiency virus type 1 selected during therapy. J Virol 1994; 68:1660–1666.

230. Larder BA, 3′-Azido-3′-deoxythymidine resistance suppressed by a mutation conferring human immunodeficiency virus type 1 resistance to nonnucleoside reverse transcriptase inhibitors. Antimicrob Agents Chemother 1992; 36:2664–2669.

231. Byrnes VW, Emini EA, Schleif WA, Condra JH, Schneider CL, Long WJ, Wolfgang JA, Graham DJ, Gotlib L, Schlabach AJ, Wolanski BS, Blahy OM, Quintero JC, Rhodes A, Roth E, Titus DL, Sardana VV. Susceptibilities of human immunodeficiency virus type 1 enzyme and viral variants expressing multiple resistance-engendering amino acid substitutions to reverse transcriptase inhibitors. Antimicrob Agents Chemother 1994; 38:1404–1407.

232. Balzarini J, Pelemans H, Riess G, Roesner M, Winkler I, De Clercq E, Klaim J-P. Zidovudine-resistant human immunodeficiency virus type 1 strains subcultured in the presence of both lamivudine and quinoxaline HBY 097 retain marked sensitivity to HBY 097 but not to lamivudine. J Infect Dis 1997; 176:1392–1397.

233. Wainberg MA, Drosopoulos WC, Salomon H, Hsu M, Borkow G, Parniak MA, Gu Z, Song Q, Manne J, Islam S, Castriota G, Prasad VR. Enhanced fidelity of 3TC-selected mutant HIV-1 reverse transcriptase. Science 1996; 271:1282–1285.

234. Wei X, Ghosh SK, Taylor ME, Johnson VA, Emini EA, Deutsch P, Lifson JD, Bonhoeffer S, Nowak MA, Hahn BH, Saag MS, Shaw GM. Viral dynamics in human immunodeficiency virus type 1 infection. Nature 1995; 373:117–122.

235. Ho DD, Neumann AU, Perelson AS, Chen W, Leonard JM, Markowitz M. Rapid turnover of plasma virions and CD4 lymphocytes in HIV-1 infection. Nature 1995; 373:123–126.

236. Perelson AS, Neumann AU, Markowitz M, Leonard JM, Ho DD. HIV-1 dynamics in vivo: virion clearance rate, infected cell life-span, and viral generation time. Science 1996; 271:1582–1586.

237. Cao Y, Qin L, Zhang L, Safrit J, Ho DD. Virologic and immunologic characterization of long-term survivors of human immunodeficiency virus type 1 infection. N Engl J Med 1995; 332:201–208.

238. Pantaleo G, Menzo S, Vaccarezza M, Graziosi C, Cohen OJ, Demarest JF, Montefiori D, Orenstein JM, Fox C, Schrager LK, Margolick JB, Buchbinder S, Giorgi JV, Fauci AS. Studies in subjects with long-term nonprogressive human immunodeficiency virus infection. N Engl J Med 1995; 332:209–216.

239. O'Brien WA, Hartigan PM, Martin D, Esinhart J, Hill A, Benoit S, Rubin M, Simberkoff MS, Hamilton JD, the Veterans Affairs Cooperative Study Group on AIDS. Changes in plasma HIV-1 RNA and CD4+ lymphocyte counts and the risk of progression to AIDS. N Engl J Med 1996; 334:426–431.

240. Saag MS, Holodniy M, Kuritzkes DR, O'Brien WA, Coombs R, Poscher ME, Jacobson DM, Shaw GM, Richman DD, Volberding PA. HIV viral load markers in clinical practice. Nat Med 1996; 2:625–629.

241. Mellors JW, Rinaldo Jr CR, Gupta P, White RM, Todd JA, Kingsley LA. Prognosis in HIV-1 infection predicted by the quantity of virus in plasma. Science 1996; 272:1167–1170.

242. Craib KJP, Strathdee SA, Hogg RS, Leung B, Montaner JSG, O'Shaugnessy MV, Schechter MT. Serum levels of human immunodeficiency virus type 1 (HIV-1) RNA after seroconversion: a predictor of long-term mortality in HIV infection. J Infect Dis 1997; 176:798–800.

243. Wong JK, Hezareh M, Günthard HF, Havlir DV, Ignacio CC, Spina CA, Richman DD. Recovery of replication-competent HIV despite prolonged suppression of plasma viremia. Science 1997; 278:1291–1295.

244. Finzi D, Hermankova M, Pierson T, Carruth LM, Buck C, Chaisson RE, Quinn TC, Chadwick K, Margolick J, Brookmeyer R, Gallant J, Markowitz M, Ho DD, Richman DD, Siliciano RF. Identification of a reservoir for HIV-1 in patients on highly active antiretroviral therapy. Science 1997; 278:1295–1300.

5

Inhibitors of HIV Protease

Sally Redshaw and Gareth J. Thomas
Roche Discovery Welwyn, Welwyn Garden City, Hertfordshire, England

I. INTRODUCTION

In the early 1980s, there were several reports of apparently healthy young individuals falling prey to pathogens that would normally be controlled easily by a healthy immune system. As these reports became more frequent, the new and alarming syndrome came to be known as the acquired immunodeficiency syndrome, or AIDS. It was quickly established that this disease was caused by an infectious agent and that this agent was a previously unknown retrovirus (1–3), which has come to be universally known as the human immunodeficiency virus, or HIV. Shortly after the discovery of the new virus, by analogy with other retroviruses, it was suggested (4) that HIV might encode a protease. This was confirmed, and HIV protease activity was shown to be crucial for maturation of infectious virions (5–7). When HIV enters a cell, the single-stranded viral RNA is copied to produce double-stranded DNA. The viral DNA becomes integrated into the host cell genome and is subsequently transcribed and translated by cellular enzymes to produce the viral polyproteins. These large molecules are not functional and must be cleaved by the viral protease before new infectious viral particles can be produced.

Groups in both industry and academia were swift to recognize an exciting new therapeutic target, and a large effort was devoted to characterizing the enzyme. It soon became clear that retroviral proteases, including HIV protease, were mechanistically similar to the aspartic proteases of mammalian and fungal origin, which had been known for some time (5,8–11). Much work had been devoted to identifying inhibitors of renin for the treatment of hypertension, and it had been found that compounds capable of mimicking the transition state of the enzymatic reaction were able to prevent substrate hydrolysis.

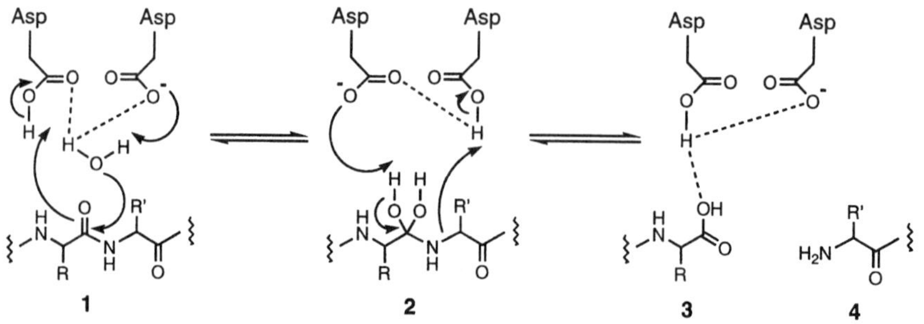

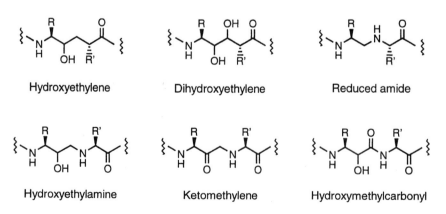

Figure 1   Mechanism of cleavage by aspartic proteases.

Proteases act as "molecular scissors," snipping large proteins into smaller pieces. A simplified diagram of how this is achieved by aspartic proteases, such as renin or HIV protease, is shown in Figure 1. Two aspartic acid residues in the active site of the protease deliver a water molecule to the amide bond that is to be cleaved. This creates a tetrahedral species (view 2, Fig. 1), which is referred to as the transition state. This unstable species rapidly falls apart to give the products: a C-terminal acid (view 3, Fig. 1) and an N-terminal amine (view 4, Fig. 1). Stable compounds that resemble the transition state but cannot be cleaved bind tightly to the active site of the protease and so act as powerful inhibitors.

Many different transition-state mimetics have been devised, some of which are illustrated in Figure 2. These are able to mimic some, but not all, of the supposed aspects of the transition state. They all feature tetrahedral geometry at the center that would have formed the scissile carbonyl group, but match other char-

Hydroxyethylene

Dihydroxyethylene

Reduced amide

Hydroxyethylamine

Ketomethylene

Hydroxymethylcarbonyl

Figure 2   Stable transition state mimetics.

acteristics with varying degrees of success. Once a particular transition-state mimetic has been chosen, it must be incorporated into a suitable peptide sequence. Initial sequences are usually selected to reflect the natural substrates of the protease.

HIV protease catalyzes cleavage of its polyprotein substrates at eight distinct sites (12) (Fig. 3). A striking feature of these amino acid sequences is their lack of homology, showing that HIV protease must be particularly versatile in its mode of substrate recognition. This, in turn, allows a variety of structural possibilities to be considered for the design of structure-based inhibitors (vide infra). The amino acid sequences that are cleaved by HIV protease may be grouped broadly into three categories, two of which are somewhat unusual. Class 1 cleavage sites (13,14) (sites 1, 5, and 6, Fig 3) involves hydrolysis of an amide bond between a phenylalanine or tyrosine residue and a proline. Although other retroviral proteases had been shown to be able to carry out this type of cleavage, there was no evidence that mammalian enzymes could also do so. This led to the suggestion that inhibitors based on Phe/Tyr-Pro sequences might be selective for the viral enzymes (15). Sites 3, 4, 7, and 8 (class 2) of Figure 3 are also interesting in that they show an element of symmetry. This, together with the symmetry of the dimeric protease, suggested

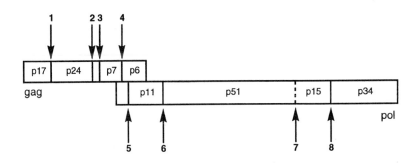

Class 1.   Tyr/Phe * Pro   Class 2.   Pseudosymmetrical

1.   Gln.Asn.Tyr * Pro.Ile.Val   3.   Thr.Ile.Met * Met.Gln.Arg
5.   Phe.Ser.Phe * Pro.Gln.Ile   4.   Gly.Asn.Phe * Leu.Gln.Ser
.6. Leu.Asn.Phe * Pro.Ile.Ser   7.   Glu.Thr.Phe * Tyr.Val.Asp
                                     8.   Lys.Val.Leu * Phe.Leu.Asp

                                     Class 3.   Renin-like

                                     2.   Arg.Val.Leu * Ala.Glu.Ala

Figure 3   Cleavage of viral polyproteins by HIV protease.

that it might be possible to design symmetrical inhibitors that would also be selective for the viral enzymes (16–20). There is only one example of the class 3 cleavage sequence. This cleavage (site 2, Fig. 3), which is between a leucine residue and an alanine, is somewhat reminiscent of the cleavage of angiotensinogen by renin, where the cleaved bond is between a leucine residue and valine.

II. APPROACHES TO INHIBITORS OF HIV PROTEASE

The first challenge in any new medicinal chemistry program is to identify a lead compound. This problem can be addressed in a number of ways:

> Random screening of samples
> Screening of compounds known to inhibit related targets (e.g., renin)
> De novo design using mechanistic and/or structural details
> Computer-aided design

All of these strategies have been applied to the search for lead compounds as inhibitors of HIV protease, and much of this work has been reviewed (14,21–28). The identification of a lead structure, from whichever source, is usually followed by a program of medicinal chemistry instituted to define structure–activity relationships, and to optimize activity. Knowledge gained from these studies may then be applied to the computer-assisted design of new structural types, especially once x-ray crystallographic structures of the native enzyme and, more particularly, of enzyme-inhibitor complexes are solved.

A. Random Screening of Samples

A number of groups have established high throughput assays for inhibition of HIV protease and have tested large numbers of samples derived from microbial (29–31) or plant (32,33) sources, or from existing compound libraries (34–36). One of the attractions of this approach is the possibility of discovering inhibitors that do not have the poor pharmacokinetic properties often associated with the peptidomimetic structures likely to arise from other strategies.

Screening of approximately 12,000 fermentation broths derived mostly from actinomycetes or fungi led to the identification of the known α-MAPI (5, Table 1), which is produced by a member of the genus *Streptomyces* (29,30). Somewhat surprisingly, because this compound had previously been characterized as an inhibitor of alkaline proteases with no activity against aspartic proteases, α-MAPI was found to inhibit HIV-1 protease with an IC_{50} of 2.0 μM. The analogous alcohol (6, Table 1) was later obtained from samples of *Streptomyces chromofuscus* isolated from soil, but was found to be less active than the aldehyde (5, Table 1) (31).

Screening of fungal metabolites led to the identification of the known iso-cochliodinol (7, Table 1), as well as other closely related novel asterriquinones

Table 1

Compound	Structure	IC$_{50}$ (or K$_i$) μM
5 R = CHO		2.0
6 R = CH$_2$OH		17.8
7		0.18
8		3.0
9		(< 0.00001)
10 R = COCH$_3$		30
11 R = CH$_3$		(0.8)
12		3.0
13		0.068

from *Chrysosporium merdarium* (37). Modeling of isocochliodinol into HIV protease suggested that the quinone moiety can bridge the gap between the active site aspartic acids and the flap region of the enzyme, and thus displace the water molecule that is present in other HIV protease-inhibitor complexes. A number of other groups have screened fungal metabolites for inhibition of HIV protease. Research workers at Merck isolated the novel cytochalasin (8, Table 1) from *Hypoxolon fragiforme*, a fungus found on the bark of American beech trees (38). However, further screening of products from closely related *Hypoxolon* species, or from other fungi known to produce cytochalasins, failed to yield additional inhibitors, and only one (cytochalasin A) of eight commercially available cytochalasins was found to show activity (39).

Although a diverse range of inhibitors have been identified by these means, few have been pursued as far as the clinic. One exception is the dihydropyrone (9, Table 1) (PNU140690) (40,41), which is currently undergoing early clinical evaluation. It is a potent inhibitor of both HIV-1 and HIV-2 proteases (40), and inhibits viral replication of HIV-1 in vitro with an average EC_{90} value of 180 nM against clinically isolated strains of HIV (41). PNU140690 also retains good activity against a variant of HIV that is broadly resistant to peptidomimetic inhibitors. The group at Pharmacia Upjohn began their program by screening 5000 dissimilar compounds from their compound collection. This search led to the identification of 4-hydroxycoumarin (warfarin) (10, Table 1) as a weak inhibitor ($IC_{50} \sim 30$ µM) (34). Similar compounds were then tested, and compound 11, Table 1, was found to have improved potency. A subsequent crystal structure of compound 11, Table 1, complexed with HIV protease provided the basis for the design of more potent inhibitors, and ultimately item 9 (40).

In a similar mass screening exercise, the Parke-Davis group independently identified several series of inhibitors, amongst them the 4-hydroxypyranone (12, Table 1) (35,36). The crystal structure of a close analogue complexed with HIV protease was used in the design of more potent inhibitors, leading to compounds such as 13, Table 1, which has an IC_{50} of 68 nM against HIV protease. Unfortunately, the antiviral activity of these compounds correlated poorly with their enzyme inhibitory activity and they also showed significant cytotoxicity, which made interpretation of antiviral activity difficult. It is speculated (36) that the relatively poor antiviral activity may be attributable to the protonation state of the 4-hydroxyl substituent. Compounds such as 13 do, however, show good pharmacokinetic properties and further studies are in progress to improve their antiviral activity (42).

B. Screening of Compounds Known to Inhibit Related Targets

In a more focused approach, many groups that had previously identified inhibitors of renin have tested these compounds for inhibition of HIV protease. For example, early work at Upjohn identified the hydroxyethylene derivative (14, Table 2), a potent inhibitor of renin, as a good inhibitor of HIV protease (43) with a K_i of 10 nM. Although a potent inhibitor of the isolated enzyme, compound 14 showed only weak antiviral activity in cell culture. A number of structural modifications led to compounds such as the dihydroxyethylene (15, Table 2) (44,45), which showed significant antiviral activity (EC_{50} = 3 nM) against HIV-1 infected human peripheral blood lymphocytes. Although a potent antiviral in cell culture, com-

Table 2

Compound	Structure	IC$_{50}$ (or K$_i$) nM	
		renin	HIV protease

Compound	renin	HIV protease
14	(0.07)	(10)
15	2	(< 1)
16 R = Boc.Phe.Phe	73	1
17 R = Boc	>10,000	0.6
18 R=H		110
19 R=CH$_2$OH		40
20 R=H		19
21 R=OH		0.3
22		7.8
23		0.56

pound 15, Table 2, was not significantly orally bioavailable and showed an inhibitory effect on simian immunodeficiency virus (SIV) in rhesus monkeys only after continuous intravenous infusion (46).

The group at Merck also began their program on HIV protease inhibitors by screening compounds that had originally been synthesized for their renin inhibitor program. They identified compound 16, Table 2, a hydroxyethylene transition state mimetic, as an interesting lead structure with IC_{50} values of 73 nM against renin and 1 nM against HIV protease (47). Their objective was then to reduce activity against renin while retaining activity against the viral enzyme. This was achieved by removing the two phenylalanine residues from the N-terminus of the inhibitor to give compound 17, Table 2, which was essentially devoid of renin inhibitory activity. They went on to develop a series of compounds (e.g., 18 and 19, Table 2), which were related to compound 17, Table 2, but contained only a benzyl amide residue at the C-terminus (48,49). Conformational restriction then led to the amino indanes, compounds 20 and 21, Table 2. In both cases, an α-hydroxymethyl group was seen to confer greater potency (48). Compound 21 was not developed further because of poor bioavailability, and at this point its similarity with saquinavir (compound 67, see Table 6) was considered. Because the active site is symmetrical and inhibitors can bind in both directions, it seemed likely to the group at Merck that the decahydroisoquinoline part of saquinavir occupied the same region of the active site as the Boc.Phe portion of inhibitors such as compound 20 or 21, Table 2. To test this hypothesis, hybrid structures were designed. The first of these (22, Table 2), was a good inhibitor with an IC_{50} of 7.8 nM (50). Further modifications gave the more potent compound (23, Table 2) (L-735,524, MK-639, indinavir) (50), which showed potent in vitro anti-HIV activity ($EC_{95} = 50$ nM), and was later to be launched as Crixivan.

Although random or focused screening to identify lead compounds have certain attractions (and in the latter case has led to a successful drug launch), the majority of HIV protease inhibitors described to date, including two of the three that were first to market, have arisen more directly from design using the transition-state mimetic approach.

C. De Novo Design Using Mechanistic and/or Structural Details

1. Symmetrical Inhibitors

A very elegant approach to the design of HIV protease inhibitors that exploited the two-fold rotational symmetry of the native enzyme was adopted by researchers at Abbott. An axis of symmetry was defined at or near to the carbon bearing the hydroxyl groups in the transition state (24, Fig. 4) of cleavage of Phe-Pro (16,17). Theoretically, either portion of the transition state could then be deleted and a C_2 symmetry operation performed on the remaining residues to generate a symmet-

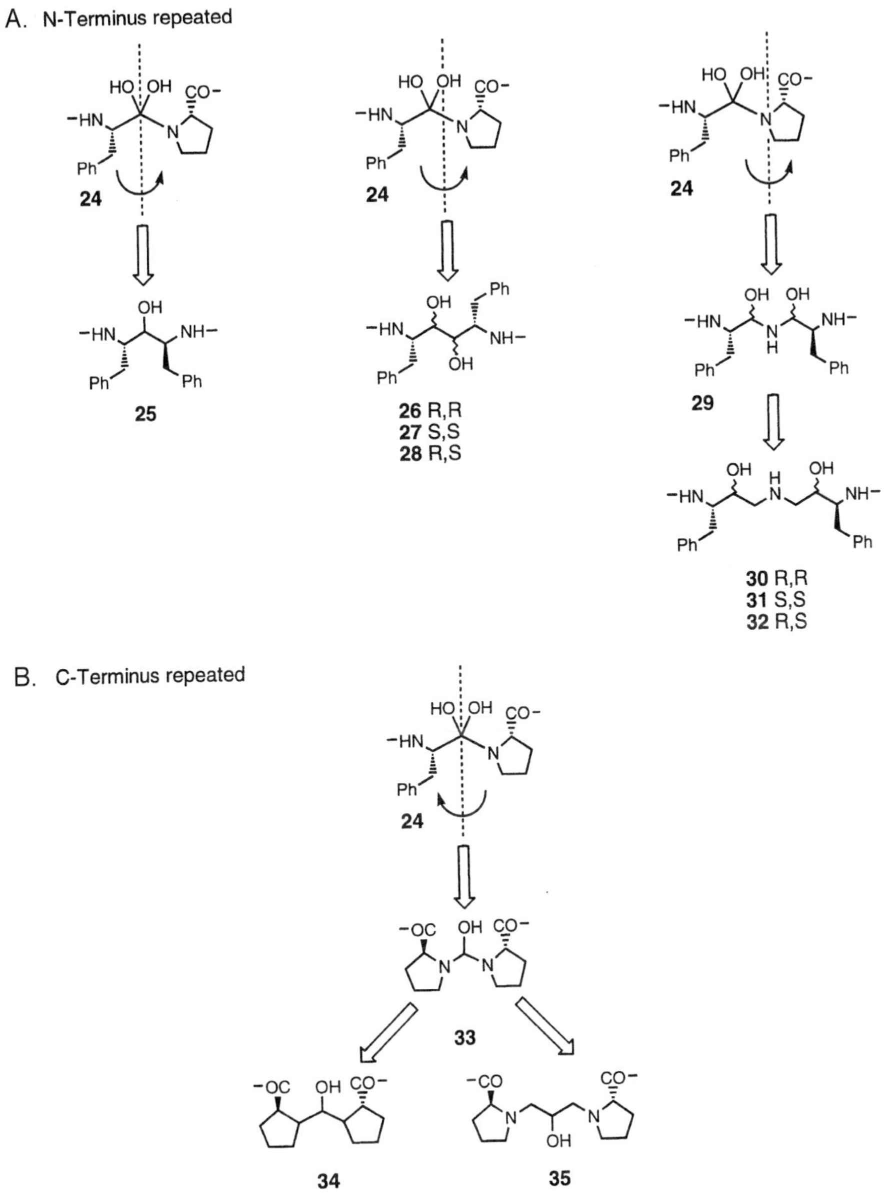
A. N-Terminus repeated
24
25
24
26 R,R
27 S,S
28 R,S
24
29
30 R,R
31 S,S
32 R,S
B. C-Terminus repeated
24
33
34
35

Figure 4 Symmetry operations performed on (A) "non–prime-side" and (B) "prime-side" residues.

rical species. The Abbott group chose to delete the "prime side" portion of structure 24, Fig. 4) to give either a diamino alcohol (25, Fig 4), or one of three stereodistinct diaminodiols (26–28, Fig. 4). Incorporation of any of these species into a suitable peptide sequence produced very potent inhibitors (Table 3). In contrast

Table 3

Compound	Structure	IC$_{50}$ (or K$_i$) nM
36		3.0
37 38 39		R,R 0.22 S,S 0.38 R,S 0.22
40		< 1
41		(0.25)
42		(< 1)
43 44 45		R,R 125 R,S 4,500 S,S >>10,000
46		0.7
47		> 1000

to more traditional hydroxyl-containing inhibitors, the configuration of the alcohol functions in compounds 37 to 39, Table 3, has little effect on potency, possibly indicating a high degree of flexibility of the central core structure. X-ray crystallography of the pseudosymmetric R,S-diol (40, Table 3) (19) complexed with HIV protease shows it to bind in an asymmetric mode (51). The R-hydroxyl group is situated close to the C_2-symmetry axis of the enzyme, within hydrogen-bonding distance of both catalytic aspartic acid residues, whereas the S-hydroxyl group can form a hydrogen bond with only one aspartic acid residue. The asymmetry of binding cannot, however, be attributed to the pseudosymmetric nature of compound 40, Table 3, because the corresponding symmetric R,R-diol binds in an asymmetric mode while the S,S-diastereomer binds symmetrically. In addition, the pseudosymmetric monohydroxy derivative (36, Table 3) binds in a symmetrical fashion (16). Clearly, the precise mode of binding is determined by how well each inhibitor can simultaneously optimize hydrogen bonding with the active site aspartic acid residues and also maintain favorable contacts with the enzyme subsites. The low solubility of prototype inhibitors (36–39, Table 3) made in vivo evaluation difficult, and the terminal benzyloxycarbonyl groups were modified in an attempt to obtain more soluble compounds. One of the new compounds, A77003 (40, Table 3) (19,20), showed good antiviral activity (EC_{50} 30–300 nM) in a range of in vitro systems and was Abbott's first clinical candidate. Despite reasonable aqueous solubility, however, A77003 had poor oral bioavailability and had to be administered by continuous intravenous infusion, which caused local phlebitis in some patients. The compound also had a very short half-life and, partly because of difficulties with the protocol, adequate levels to achieve a conclusive antiviral effect could not be maintained. Further studies (52,53) identified A80987 (41, Table 3) as a potent (K_i 0.25 nM) inhibitor, which, although much better absorbed, still had a very short duration of action. This was found to be caused by extensive oxidative metabolism of the pyridyl groups. A study of analogues of compound 41, Table 3, in which the pyridyl groups were replaced by other heterocyclic residues resulted in the discovery of ABT-538 (ritonavir) (42, Table 3) (53). Ritonavir is a potent inhibitor of HIV protease with enhanced antiviral activity and oral pharmacokinetics and potent anti-HIV activity ($EC_{50} = 25$ nM). This compound was launched in 1996 as Norvir.

In another approach, location of the axis of symmetry at the nitrogen atom of the transition state (24, Fig. 4) and deletion of the "prime side" portion led to the unstable aminodiol (29, Fig. 4). Insertion of methylene groups between the nitrogen atom and the hydroxy-bearing carbons gave the more stable extended aminodiols (30–32, Fig. 4), which have been incorporated into inhibitors (43–45, Table 3) (54). In contrast to the diols (37–39, Table 3), the stereochemistry of the hydroxyl functions in compounds 43 to 45, Table 3, is critical for activity, with the R,R-diastereomer (43, Table 3) being substantially more potent than the other isomers.

An alternative strategy for the design of symmetrical inhibitors involves a C_2 axis at the hydroxyl-bearing carbon of the transition state (24, Fig. 4), but performs the symmetry operation on "prime" rater than "non-prime" residues. This results in the diaminomethanol (33, Fig. 4), which is not chemically stable. Stable analogues have been prepared by replacing the nitrogen atoms by carbon, giving compound 34, Figure 4, or by inserting methylene groups between the nitrogen atoms and the hydroxyl-bearing carbon atom as described, to give compound 35, Figure 4. Performance of the former operation on the Merck compound L-685,4343 (21, Table 2) gave the potent pseudosymmetric inhibitor, compound 46, Table 3 (18). The second approach has, however, been less successful. Compounds such as compound 47, Table 3, which contain a 1,3-diamino-2-propanol moiety analogous to compound 35, Figure 4, are poor inhibitors (55).

2.   Transition-State Mimetics Based on Scissile Tyr/Phe-Pro

The Roche group were intrigued by the ability of retroviral proteases, and particularly HIV protease, to cleave amide bonds between aromatic amino acids and proline. Because mammalian enzymes are unable to carry out this specific cleavage, and, by implication, do not recognize and bind proteins containing this motif, it seemed likely that inhibitors based on this sequence would be selective for the viral enzyme. Such inhibitors should not, therefore, cause side effects through inhibition of human aspartic proteases. Of the possible transition-state mimetics, the reduced amides, ketomethylene derivatives, and hydroxyethylamines (see Fig. 2) seemed particularly suited to mimic scissile Tyr/Phe-Pro. In a preliminary study (15), compounds 48 to 51, Table 4, based on the Asn.Phe-Pro cleavage sequence in the *pol* polyprotein (6, Fig. 3) were evaluated. The reduced amide (48, Table 4) proved to be a rather poor inhibitor of HIV protease, and similar findings have also been reported by other laboratories (56–58). The ketomethylene derivative (49, Table 4) was more active but less potent than the diastereomeric hydroxyethyl-

Table 4

Compound	Structure	IC_{50} μM
48		50
49		0.87
50, 51		0.14, 0.3

Table 5

Phe-ψ[CH(OH)CH$_2$N]Pro

Compound	Structure	IC$_{50}$ nM
52 and **53**	Cbz.Pheψ[CH(OH)CH$_2$N]Pro.O^{t}Bu	6500 and 30000
50 and **51**	Cbz.Asn.Pheψ[CH(OH)CH$_2$N]Pro.O^{t}Bu	140 and 300
54 and **55**	Cbz.Leu.Asn.Pheψ[CH(OH)CH$_2$N]Pro.O^{t}Bu	600 and 1100
56 and **57**	Cbz.Asn.Pheψ[CH(OH)CH$_2$N]Pro.Ile.NH^{i}Bu	130 and 2400
58 and **59**	Cbz.Leu.Asn.Pheψ[CH(OH)CH$_2$N]Pro.Ile.NH^{i}Bu	750 and 10000

amines (50 and 51, Table 4). The next task was to determine the minimum size of molecule needed for potent inhibition. The protected dipeptide mimetics (52 and 53, Table 5) showed much reduced activity (15) compared with compounds 50 and 51. Extension toward the N-terminus (compounds 54 and 55, Table 5), the C-terminus (compounds 56 and 57, Table 5), or indeed, in both directions (compounds 58 and 59, Table 5), gave no improvement in potency. The more potent (50 and 51, Table 4) was shown to have the *R*-configuration at the secondary alcohol function, and this compound was chosen for further investigation of structure–activity relationships and optimization of activity. At the time, no x-ray crystallographic data were available and, in the absence of structural information that might help in the design of more potent inhibitors, structure–activity relationships were explored through systematic modification of each amino acid residue in turn.

Replacement of the N-terminal Cbz group by nonaromatic groups such as acetyl or Boc gave compounds with significantly reduced activity. Introduction of bicyclic aromatic groups such as β-naphthoyl or, especially, quinoline-2-carbonyl (compound 61, Table 5), on the other hand, led to compounds with improved potency compared with the parent compound. At the P$_2$ position, conservative changes were found to be tolerated, but no improvement over asparagine itself was identified. At the P$_1$ position, aromatic groups were strongly preferred, but again no significant improvement over the parent compound was identified. The most dramatic changes in potency were achieved by modifying the prolyl residue that occupies the S$_1$´ subsite. Within a series of imino acids, ring size was found to be very important for activity. Replacing the proline five-membered ring by a four-membered azetidine ring almost abolished activity, whereas incorporation of a six-membered ring improved potency approximately 12-fold (62, Table 6). Replace-

Table 6

Compound	Structure	HIV-1 protease IC$_{50}$ nM	HIV-2 protease IC$_{50}$ nM
60		210	330
61		52	50
62		18	ND
63		2.7	ND
64		2	10
65		< 0.4	< 0.8
66		4	10
67		6.5	ND

ment of proline by fused bicyclic imino acids led to the greatest enhancement of activity, and *S,S,S*-decahydroisoquinoline carboxylic acid was the best replacement for proline that was identified (63, Table 6). At the carboxyl terminus, medium size lipophilic residues appeared to be preferred, with little difference between esters and amides (compounds 50, Table 4, and 60, Table 6). The ^{t}butylamide group was chosen as the C-terminal residue on the basis of chemical, and possibly metabolic, stability.

Having located two regions of the molecule in which changes substantially altered binding affinities, further syntheses were undertaken to determine whether the combined effects of individual changes were additive. The compounds synthesized in this process (64 and 65, Table 6) showed that the effects of beneficial changes were frequently more than additive. The compounds, moreover, showed the same order of potencies against HIV-2 protease, although they were somewhat more active against the HIV-1 enzyme. Within this series of compounds, the order of potencies in a preliminary antiviral assay also closely paralleled the enzyme inhibitory potency, probably indicating good penetration into cells (15). One of the most potent (EC_{50} = 10 nM) of these hydroxyethylamine derivatives was Ro 31-8959, saquinavir (65, Table 6). Because one of the aims of this program had been to identify highly selective inhibitors of the viral protease, it was of interest to test selected compounds for inhibition of mammalian proteases. Saquinavir inhibited the human aspartic proteases, renin, pepsin, gastricsin, cathepsin D, and cathepsin E by less than 50% at 10 μM. When tested against representative members of the three other mechanistic classes of mammalian proteases (serine, cysteine, and metallo), the compound also showed less than 50% inhibition at 50 μM Concentrations of saquinavir at least 10^5 higher than the K_i against the viral enzyme were thus needed to inhibit any of the mammalian enzymes, confirming that, as intended, the compound was an extremely selective inhibitor of the HIV proteases. On the basis of these and other data, saquinavir was selected for clinical evaluation and, as Invirase, was later to become the first inhibitor of HIV protease to be licensed for the treatment of AIDS.

Research workers at Bio-Méga Boehringer Ingelheim have recently described the substituted piperidine (66, Table 6) (palinavir) (59), a close analogue of the Phe-Pro transition-state mimetics synthesized in the Roche laboratories. Palinavir is a potent and selective inhibitor of both HIV-1 and HIV-2 proteases and shows good in vitro antiviral activity (EC_{50} = 0.5–30 nM) against a number of laboratory and clinical strains of HIV. This compound is currently undergoing in-depth preclinical evaluation.

Kiso and coworkers (60) also noted the unique ability of HIV protease to cleave the Phe-Pro bond. They chose the hydroxymethylcarbonyl transition state mimetic (see Fig. 2) as the core structure of their inhibitors. In contrast to the hydroxyethylamine derivatives described by the Roche group, a decrease in potency in the order proline > piperidine-2-carboxylic acid > decahydroquinoline-3-carboxylic acid (the imino acids of structures 61, 62, and 63, Table 6, respectively) is seen. The need for specific interactions with the carbonyl group of the carboxamide or intrinsic conformational differences may explain these intriguing differences between seemingly closely related series of compounds. Replacement of the pyrrolidine ring of proline by other heterocyclic five-membered rings, especially thiazolidine or dimethylthiazolidine, led to significantly more potent inhibitors.

Subsequent modification of P_2 and P_3 residues has led to very active and, again, very selective inhibitors of HIV protease such as KNI-272, kynostatin (67, Table 6). Kynostatin also shows good antiviral activity (EC_{50} = 20–100 nM) in cell culture experiments (61).

D. Computer-Aided Design

A large number of crystal structures of HIV protease complexed to different inhibitors has provided a wealth of information concerning binding interactions. All of the inhibitors bind in a similar fashion and one interesting feature is a "structural" water molecule that links the flaps to the inhibitor. In the native enzyme, the flaps are in an "open" position but "close" when a substrate or inhibitor is bound (Fig. 5). The hydrogen bonds between the inhibitors and the flap are mediated through the so-called structural water molecule. This structural walter molecule accepts two hydrogen bonds from the backbone amide hydrogens of residues Ile^{50} and $Ile^{50'}$ in the flap and donates two hydrogen bonds to the carbonyl oxygens flanking the transition-state mimetic (Fig. 6). A group at DuPont Merck decided to incorporate this water molecule into inhibitors for a number of reasons. Displacement of the water molecule should be energetically favorable, and because the water molecule is unique to retroviral proteases, incorporation of a water mimic into an inhibitor should give selectivity for the viral enzyme. The group wanted to explore rigid, nonpeptide, cyclic structures, and decided to use the structure–activity relationships developed for linear C_2 symmetrical diols to generate several pharmacophore models. This approach (62 and references therein) led to the identification of a series of cyclic ureas exemplified by DMP 323 (68, Table 7) and DMP 450 (69, Table 7). High resolution X-ray structures of the complexes of these inhibitors with HIV protease show that the urea oxygen hydrogen bonds directly to the flap residues Ile^{50} and $Ile^{50'}$ with exclusion of the "structural" water molecule as had been predicted from the design of the molecules. As a class, the cyclic ureas are significantly bioavailable. Poor solubility, first-pass metabolism, and limited formulation possibilities cut short clinical trials with DMP 323. DMP 450, however, combines good antiviral potency (average ED_{50} = 144 nM) with attractive physical properties (63) and this compound was chosen as a second clinical candidate.

Research workers at Gilead Sciences and at Abbott have pursued similar strategies. The Gilead group have synthesized a series of cyclic sulphones such as compound 70, Table 7 (64). The presence of amino functions in the P_2 and $P_{2'}$ aryl rings in compound 70, Table 7, confers good water solubility and bioavailability, and this compound, which shows potent anti-HIV activity (EC_{50} = 9 nM) is undergoing preclinical studies. The Abbott group have introduced an additional nitrogen atom into the seven-membered ring, giving azacyclic ureas such as compound 71, Table 7 (65). These derivatives have the synthetic advantage that two the chiral centers present in earlier analogues are replaced by a nonchiral methyl-

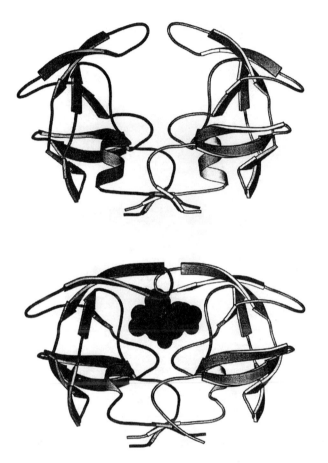

Figure 5 Crystal structure of (top) native HIV protease showing open flaps and (bottom) HIV protease-inhibitor complex showing closed flaps.

ene unit and a nitrogen atom. Compound 71 has reasonable bioavailability and similar antiviral activity to earlier cyclic ureas (EC_{50} = 150 nM).

A collaboration between Agouron and Lilly led to the discovery of AG-1343, nelfinavir (72, Table 7). The compound was identified (66) by a combination of iterative structure-based design and an analysis of oral pharmacokinetics and antiviral activity. The structure is closely related to that of saquinavir, with the P_3-P_2 fragment replaced by a hydroxytoluidic acid residue and the phenylalanine side chain homologated to include a sulphur atom. Nelfinavir is a potent enzyme inhibitor (K_i = 2 nM) and antiviral agent (HIV-1, EC_{50} = 14 nM). In vivo studies indicated that AG-1343 was well absorbed orally in a variety of species and possessed favorable pharmacokinetic properties in humans. Nelfinavir, under the

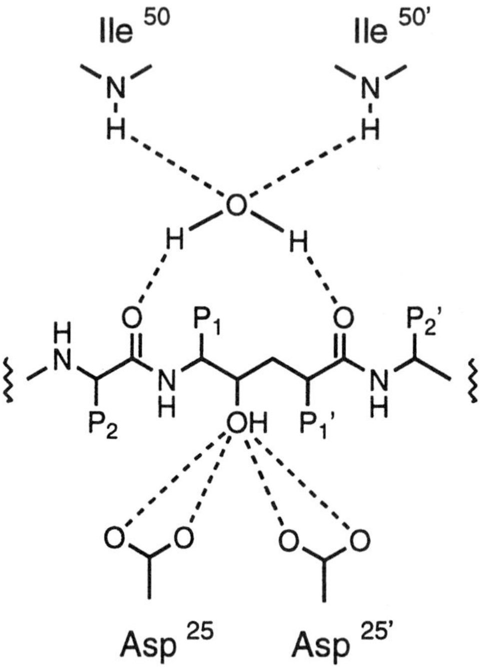

Figure 6   Binding of peptidomimetic inhibitors via a "structural" water molecule.

tradename Viracept, was the fourth protease inhibitor to be approved for the treatment of AIDS.

Another HIV protease inhibitor, 73, Table 7 (67,68), is in late-stage clinical trials. The compound was discovered by researchers at Vertex and was subsequently licensed to Glaxo Wellcome where it is currently undergoing phase III development as 141W94 (amprenavir). The compound is the result of a focused program of structure-based inhibitor design, which sought to maintain potency while reducing inhibitor size and complexity. 141W94 is a potent inhibitor of HIV protease ($K_i = 0.6$ nM) and shows good antiviral activity in cell culture ($EC_{50} = 80$ nM).

III.   CLINICAL USE OF PROTEASE INHIBITORS

The clinical care of people infected with HIV has been dramatically influenced by the introduction of the first protease inhibitors. The four available drugs, saquinavir (69), ritonavir (70,71), indinavir (72), and nelfinavir (73) have all been shown to have a beneficial effect on viral load and/or CD4+ cell counts, with higher doses giving a bigger effect in all cases in which this has been examined (74–77).

Table 7

Compound	Structure	IC$_{50}$ (or K$_i$) nM
68		(0.26)
69		(0.22)
70		1.0
71		1
72		2
73		0.6

Prompted by the increased antiviral effect achieved in the Stanford University high-dose study (74) with Invirase, the Roche group have developed a new, soft gelatin formulation of saquinavir to improve the clinical efficiency of the compound. This formulation, which was assigned the trade name Fortovase, gives increased exposure levels and antiviral potency in the clinic, and has been approved in the United States. At the approved does (1200 mg t.i.d.), Fortovase gives an exposure to saquinavir eight-fold higher than that achieved with Invirase (600 mg t.i.d.).

In many studies (78–84), the combination of a protease inhibitor with one or more reverse transcriptase inhibitors has been shown to produce a greater and more prolonged effect on surrogate markers than can be achieved with either agent alone. Indeed, although indinavir and ritonavir are licensed for monotherapy of HIV infection, current clinical practice would be to use all of the protease inhibitors as part of combination therapy.

As well as beneficial effects on surrogate markers, extended studies have demonstrated that the inclusion of a protease inhibitor into treatment regimens can substantially reduce mortality rate and clinical progression of disease (85–89). Resolution of complications such as Kaposi' sarcoma (90–93), oral candidiasis (94), and cytomegalovirus retinitis (95) has also been observed.

Development of resistance is seen as the main barrier to long-term efficacious use of the protease inhibitors. Recent studies (96) show that the replication rate of HIV is very high, with ~10^{10} viral particles produced each day. HIV reverse transcriptase is also error-prone, resulting in very high levels of genetic variation (97). These factors together allow a high rate of mutation, which favors the development of resistant mutants under the selective pressure of antiretroviral therapies. Mutations within the protease gene conferring resistance have been described for all of the currently available protease inhibitors (98–105). Each inhibitor selects for a particular pattern of mutations within the protease gene, leading to structural changes in the enzyme and subsequent drug resistance. The extent to which resistance to one of the protease inhibitors is likely to limit sustained suppression of viral replication by other members of the class appears to vary (103,106–109). Because of this, it is possible that sequential therapy, starting with those inhibitors that induce less "cross-resistance," will become normal practice (110). Full understanding of the controversial issue of resistance is complicated by the fact that mutations generated during in vitro experiments may differ from those arising during patient treatment.

In some instances, the viability of virions with resistant protease is diminished compared with wild-type virus (111) and it has been observed (112) that, in some cases, the emergence of resistant strains during treatment with a protease inhibitor may be associated with the selection of viral strains with less cytopathogenicity. Although the precise clinical implications of specific mutations may still be unclear, it is becoming evident that resistance emerges most readily when HIV is exposed to subtherapeutic levels of drug, which allow continuing viral replication (102,113). In line with this observation, patients receiving combination therapy in which viral replication is more effectively inhibited, are at lower risk of acquiring resistant virus. This also means that noncompliance and "drug holidays" should be strongly discouraged in patients receiving antiretroviral therapy.

IV. CONCLUSION

The use of protease inhibitors in combination with other antiretrovirals such as nucleoside analogues has had a large impact on the expectations of both physicians and patients, and has resulted in widespread optimism that HIV infection can become a long-term manageable disease. A population of patients with what was an incurable, progressive, and ultimately fatal disease has been offered the prospect of extended survival and enhanced quality of life. In view of the advantages offered by combination therapy, it seems likely (114) that aggressive intervention will, in the future, be initiated much earlier in the disease.

REFERENCES

1. Barré-Sinoussi F, Chermann JC, Rey F, Nugeyre MT, Chamaret S, Gruest J, Dauguet C, Axler-Blin C, Vézinet-Brun F, Rouzioux C, Rozenbaum W, Montagnier L. Isolation of a T-lymphotropic retrovirus from a patient at risk for acquired immune deficiency syndrome (AIDS). Science 1983; 220:868–871.
2. Popovic M, Sarngadharan MG, Read E, Gallo RC. Detection and continuous production of cytopathic retroviruses (HTLV-III) from patients with AIDS and pre-AIDS. Science 1984; 224:497–500.
3. Gallo RC, Salahuddin SZ, Popovic M, Shearer GM, Kaplan M, Haynes BF, Palker TJ, Redfield R, Oleske J, Safai B, White G, Foster P, Markham PD. Frequent detection and isolation of cytopathic retroviruses (HTLV-III) from patients with AIDS and at risk of AIDS. Science 1984; 224:500–503.
4. Ratner L, Haseltine W, Patarca R, Livak KJ, Starcich B, Josephs SF, Doran ER, Rafalski JA, Whitehorn EA, Baumeister K, Ivanoff L, Petteway SR Jr, Pearson ML, Lautenberger JA, Papas TS, Ghrayeb J, Chang NT, Gallo RC, Wong-Staal F. Complete nucleotide sequence of the AIDS virus, HTLV-III. Nature 1985; 313:277–284.
5. Kohl NE, Emini EA, Schlief WA, Davis LJ, Heimbach JC, Dixon RA, Scolnick EM, Sigal IS. Active human immunodeficiency virus protease is required for viral infectivity. Proc Natl Acad Sci U S A 1988; 85:4686–4690.
6. Gottlinger HG, Sodroski JG, Haseltine WA. Role of capsid precursor processing and myristoylation in morphogenesis and infectivity of human immunodeficiency virus type 1. Proc Natl Acad Sci U S A 1989; 86:5781–5785.
7. Peng C, Ho BK, Chang TW, Chang NT. Role of human immunodeficiency virus type 1-specific protease in core protein maturation and infectivity. J Virol 1989; 63:2550–2556.
8. Toh H, Ono M, Saigo K, Miyata T, Retroviral protease-like sequence in the yeast transposon Ty 1. Nature 1985; 315:691–692.
9. Le Grice SFJ, Mills J, Mous J. Active site mutagenesis of the AIDS virus protease and its alleviation by *trans* complementation. EMBO J 1988; 7:2547–2553.
10. Darke PL, Leu C-T, Davis LJ, Heimbach JC, Diehl RE, Hill WS, Dixon RAF, Sigal IS. Human immunodeficiency protease. Bacterial expression and characterisation of the purified aspartic protease. J Biol Chem 1989; 264:2307–2312.
11. Seelmeier S, Schmidt H, Turk V, von der Helm K. Human immunodeficiency virus has an aspartic-type protease that can be inhibited by pepstatin. Proc Natl Acad Sci U S A 1988; 85:6612–6616.
12. Pettit SC, Michael SF, Swanstrom R. The specificity of HIV-1 protease. Perspect Drug Discovery Design 1993; 1:69–83.

13. Henderson LE, Benveniste RE, Sowder R, Copeland TD, Schulz AM, Oroszlan S. Molecular characterization of *gag* proteins from simian immunodeficiency virus (SIV$_{Mne}$). J Virol 1988; 62:2587–2795.

14. Martin JA. Recent advances in the design of HIV proteinase inhibitors. Antiviral Res 1992; 17:265–278.

15. Roberts NA, Martin JA, Kinchington D, Broadhurst AV, Craig JC, Duncan IB, Galpin SA, Handa BK, Kay J, Krohn A, Lambert RW, Merrett HJ, Mills JS, Parkes KEB, Redshaw S, Ritchie AJ, Taylor DL, Thomas GJ, Machin PJ. Inhibitors of HIV proteinase. Science 1990; 248:358–361.

16. Erickson J, Niedhart DJ, Vandrie J, Kempf DJ, Wang XC, Norbeck DW, Plattner JJ, Rittenhouse JW, Turon M, Wildeburg N, Kohlbrenner WE, Simmer R, Helfrich R, Paul DA, Knigge M, Design, activity, and 2.8Å crystal structure of a C$_2$ symmetric inhibitor complexed to HIV-1 protease. Science 1990; 249:527–533.

17. Kempf DJ, Norbeck DW, Codacovi L, Wang XC, Kohlbrenner WE, Widenburg NE, Paul DA, Knigge MF, Vasavanonda S, Craig-Kennard A, Saldivar A, Rosenbrook WM Jr, Clement JJ, Plattner JJ, Erickson J. Structure based C$_2$ symmetric inhibitors of HIV protease. J Med Chem 1990; 33:2687–2689.

18. Bone R, Vacca JP, Anderson PS, Holloway, MK. X-ray crystal structure of the HIV protease complex with L-700,417, an inhibitor with pseudo C$_2$ symmetry. J Am Chem Soc 1991; 113:9382–9384.

19. Kempf DJ, Codacovi L, Wang XC, Kohlbrenner WE, Wideburg NE, Saldivar A, Vasavanonda S, Marsh KC, Bryant P, Sham HL, Green BE, Betebenner DA, Erickson J, Norbeck DW. Symmetry-based inhibitors of HIV protease. Structure-activity studies of acylated 2,4-diamino-1,5-diphenyl-3-hydroxypentane and 2,5-diamino 1,6-diphenylhexane-3,4-diol. J Med Chem 1993; 36:320–330.

20. Kempf DJ, Marsh KC, Paul DA, Knigge MF, Norbeck DW, Kohlbrenner WE, Codacovi L, Vasavanonda S, Bryant P, Wang XC, Wideburg NE, Clement JJ, Plattner JJ, Erickson J. Antiviral and pharmacokinetic properties of C$_2$ symmetric inhibitors of the human immunodeficiency virus type 1 protease. Antimicrob Agents Chemother 1991; 35:2209–2214.

21. Tomasselli AG, Thaisrivongs S, Heinrikson RL. Discovery and design of HIV protease inhibitors as drugs for the treatment of AIDS. Adv Antiviral Drug Design 1996; 2:173–228.

22. Thomas GJ. The design and synthesis of inhibitors of HIV proteinase. In: Choudhary MI, ed. Biological Inhibitors. Vol. 2. Langhorne, PA: Harwood Academic Publishers, 1996:161–211.

23. Martin JA, Redshaw S, Thomas GJ. Inhibitors of HIV proteinase. In: Ellis GP, Luscombe DK, eds. Progress in Medicinal Chemistry. Vol. 32. Amsterdam: Elsevier, 1995: 239–287.

24. Meek TD. Inhibitors of HIV-1 protease. J Enz Inhib 1992; 6:65–98.

25. Debouck C. The HIV-1 protease as a therapeutic target for AIDS. AIDS Res Human Retroviruses 1992; 8:153–164.

26. Huff JR. HIV protease: a novel chemotherapeutic target for AIDS. J Med Chem 1991; 34:2305–2314.

27. Norbeck DW, Kempf DJ. HIV protease inhibitors. Ann Rep Med Chem 1991; 26:141–150.

28. Tomasselli AG, Howe WJ, Sawyer TK, Wlodawer A, Heinrikson RL. The complexities of AIDS: an assessment of the HIV protease as a therapeutic target. Chimica Oggi May 1991:6–27.

29. Sarubbi E, Nolli ML, Andronico F, Stella S, Saddler G, Selva E, Siccardi A, Denaro M. A high throughput assay for inhibitors of HIV-1 protease. FEBS Lett 1991; 279: 265–269.

30. Stella S, Saddler G, Sarubbi E, Colombo L, Stefanelli S, Denaro M, Selva E. Isolation of 1-MAPI from fermentation broths during a screening program for HIV-1 protease inhibitors. J Antibiot 1991; 44:1019–1022.

31. Kaneto R, Chiba H, Dobashi K, Kojima I, Sakai K, Shibamoto N, Nishida H, Okamoto R, Akagawa H, Mizuno S. Mer-N5075A, a potential HIV-1 protease inhibitor, produced by *Streptomyces chromofuscu*. J Antibiot 1993; 46:1622–1624.

32. Xu H-X, Zeng F-Q, Wan M, Sim K-Y. Anti-HIV triterpene acids from *Geum japonicum*. J Nat Proc 1996; 59:643–645.

33. Kusumoto IT, Nakabayashi T, Kida H, Miyashiro H, Hattori M, Namba T. Screening of various plant extracts used in Ayurvedic medicine for inhibitory effects on human immunodeficiency virus type 1 (HIV-1) protease. Phytother Res 1995; 9:180– 184.

34. Thaisrivongs S, Tomich PK, Watenpaugh KD, Chong K-T, Howe WJ, Yang C-P, Strohbach JW, Turner SR, McGrath JP, Bohanon MJ, Lynn JC, Mulichak AM, Spinelli PA, Hinshaw RR, Pagano PJ, Moon JB, Ruwart MJ, Wilkinson KF, Rush BD, Zipp GL, Dalga RJ, Schwende FJ, Howard GM, Padbury GE, Toth LN, Zhao Z, Koepelinger KA, Kakuk TJ, Cole SL, Zaya RM, Piper RC, Jeffrey P. Structure-based design of HIV protease inhibitors: 4-hydroxycoumarins and 4-hydroxy 2-pyrones as non-peptidic inhibitors. J Med Chem 1994; 37:3200–3204.

35. Tummino PJ, Ferguson D, Hupe L, Hupe D. Competitive inhibition of HIV-1 protease by 4-hydroxy-benzypyran-2-ones and by 4-hydroxy-6-phenylpyran-2-ones. Biochem Biophys Res Comm 1994; 200:1658–1664.

36. Tummino PJ, Prasad JVNV, Ferguson D, Nouhan C, Graham N, Domagala JM, Ellsworth E, Gajda C, Hagen SE, Lunney EA, Para KS, Tait BD, Pavlovsky A, Erickson JW, Gracheck S, McQuade TJ, Hupe DJ. Discovery and optimisation of non-peptide HIV-1 protease inhibitors. Bioorg Med Chem 1996; 4:1401–1410.

37. Fredenhagen A, Petersen F, Tintelnot-Blomley M, Rosel J, Mett H, Hug P. Semicochliodinol A and B: inhibitors of HIV-1 protease and EGF-R protein tyrosine kinase related to asterriquinones produced by the fungus *Chrysosporium merdarium*. J Antibiot 1997; 50:395–401.

38. Dombrowski AW, Bills GF, Sabnis G, Koupal LR, Meyer R, Ondeyka JG, Giacobbe RA, Monaghan RL, Lingham RB. L-696,474, a novel cytochalasin as an inhibitor of HIV-1 protease 1. The producing organism and its fermentaiton. J Antibiot 1992; 45: 671–678.

39. Lingham RB, Hsu A, Silverman KC, Bills GF, Dombrowski A, Goldman ME, Darke PL, Huang L, Koch G, Ondeyka JG, Goetz MA. L-696,474, a novel cytochalasin as an inhibitor of HIV-1 protease III. Biological activity. J Antibiot 1992; 45:686–691.

40. Thaisrivongs S, Skulnick HI, Turner SR, Strohbach JW, Tommasi RA, Johnson PD, Aristoff PA, Judge TM, Gammill RB, Morris JK, Romines KR, Chrusciel RA, Hinshaw RR, Chong K-T, Tarpley WG, Poppe SM, Slade DE, Lynn JC, Horng M-M, Tomich PK, Seest EP, Dolak LE, Howe WJ, Howard GM, Schwende FJ, Toth LN,

Padbury GE, Wilson GJ, Shiou L, Zipp GL, Wilkinson KF, Rush BD, Ruwart MJ, Koepelinger KA, Zhao Z, Cole S, Zaya RM, Kakuk TJ, Janakiraman MN, Watenpaugh KD. Structure-based design of HIV protease inhibitors: sulfonamide-containing 5,6-dihydro-4-hydroxy-2-pyrones as non-peptidic inhibitors. J Med Chem 1996; 39:4349–4353.

41. Poppe SM, Slade DE, Chong K-T, Hinshaw RR, Pagano PJ, Markowitz M, Ho DD, Gorman RR III, Dueweke TJ, Thaisrivongs S, Tarpley WG. Antiviral activity of the dihydropyrone PNU-140690, a new nonpeptidic human immunodeficiency virus protease inhibitor. Antimicrob Agents Chemother 1997; 41:1058–1063.

42. Prasad JVNV, Tummino PJ, Ferguson D, Saunders J, Vander Roest S, McQuade TJ, Heldsinger A, Reyner EL, Stewart BH, Guttendorf RJ, Para KS, Lunney EA, Gracheck SJ, Domagala JM. Nonpeptidic HIV protease inhibitors: 4-hydroxy-pyran-2-one inhibitors with functional tethers to P_1 phenyl ring to reach S_3 pocket of the enzyme. Biochem Biophys Res Comm 1996; 221:815–820.

43. Tomasselli AG, Hui JO, Sawyer TK, Staples DJ, Bannow C, Reardon IM, Howe WJ, DeCamp DL, Craik CS, Heinrikson RL. Specificity and inhibition of proteases from human immunodeficiency viruses 1 and 2. J Biol Chem 1990; 256:14675–14683.

44. Thaisrivongs S, Thomasselli AG, Moon JB, Hui J, McQuade TJ, Turner SR, Strohbach JW, Howe WJ, Tarpley WG, Heinrikson RL. Inhibitors of the protease from human immunodeficiency virus: design and modeling of a compound containing a dihydroxyethylene isostere insert with high binding affinity and effective antiviral activity. J Med Chem 1991; 34:2344–2356.

45. Ashorn P, McQuade TJ, Thaisrivongs S, Tomasselli AG, Tarpley WG, Moss B. An inhibitor of the protease blocks maturation of human and simian immunodeficiency viruses and spread of infection. Proc Natl Acad Sci U S A 1990; 87:7472–7476.

46. Martin LN, Soike KF, Murphey-Corb M, Bohm RP, Roberts ED, Kakuk TJ, Thaisrivongs S, Vidmar TJ, Ruwart MJ, Davio SR, Tarpley WG. Effects of U-75875, a peptidomimetic inhibitor of retroviral protease, on simian immunodeficiency virus infection in rehsus monkeys. Antimicrob Agents Chemother 1994; 38:1277–1283.

47. Vacca JP, Guare JP, deSolms SJ, Sanders WM, Giuliani EA, Young SD, Darke PL, Zugay J, Sigal IS, Schlief WA, Quintero JC, Emini EA, Anderson PS, Huff JR. L-687,908, a potent hydroxyethylene-containing HIV protease inhibitor. J Med Chem 1991; 34:1225–1228.

48. Lyle TA, Wiscount CM, Guare JP, Thompson WJ, Anderson PS, Darke PL, Zugay JA, Emini EA, Schlief WA, Quintero JC, Dixon RAF, Sigal IS, Huff JR. Benzocycloalkyl amines as novel C-termini for HIV protease inhibitors. J Med Chem 1991; 34:1228–1230.

49. Holloway MK, Wai HM, Halgren TA, Fitzgerald PMD, Vacca JP, Dorsey BD, Levin RB, Thompson WJ, Chen LJ, deSolms J, Gaffin N, Ghosh AK, Giuliani EA, Graham SL, Guare JP, Hungate RW, Lyle TA, Sanders WM, Tucker TJ, Wiggins M, Wiscount CM, Woltersdorf OW, Young SD, Darke PL, Zugay JA. A priori prediction of activity for HIV-1 protease inhibitors employing energy minimization in the active site. J Med Chem 1995; 38:305–317.

50. Dorsey BD, Levin RB, McDaniel SL, Vacca JP, Guare JP, Darke PL, Zugay JA, Emini EA, Schlief WA, Quintero JC, Lin JH, Chen I-W, Holloway MK, Fitzgerald PMD, Axel MG, Ostovic D, Anderson PS, Huff JR. L-735,524: the design of a potent and orally bioavailable HIV protease inhibitor. J Med Chem 1994; 37:3443–3451.

51. Hosur MV, Bhat N, Kempf DJ, Baldwin ET, Liu B, Gulnik S, Wideburg NE, Norbek DW, Appelt K, Erickson JW. Influence of stereochemistry on activity and binding modes for C_2 symmetry-based diol inhibitors of HIV-1 protease. J Am Chem Soc 1994; 116:847–855.

52. Kempf DJ, Marsh KC, Fino LC, Bryant P, Graig-Kennard A, Sham HL, Chen Z, Vasavanonda S, Kohlbrenner WE, Wideburg NE, Saldivar A, Green BE, Herrin T, Norbeck DW. Design of orally bioavailable, symmetry-based inhibitors of HIV protease. Bioorg Med Chem 1994; 2:847–858.

53. Kempf DJ, Marsh KC, Denissen JF, McDonald E, Vasavanonda S, Flentge CA, Green BE, Fino L, Park CH, Kong X-C, Wideburg NE, Saldivar A, Ruiz L, Kati WM, Sham HL, Robins T, Stewart KD, Hsu A, Plattner JJ, Leonard JM, Norbeck DW. ABT-538 is a potent inhibitor of human immunodeficiency virus protease and has high oral bioavailability in humans. Proc Natl Acad Sci U S A 1995; 92:2484–2488.

54. Barrish JC, Gordon E, Alam M, Lin P-F, Bisacchi BS, Chen P, Cheng PTW, Fritz AW, Greytok JA, Hermsmeier MA, Humphreys WG, Lis KA, Marella MA, Merchant Z, Mitt T, Morrison RA, Obermeier MT, Pluscec J, Skoog M, Slusarchyk WA, Spergel SH, Stevenson JM, Sun C-Q, Sundeen JE, Taunk P, Tino JA, Warrack BM, Colonno RJ, Zahler R. Aminodiol HIV protease inhibitors. 1. Design, synthesis, and preliminary SAR. J Med Chem 1994; 37:1758–1768.

55. Yu KL, Harte WE, Spinazze P, Martin JC, Mansuri MM. Synthesis of 1,3-diamino-2-hydroxypropane derivatives as pseudosymmetric HIV protease inhibitors. Bioorg Med Chem 1993; 3:535–538.

56. Moore ML, Bryan WM, Fakhoury SA, Magaard VW, Huffman WF, Dayton BD, Meek TD, Myland L, Dreyer GB, Metcalf BW, Strickler JE, Gorniak J, Debouck C. Peptide substrates and inhibitors of the HIV-1 protease. Biochem Biophys Res Comm 1989; 159:420–425.

57. Tomasseli AG, Olsen MK, Hui JO, Staples DJ, Sawyer TK, Henrikson RL, Tomich C-SC. Substrate analogue inhibition and active site titration of purified recombinant HIV-1 protease. Biochem 1990; 29:264–269.

58. Dreyer GB, Metcalf BW, Tomaszek TA Jr, Carr TA, Chandler AC III, Hyland L, Fakhoury SA, Magaard VW, Moore ML, Strickler JE, Debouk C, Meek TD. Inhibition of human immunodeficiency virus 1 protease in vitro: rational design of substrate analogue inhibitors. Proc Natl Acad Sci U S A 1989; 86:9752–9756.

59. Lamarre D, Croteau G, Wardrop E, Bourgon L, Thibeault D, Clouette C, Vaillancourt M, Cohen E, Pargellis C, Yoakim C, Anderson PC. Antiviral properties of Palinavir, a potent inhibitor of the human immunodeficiency virus type 2 protease. Antimicrob Agents Chemother 1997; 41:965–971.

60. Mimoto T, Imai J, Kisanuki S, Enomoto H, Hattori N, Akaji K, Kiso Y. Kynostatin (KNI)-227 and -272, highly potent anti-HIV agents: conformationally constrained tripeptide inhibitors of HIV protease containing allophenylnorstatine. Chem Pharmacol Bull 1992; 40:2251–2253.

61. Kageyama S, Mimoto T, Murakawa Y, Nomizu M, Ford H Jr, Shirasaka T, Gulnik S, Erickson J, Takada K, Hayashi H, Broder S, Kiso Y, Mitsuya H. In vitro anti-human immunodeficiency virus (HIV) activities of transition state mimetic HIV protease inhibitors containing allophenylnorstatine. Antimicrob Agents Chemother 1993; 37: 810–817.

62. De Lucca GV, George V, Erickson-Viitanen S, Lam PYS. Cyclic HIV protease in-

hibitors capable of displacing the active site structural water molecule. Drug Discovery Today 1997; 2:6–18.

63. Hodge CN, Aldrich PE, Bacheler LT, Chang C-H, Eyermann CJ, Garber S, Grubb M, Jackson DA, Jadhav PK, Korant B, Lam PYS, Maurin MB, Meek JL, Otto MJ, Rayner MM, Reid C, Sharpe TR, Shum L, Winslow DL, Erickson-Viitanen S. Improved cyclic urea inhibitors of the HIV-1 protease: synthesis, potency, resistance profile, human pharmacokinetics and X-ray crystal structure. Chem Biol 1996; 3: 301–314.

64. Kim CU, McGee LR, Krawczyk SH, Harwood E, Harada Y, Swaminathan S, Bischofberger N, Chen MS, Cherrington JM, Xiong SF, Griffin L, Cundy KC, Lee A, Yu B, Gulnik S, Erickson JW. New series of potent, orally bioavailable, non-peptidic cyclic sulfones as HIV-1 protease inhibitors. J Med Chem 1996; 39:3431–3434.

65. Sham HL, Zhao C, Marsh KC, Betebenner DA, Lin S, Rosenbrook W Jr, Herrin T, Li L, Madigan D, Vasavanonda S, Molla A, Saldivar A, McDonald E, Wideburg NE, Kempf D, Norbeck DW, Plattner JJ. Novel azacyclic ureas that are potent inhibitors of HIV-1 protease. Biochem Biophys Res Comm 1996; 225:436–440.

66. Kaldor SW, Stephen W, Kalish VJ, Vincent J, Davies JF II, Shetty BV, Bhasker V, Fritz JE, James E, Appelt K, Burgess JA, Jeffrey A, Campanale KM, Chirgadze NY, Clawson DK, Dressman BA, Hatch SD, Khalil DA, Kosa MB, Lubbehusen PP, Muesing MA, Patick AK, Reich SH, Su KS, Tatlock JH. Viracept (nelfinavir mesylate, AG1343): a potent, orally bioavailable inhibitor of HIV-1 protease. J Med Chem 1997; 40:3979–3985.

67. Kim EE, Baker CT, Dwyer MD, Murcko MA, Rao BG, Tung RD, Navia MA. Crystal structure of HIV-1 protease in complex with VX-478, a potent and orally bioavailable inhibitor of the enzyme. J Am Chem Soc 1995; 117:1181–1182.

68. Painter GR, Ching S, Reynolds D, St Clair M, Sadler BM, Elkins M, Blum R, Dornsife R, Livingston DJ, Partaledis JA, Pazhanisamy S, Tung RD, Tisdale M. 141W94. Anti-HIV. VX-478. KVX-478. Drugs Future 1996; 21:347–350.

69. Kitchen VS, Skinner C, Ariyoshi K, Lane EA, Duncan IB, Burckhardt J, Burger HU, Bragman K, Pinching AJ, Weber JN. Safety and activity of saquinavir in HIV infection. Lancet 1995; 345:952–955.

70. Danner SA, Carr A, Leonard JM, Lehman LM, Gudiol F, Gonzales J, Raventos A, Rubio R, Bouza E, Pintado V, Aguado AG, Garcia de Lomas J, Delgado R, Borleffs JCC, Valdes JM, Boucher CAB, Cooper DA. A short-term study of the safety, pharmacokinetics, and efficacy of ritonavir, an inhibitor of HIV-1 protease. N Engl J Med 1995; 333;1528–1533.

71. Markowitz M, Saag M, Powderly WG, Hurley AM, Hsu A, Valdes JM, Henry D, Sattler F, La Marca A, Leonard JM, Ho DD. A preliminary study of ritonavir, an inhibitor of HIV-1 protease, to treat HIV-1 infection. N Engl J Med 1995; 333:1534–1539.

72. Stein D, Fish DG, Bilello JA, Preston SL, Martineau GL, Drusano GL. A 24-week open-label phase I/II evaluation of the HIV protease inhibitor MK-639 (indinavir). AIDS (London) 1996; 10:485–492.

73. Moyle GJ, Youle M, Higgs C, Monaghan J, Peterkin J, Chapman S, Nelson M. Extended follow-up of safety and efficacy of Agouron's HIV proteinase inhibitor AG1343 (Viracept) in virological responders from the UK phase I/II dose finding

study. 11th International Conference on AIDS, Vancouver, Canada, Jul 7–12, 1996; Abstr Mo B 173.

74. Schapiro JM, Wimters MA, Steart F, Efron B, Norris J, Kozal MJ, Merigan TC. The effect of high-dose saquinavir on viral load and CD4+ T-cell counts in HIV-infected patients. Ann Int Med 1996; 124:1039–1050.

75. Hicks CB, Lehman L, Eron HJ, Jemsek J, Kelly N, Leonard J. Safety and efficacy of ritonavir administered at two potentially maximum tolerated doses. 11th International Conference on AIDS, Vancouver, Canada, Jul 7–12, 1996; Abstr Mo B 415.

76. Steigbigel R, Berry P, Teppler H, Mellors J, Drusano G, Leavitt R, Hildebrand C, Jonas L, Nessly M, Deutsch P, Chodakewitz J. Extended follow-up of patients in a study of indinavir at 800 mg q8h (2.4 g/d), 1000 mg q8h (3.0 g/d) and 800 mg q6h (3.2 g/d). 11th International Conference on AIDS, Vancouver, Canada, Jul 7–12, 1996; Abstr Mo B 412.

77. Conant M, Markowitz M, Hurley A, Ho D, Peterkin J, Chapman S. A randomised phase II dose range-finding study of the HIV protease inhibitor Viracept as monotherapy in HIV positive patients. 11th International Conference on AIDS, Vancouver, Canada, Jul 7–12, 1996; Abstr Tu B 2129.

78. Collier AC, Coombs RW, Schoenfeld DA, Bassett RL, Timpone J, Baruch A, Jones M, Facey K, Whitacre C, McAuliffe VJ, Friedman HM, Merigan TC, Reichman RC, Hooper C, Corey L. Treatment of human immunodeficiency virus infection with saquinavir, zidovudine, and zalcitabine. N Engl J Med 1996; 334:1011–7.

79. Rutschmann OT, Kaiser L, Gabriel V, Fathi M, Perrin L, Hirschel B. Adding saquinavir to d4T in advanced HIV infection. 11th International Conference on AIDS, Vancouver, Canada, Jul 7–12, 1996; Abstr Th B 945.

80. Markowitz M, Cao Y, Hurley A, O'Donovan R, Heath-Chiozzi M, Leonard J, Smiley L, Keller A, Johnson D, Johnson P, Ho DD. Triple therapy with AZT, 3TC, and ritonavir in 12 subjects newly infected with HIV-1. 11th International Conference on AIDS, Vancouver, Canada, Jul 7–12, 1996; Abstr Th B 933.

81. Mathez D, Bagnarelli P, De Truchis P, Gorin I, Katlama C, Pialoux G, Ruggeri C, Saimot AG, Tubiana R, Chauvin JP, Clementi M, Leibowitch J. A triple combination of ritonavir + AZT + ddC as a first line treatment of patients with AIDS: update. 11th International Conference on AIDS, Vancouver, Canada, Jul 7–12, 1996; Abstr Mo B 175.

82. Gathe J Jr, Burkhardt B, Hawley P, Conant M, Peterkin J, Chapman S. A randomised phase II study of Viracept, a novel HIV protease inhibitor, used in combination with stavudine (d4T) vs. stavudine (d4T) alone. 11th International Conference on AIDS, Vancouver, Canada, Jul 7–12, 1996; Abstr Mo B 413.

83. Markowitz M, Cao Y, Hurley A, O'Donovan R, Peterkin J, Anderson B, Smiley L, Keller A, Johnson P, Johnson D, Ho DD. Triple therapy with AZT and 3TC in combination with nelfinavir mesylate in 12 antiretroviral-naive subjects chronically infected with HIV-1. 11th International Conference on AIDS, Vancouver, Canada, Jul 7–12, 1996; Abstr LB B 6031.

84. Workman C, Downie J, Sutherland D, Smith DE, Dyer W, Shen J, Sullivan J. Rapid viral load decrease in primary infection associated with aggressive therapy. 11th International Conference on AIDS, Vancouver, Canada, Jul 7–12, 1996; Abstr LB B 6021.

85. Lalezari J, Haubrich R, Burger HU, Beattie D, Donatacci L, Salpo MP, NV14256 Study Team. Improved survival and decreased progression of HIV in patients treated with saquinavir (Invirase, SQV) plus Hivid (zalcitabine, ddC). 11th International Conference on AIDS, Vancouver, Canada, Jul 7–12, 1996; Abstr LB B 6033.
86. James JS. Saquinavir: major study shows survival benefit in treatment-naive patients. AIDS Treat News 1997; 274:6.
87. Cameron DW, Heath-Chiozzi M, Kravcik S, Mills R, Potthoff A, Henry D, the Advanced HIV Ritonavir Study Group, Leonard J. Prolongation of life and prevention of AIDS Complications in advanced HIV immunodeficiency with ritonavir: an update. 11th International Conference on AIDS, Vancouver, Canada, Jul 7–12, 1996; Abstr Mo B 411.
88. Hammer SM, Squires KE, Hughes MD, Grimes JM, Demeter LM, Currier JS, Eron JJ, Feinberg JE, Balfour HH, Deyton LR, Chodakewitz JA, Fischl MA. A controlled trial of two nucleoside analogs plus indinavir in persons with human immunodeficiency virus infection and CD4 cell counts of 200 per cubic millimeter or less. N Engl J Med 1997; 337:725–733.
89. Baker R. 3-Drug therapy reduces death and new AIDS-related illnesses by 50%. BETA 1997; Mar 3–4.
90. Workman C, Lewis C, Smith DO. Resolution of Kaposi's sarcoma associated with saquinavir therapy—case report. 11th International Conference on AIDS, Vancouver, Canada, Jul 7–12, 1996; Abstr Tu B 2217.
91. Conant MA, Opp KM, Poretz D, Mills RG. Reduction of Kaposi's sarcoma lesions following treatment of AIDS with ritonovir [letter]. AIDS 1997; 11:1300–1301.
92. Murphy M, Armstrong D, Sepkowitz KA, Ahkami RN, Myskowski PL. Regression of AIDS-related Kaposi's sarcoma following treatment with an HIV-1 protease inhibitor [letter]. AIDS 1997; 11:261–262.
93. Burdick AE, Carmichael C, Rady PL, Tyring SK, Badiavas E. Resolution of Kaposi's sarcoma associated with undetectable level of human herpes virus 8 DNA in a patient with AIDS after protease inhibitor therapy. J Am Acad Dermatol 1997; 37:648–649.
94. Zingman BS. Resolution of refractory AIDS-related mucosal candidiasis after initiation of didanosine plus saquinavir. N Engl J Med 1996; 334:1674–1675.
95. Reed JB, Schwab IR, Gordon J, Morse LS. Regression of cytomegalovirus retinitis associated with protease-inhibitor treatment in patients with AIDS. Am J Ophthalmol 1997; 124:199–205.
96. Perelson S, Neumann AU, Markowitz M, Leonard JM, Ho D. HIV-1 dynamics in vivo: virion clearance rate, infected cell life-span, and viral generation time. Science 1996; 271:1582–1586.
97. Coffin M. HIV population dynamics in vivo: implications for genetic variation, pathogenesis, and therapy. Science 1995; 267:483–489.
98. Vella S, Galluzzo C, Giannini G, Pirillo MF, Duncan I, Jacobsen H, Andreoni M, Sarmati L, Ercoli L. Saquinavir/zidovudine combination in patients with advanced HIV infection and no prior antiretroviral therapy: CD4+ lymphocyte/plasma RNA changes, and emergence of HIV strains with reduced phenotypic sensitivity. Antiviral Res 1996; 29:91–93.
99. Jacobsen H, Haenggi M, Ott M, Duncan IB, Andreoni M, Vella S, Mous J. Reduced sensitivity to saquinavir: an update on genotyping from phase I/II trials. Antiviral Res 1996; 29:95–97.

100. Jacobsen H, Haenggi M, Ott M, Duncan IB, Owen S, Andreoni M, Vella S, Mous J. In vivo resistance to a human immunodeficiency virus type 1 proteinase inhibitor: mutations, kinetics, and frequencies. J Infect Dis 1996; 173:1379–1387.

101. Ives KJ, Jacobsen H, Galpin SA, Garaev MM, Dorrell L, Mous J, Bragman K, Weber JN. Emergence of resistant variants of HIV in vivo during monotherapy with the proteinase inhibitor saquinavir. J Antimicrob Chemother 1997; 39:771–779.

102. Molla A, Korneyeva M, Gao Q, Vasavanonda S, Schipper PJ, Mo H-M, Markowitz M, Chernyavskiy T, Niu P, Lyons N, Hsu A, Grannemen GR, Ho DD, Boucher CAB, Leonard JM, Norbeek DW, Kempf DJ. Ordered accumulation of mutations in HIV protease confers resistance to ritonavir. Nat Med 1996; 2:760–766.

103. Condra JH, Schleif WA, Blahy OM, Gabryelski LJ, Graham DJ, Quintero JC, Rhodes A, Robbins HL, Roth E, Shivaprakash M, Titus D, Yang T, Teppler H, Squires KE, Deutsch PJ, Emini EA. In vivo emergence of HIV-1 variants resistant to multiple protease inhibitors. Nature 1995; 374:569–571.

104. Condra JH, Holder DJ, Schleif WA, Blahy OM, Danovich RM, Gabryelski LJ, Graham DJ, Laird D, Quintero JC, Rhodes A, Robbins HL, Roth E, Shivaprakash M, Yang T, Chodakewitz JA, Deutsch PJ, Leavitt RY, Massari FE, Mellors JW, Squires KE, Steigbigel RT, Teppler H, Emini EA. Genetic correlates of in vivo viral resistance to indinavir, a human immunodeficiency virus type 1 protease inhibitor. J Virol 1996; 70:8270–8276.

105. Patick AK, Duran M, Cao Y, Ho T, Pei Z, Keller MR, Peterkin J, Chapman S, Anderson B, Ho D, Markowitz M. Genotypic and phenotypic characterization of HIV-1 variance isolated from in vitro selection studies and from patients treated with the protease inhibitor, nelfinavir. 5th International Workshop on HIV Drugs Resistance, Whistler, Canada, Jul 3–6, 1996; Abstr 29.

106. Tisdale M, Myers RE, Maschera B, Parry NR, Oliver NM, Blair ED. Cross-resistance analysis of human immunodeficiency virus type 1 variants individually selected for resistance to five different protease inhibitors. Antimicrob Agents Chemother 1995; 39:1704–1710.

107. St Clair MH, Millard J, Rooney J, Tisdale M, Parry N, Sadler BM, Blum MR, Painter G. In vitro antiviral activity of 141W94 (VX-478) in combination with other antiretroviral agents. Antiviral Res 1996; 29:53–56.

108. Schmit JC, Ruiz L, Clotet B, Raventos A, Tor J, Leonard J, Desmyter J, De Clercq E, Vandamme AM. Resistance-related mutations in the HIV-1 protease gene of patients treated for 1 year with the protease inhibitor ritonavir (ABT-538). AIDS 1996; 10:995–999.

109. Craig JC, Duncan IB, Gilbert S, Jacobsen H, Jupp R, Moffatt A, Race E, Roberts NA, Mills JS, Mous J, Sheldon J, Tomlinson PW, Whittaker LN. Treatment with saquinavir (Invirase) should leave the majority of patients with the option to use other HIV proteinase inhibitors. 5th International Workshop on HIV Drug Resistance, Whistler, Canada, Jul 3–6, 1996; Abstr 32.

110. Boucher C. Rational approaches to resistance: using saquinavir. AIDS 1996; 10:S15–S19.

111. Croteau G, Doyon L, Thibeault D, McKercher G, Pilote L, Lamarre D. Impaired fitness of human immunodeficiency virus type 1 variants with high-level resistance to protease inhibitors. J Virol 1997; 71:1089–1096.

112. Ercoli L, Sarmati L, Nicastri E, Giannini G, Galluzzo C, Vella S, Andreoni M. HIV

phenotype switching during antiretroviral therapy: emergence of saquinavir-resistant strains with less cytopathogenicity. AIDS 1997; 11:1211–1217.
113. Nijhuis M, Schuurman R, Boucher CAB. Homologous recombination for rapid phenotyping of HIV. Curr Opin Infect Dis 1997; 10:475–479.
114. Nadler JP. Early initiation of antiretroviral therapy for infection with human immunodeficiency virus: considerations in 1996. Clin Infect Dis 1996; 23:227–230.

6

HIV Vaccine Research

Patricia E. Fast
Aviron, Mountain View, California

Alan M. Schultz
International AIDS Vaccine Initiative, New York, New York

I. HISTORICAL OVERVIEW

A. The Need for a Vaccine

When human immunodeficiency virus (HIV) was identified as the cause of acquired immunodeficiency syndrome (AIDS) in 1983 (1–3), it seemed that a vaccine to stop the spread of HIV was almost within reach. The need for a vaccine
was well recognized; other viral vaccines have been used to eradicate or control
diseases that formerly killed or harmed many thousands of children and adults
yearly. Soon, however, significant obstacles to HIV vaccine development were
noted (4–7). During the past decade, despite alternating optimism and pessimism
about the chances for controlling HIV through vaccination, there has been great
progress both in developing and testing candidate HIV vaccines and in understanding the challenges that will face development of an HIV vaccine. Vaccine research has been guided by a few dominant paradigms that have profoundly influenced the choices of vaccine antigens, presentation methods and immune
measurements, and animal models for the testing of efficacy. This chapter examines those paradigms and the work that supports or refutes them.

This chapter was written in part while the authors were at the Division of AIDS, National Institute of
Allergy and Infectious Diseases, National Institutes of Health, Bethesda, Maryland.

B. The Initial Concept: Antibody as a Means to Achieve Sterilizing Immunity

Immune responses against HIV, both humoral and cellular, were recognized early in the epidemic (8–12). Natural history studies of HIV infection showed that these responses are incapable of clearing or totally containing HIV infection, although a relatively few long-term nonprogressors have remained disease-free for up to 20 years without treatment (13,14). Long-term health in the face of HIV infection may be determined by the genetics of host or virus, or by immune responses of the host.

Vaccination against infectious diseases is generally thought to be best accomplished by duplicating the immune responses of those who have recovered from infection with a pathogen. The possibility that infection of a small number of cells could occur and be cleared without seroconversion or establishment of a permanent infection in the host was not initially considered. This logic led to pessimism about the possible success of a vaccine.

The first decade of HIV vaccine development addressed these concerns by aiming for a vaccine that would prevent AIDS by completely preventing infection. The paradigm of sterilizing immunity requires that antibody be able to neutralize HIV at the time of exposure, and therefore viral envelope was thought to be the critical antigen. Passively administered antibodies can protect animals against infection (by an intravenous route) provided that they can neutralize the challenge virus (15–17). Rare monoclonal antibodies can neutralize a significant fraction of primary HIV primary viruses, demonstrating that individual immunoglobulin G (IgG) molecules with sufficient avidity can prevent attachment and infection (18). However, neither HIV-infected humans and chimpanzees nor macaques infected with virulent or attenuated simian immunodeficiency virus (SIV) frequently produce broadly neutralizing antibody.

Human immunodeficiency virus is difficult to neutralize. Unlike many other viruses, HIV antisera are judged strong if they reduce the titer of 10 to 100 infectious virions by 90%. Therefore, the breadth of the spectrum of variants that would be neutralized was a strong concern (18,19). Even in HIV-infected individuals, the neutralizing antibodies seem to lag behind the continuous evolution of the virus (20). Early attempts to induce neutralizing antibodies were made with synthetic envelope peptides (21), recombinant vaccinia (22), and subunit proteins (23). The most effective antibodies raised in small animals and primates against HIV-1 were induced by envelope protein vaccines. Mammalian cell expression systems have produced better immunogens for neutralizing antibody against laboratory strains than yeast or insect cell expression systems (24). The ability of recombinant HIV gp120 produced in mammalian cells to bind to broadly neutralizing antibodies from infected patient sera provided evidence that gp120 was an important target for neutralizing antibodies (25). Eventually, phase 1 and 2 human trials evaluated recombinant products based on HIV envelope and expressed in yeast, insect, and mammalian cells (26–28). Like smaller animals and nonhuman primates, human volunteers produced neutralizing antibodies, but the antibodies were low in titer compared with sera from individuals with chronic HIV infection, and they were relatively short-lived (24,29–32).

To examine the reaction of the vaccine-induced antibodies with the HIV encountered in the community, recent isolates of HIV were used to test neutralization by the sera of immunized volunteers. It became clear that strains of HIV adapted for growth in T-cell lines, such as IIIB, MN, and SF2, on which early vaccine candidates were based, were substantially different from primary isolates of HIV with limited in vitro passage in peripheral blood mononuclear cells (PBMC). After long passage in vitro, the laboratory strains exhibit prominent and immunodominant V3 regions (33,34) and tend to be more susceptible to neutralization (35) compared to primary HIV strains. The sera from vaccinated volunteers do not neutralize primary HIV isolates effectively (27,36–38), although more sensitive methods can detect some neutralization of primary isolates (39,40). Even though the relationship of in vitro neutralization to protection is uncertain, the inability to demonstrate cross-neutralization between the sera of immunized volunteers and HIV strains currently circulating in the community led to concern about the protective value of these neutralizing antibodies. A WHO-sponsored systematic study of biological and immunological properties of HIV-1 subtypes isolated in different parts of the world was able to generate well-characterized materials and methods for further vaccine studies, but did not reveal any common principle that could be used to overcome the intrinsic problem of HIV-1 variation for developing a broadly protective vaccine (40a–g).

Several approaches are being used to improve the quality of antibodies induced. Some have assumed that the difference between primary isolates and laboratory strains relates to the presence or absence of specific antigenic structures or epitopes on the envelope protein, leading to the postulate that the best immunogens would be envelopes from primary isolates of HIV. Recently, envelope vaccines have been modified to contain recombinant gp120 based on primary isolates, and vaccines containing these isolates have entered large-scale clinical trials (41). Whether recombinants based on primary isolates induce broader or stronger neutralizing antibodies should soon be determined.

Perhaps using the native three-dimensional structure of gp120 (42) or the trimeric complex of gp120 and gp41 that is thought to comprise the glycoprotein spike will induce more effective neutralizing antibodies (43). However, in primates, current so-called "oligomeric" gp140 constructs may not consistently induce significantly better neutralizing antibodies or protection than the corresponding gp120 proteins (44,45). Either these constructs do not express "native" structures, or, alternatively, the hypothesis that "native" conformations automatically induce broadly neutralizing antibody may be flawed. Live recombinant vectors or DNA, which should allow for synthesis and assembly of native structures in the cell, have induced low antibody titers, and there is little indication that they have induced particularly broad neutralizing properties. Complexing the envelope protein with receptors on a cell surface can reveal a structure that is critical for infection, vulnerable to neutralizing antibody, and conserved in a wide spectrum of HIV strains (46). If this immunization strategy can be used in primates and eventually be adapted to make a safe vaccine for humans that is feasible to manufacture, then it holds great hope.

The high carbohydrate content of HIV gp120 led to the suggestion that shielding of the polypeptide backbone interfered with developing effective neutralizing antibodies. Recent results with SIV suggest that deletion of carbohydrate attachment sites greatly improves the titer of homologous neutralizing antibody (47). By removing immunodominant variable regions, antibodies may be directed toward conserved regions. Whether the remaining conserved structures could represent effective neutralization epitopes is under investigation.

C. A New Paradigm: Limiting or Clearing HIV Infection Through Cell-Mediated Immunity

The first decade of vaccine development had been aiming for complete prevention of infection. Currently, AIDS vaccine researchers recognize a more standard paradigm for vaccines, that is, that an immunized person who then becomes infected will be able to recover from infection. It is rare for any viral vaccine to induce "sterilizing" immunity. Other viral vaccines shift the balance between the host immune system and the pathogenic virus, allowing the immune response to occur more rapidly so that infection, it if occurs in vaccinated individuals, is quickly controlled.

Several independent observations support the concept that prior immunity might allow humans to control incipient HIV infection. First, demonstration of the high rate of HIV production and destruction in vivo has emphasized the effectiveness of the human immune response against this virus. Billions of HIV virions are cleared from the body on a daily basis (48,49). Instead of being weak and ineffectual, the immune system usually severely limits HIV replication within days or weeks of initial infection, and the immune response nearly controls HIV replication for several years (50). With vaccination, the balance might be tipped against HIV.

Second, primate experiments have demonstrated some clinical benefit of prior vaccination against even a highly pathogenic challenge virus. Macaque monkeys that were immunized with live recombinant vaccinia containing SIV env and boosted with env protein had fewer PBMCs infected with SIV after challenge than unimmunized, challenged, macaques (51). Including gag-pol as well as env in the vector and boosting with inactivated SIV left some macaques disease-free for years. SIV could not be isolated from their PBMC, even though polymerase chain reaction (PCR) continued to detect the challenge virus (52,53). Live attenuated SIV can protect against infection or modify disease caused by a chimera of HIV and SIV (SHIV) bearing an HIV envelope (50,54,55), presumably by inducing T-cell responses against gag, pol, and/or accessory proteins.

Genital exposure can apparently lead to self-limiting infection even in naive, unvaccinated animals. Both vaginally in macaques (56,57) and by way of the cervical os in chimpanzees (58), low-dose virus exposure has led to the transient presence of circulating PCR-positive PBMCs. These animals did not produce antibodies (seroconvert) and virus could not be isolated. Apparently, some cells became infected, but the infection was not sustained. If low-dose exposure without establishing infection also occurs in humans, it may occasionally act as a vaccine to create a protective state.

Epidemiological evidence has been gradually accumulating that some individuals remain uninfected with HIV, as judged by serological testing, despite extensive high-risk behavior (59,60). It appears that most are genetically capable of being infected by HIV. Perhaps such individuals have cell-mediated or nonspecific immune responses that are protective and thus hold clues to how an effective HIV vaccine would act. HIV-specific cellular immune responses have been detected in some of these individuals (61–63), suggesting that they have become transiently infected. However, it is difficult to draw definitive conclusions about correlates of immune protection from studying such exposed but uninfected populations. In addition, the appearance of $CD8^+$ cytotoxic T lymphocytes (CTLs) in the circulation often precedes a decrease in virus load. Depletion of $CD8^+$ cells in macaques greatly diminishes the ability of the animals to limit SIV replication (64–66). When HIV or SIV load increases, it sometimes coincides with the development of an escape mutant that is not a target for the predominant CTL clones (67–69).

T cells, specifically $CD8^+$ CTL, can recognize a broad spectrum of HIV strains (70,71). CTL epitopes are short linear arrays of amino acids, in contrast to some antibody epitopes that depend upon protein folding; therefore, many are conserved throughout all or most strains of HIV. Cytotoxic responses can be measured against not only env but also gag, pol, and accessory gene proteins. Both the gag- and pol-encoded proteins are more conserved than the env gene. This cross-reactivity extends across clades, not only in infected people (40a–g,71,72) but also in volunteers immunized with recombinant poxvirus vectors. CTL studies with vaccine volunteers in the United States showed killing of targets expressing HIV from clades A–F (73). In addition, $CD8^+$ CTL can lyse not only on the basis of conserved epitopes but also with epitopes mismatched in one or even two amino acids (70).

The simplest approach to obtaining breadth in the T-cell responses to vaccine candidates has been to provide genes encoding multiple polypeptides in recombinant vectors or DNA to achieve efficient CTL induction by antigens synthesized endogenously by host cells. Recognition is dependent upon major histocompatibility complex (MHC) molecules; CTL with a particular MHC genotype will recognize only certain epitopes. Inclusion of more gene products into the vaccine is the most practical way to increase the chances that all vaccinated individuals will be able to respond to the vaccine. Small proteins encoded by accessory genes such as nef and rev have also been shown to contain CTL epitopes (74–78). Including such proteins in a vaccine candidate has the theoretical advantage that these early proteins may mark the infected cell for destruction by CTL before any virus progeny emerge.

In the SIV/macaque model, when a vaccine capable of inducing CTL shows protection, detectable CTL activity is often neither necessary nor sufficient for protection in individual primates (79–84). The assay is technically difficult, and sampling only circulating cells may underestimate the immune response. Nevertheless, some studies do show a correlation between CTL induction and protection. For example, macaques were immunized with recombinant vaccinia that expressed only nef. Nef-specific CTL precursor frequency was inversely correlated with the quantity of detectable virus after challenge with a lethal dose of SIV; the macaque with the highest precursor frequency was not infected (85). In another study, macaques were immunized with recombinant vaccinia expressing env and boosted with env protein, inducing both neutralizing antibody and anti-env CTL activity (86). When challenged, the animals were protected in apparently "sterile" fashion; with no challenge, virus was detected by isolation or by PCR. Nonetheless, in one macaque, anti-gag CTL developed after challenge, suggesting that subclinical infection had occurred. The CTL against gag and other proteins lacking in the vaccine, arising de novo after challenge, may have contributed to protection.

The data confirm that cytotoxic responses can be cross-reactive against a wide variety of HIV. Animal models and natural history studies suggest that T-cell mediated immunity plays an important role in protection against lentiviruses. Evidence that vaccine-induced CTL responses will be protective against HIV will not be definitive until an efficacy trial of a CTL-inducing vaccine has been conducted. A canarypox vector carrying multiple HIV proteins is currently in phase 2 testing.

D. T-Cell Activities Other Than Cell Killing

Noncytolytic suppression of HIV and SIV by $CD8^+$ cells has been known for a long time (87,88), but little progress has been made in exploiting this observation for vaccine design. Although this suppressor activity can be found in MHC-restricted cytotoxic cells, noncytolytic suppressor cells can be effective against HIV replication in MHC-mismatched cells (89). Chemokines can block the interaction of HIV with its coreceptors and thus block infection. These effector molecules are elaborated by both $CD4^+$ and $CD8^+$ T cells, and may at times be induced by a specific immune interaction (and therefore be produced in larger quantities by vaccinated individuals on initial contact with the virus). Protection against rectal challenge with SIV, induced by a subunit vaccine targeted to lymph nodes, has been linked to chemokine secretion assessed after nonspecific stimulation with phytohemagglutinin (PHA) (90). A similar activity has been found in a long-term nonprogressing HIV-infected human (91).

T-cell help, usually assessed by antigen-specific lymphoproliferation, is essential for the development of effector responses. Most HIV vaccine candidates induce lymphoproliferative responses in humans, which may arise within weeks and last at least 1 to 2 years (92). These responses have been considered less important than CTL and neutralization, but recent studies of long-term nonprogressors and patients who initiate triple-drug therapy during acute infection suggest that maintaining T-cell help is important if HIV is to be contained (93). Studies of immunity to human cytomegalovirus in recipients of bone marrow transplants, likewise, show that $CD4^+$ help is critical for maintenance of $CD8^+$ CTL and for preventing disease (94).

Refinement of proliferation assays, through quantitation of cytokines that are produced in response to the antigen stimulation, allows for distinction between T-helper 1 and T-helper 2 classes of cells (95,96). It remains to be seen how important this aspect of immunity will prove to be.

E. Defense at the Portal of Entry

Because HIV is spread primarily by sexual contact, across mucosal surfaces, specific mucosal or regional immunity may be required for a successful HIV vaccine. At one time, there was concern that mucosal transmission would be a particular problem for protection (97). Subsequent experiments in primates have shown that vaccination can prevent mucosal transmission of SIV in macaques (56,98,99) and of HIV in chimpanzees (58). Even a vaccine that failed to protect against intravenous challenge was partially protective against rectal challenge (100).

HIV or SIV infection induces mucosal immune responses, including HIV-specific secretory IgA antibodies (multimeric IgA antibodies that are actively transported to the mucosal surface). Serum IgG antibodies passively leak through the mucosal barrier (transudate) from serum or plasma to the mucosal surface. In addition, SIV- specific T cells can be found in the submucosal tissues and in regional draining lymph nodes (57,101,102). Immunization can also induce such responses in macaques (56,103–105). Such responses may be correlated with resistance to infection.

Secretory IgA antibodies would have the same limitations in breadth of neutralization as IgG. However, the range of envelope molecules bound by IgG antibodies is much broader than the range of HIV variants neutralized. It is possible that surface IgA could be effective against HIV by binding without requiring neutralization. On the other hand, IgA theoretically could facilitate HIV entry via the M cells. However, rotavirus infection in mice can be cleared by treatment with a nonneutralizing monoclonal antibody that may block viral assembly (106) and there is in vitro evidence for a similar phenomenon in HIV (107).

Is there an effective cellular mucosal response? If HIV simply crosses the mucosal barrier and enters into the circulation, then immune responses to defend cells in these tissues could be induced by whole-body vaccination strategies. However, there may be a role for specific mucosal immunity in the local tissues below the mucosa and in the draining lymph nodes, before infection spreads. Infected primates have CTL in the vaginal submucosa and lamina propria of the gut as well as in the circulation (102). The CTL or other immune cells may reside in the mucosal tissues without being detectable in the blood. Live attenuated retrovirus, recombinant poxvirus, or regional immunization with nonliving vaccines can protect against SIV infection after an intravaginal or intrarectal challenge (90,98–100, 108–110).

Mucosal or regional immunity might consist of three kinds of responses: antibodies that are secreted locally or transudated from serum, specific T-cell responses occurring in the mucosal or submucosal tissues, and T-cell responses occurring in the draining lymph nodes, where virus would first encounter organized lymphoid tissue.

Secretory antibody responses to HIV antigens have been measured in HIV-infected individuals, particularly in semen and cervicovaginal secretions. Both IgG and secretory IgA antibodies can be found in genital secretions (111–113). The relationship of local antibodies to infectious virus in these secretions may prove to be difficult to interpret, because local HIV replication might stimulate additional antibody secretion, whereas the antibodies could serve to neutralize the virus.

Secretory immune responses induced by HIV vaccines are beginning to be assessed in human volunteers (114), and mucosal administration of particulate peptide and of particle and vectored vaccines is currently underway (Table 1). In primates, low-dose infection with pathogenic SIV in the colon of macaques can lead to the induction of SIV-specific CTL in the lamina propria of the gut; no CTLs were detected in the blood. When subsequently challenged rectally with doses of the same SIV sufficient to establish persistent infection, the macaques with local CTL were protected from infection, and the macaques that had failed to produce measurable CTL activity in the lamina propria became productively infected (103).

These results give some independent experimental credence to the possibility that protective immune responses could occur in exposed but uninfected humans. Efficient immunization of this local compartment might best be accomplished through a specific mucosal vaccination regimen (56,105).

F. Goals of Immunization

Induction of broad, highly effective neutralizing antibody in the blood could theoretically prevent infection by either parenteral or mucosal exposure. Passive immunization experiments in primates show that antibody that neutralizes the challenge virus can prevent HIV infection in chimpanzees if it is present at the time of challenge (15,16,115). Likewise, the relatively low proportion (about one fourth)

Table 1 AIDS Vaccine Candidates in Clinical Trials

Vaccine candidate	Expression system/ production method	HIV strains	Adjuvant or delivery system
Subunits			
rgp160	Baculovirus/insect cell	LAI	Alum
rgp 160	Vaccinia/monkey kidney cell	IIIB	Alum + DOC
rgp 160	Vaccinia/monkey kidney cell	MN	Alum + DOC
rgp 160	Vaccinia/mammalian cell	MN/LAI	Alum or IFA
rgp 160	Vaccinia/mammalian cell	LAI	IFA
rgp120 (Env 2-3)	Yeast	SF2	MF59+/-MTP-PE
rgp 120	Chinese hamster ovary cells	SF2	MF59+/-MTP-PE, others
rgp 120 (bivalent)	Chinese hamster ovary cells	SF2/Primary Clade E	MF59
rgp 120	Chinese hamster ovary cells	IIIB	Alum
rgp 120	Chinese hamster ovary cells	MN	Alum, QS21, QS21 + alum
rgp 120	Chinese hamster ovary cells	MN-like	QS21 + MPL, alum
rgp 120 (bivalent)	Chinese hamster ovary cells	MN/Primary Clade B	Alum
rgp 120 (bivalent)	Chinese hamster ovary cells	MN/Primary Clade E	Alum
rp24	Baculovirus/insect	LAI	Alum
rp24	Yeast	SF2	MF59

Table 1 Continued

Vaccine candidate	Expression system/ production method	HIV strains	Adjuvant or delivery system
Peptides			
V3 peptide	Synthetic peptide	MN	Alum or IFA
V3 peptide (RP400c)	Synthetic	MN	Alum
Mixed env peptides	Synthetic peptides	LAI	IFA
V3-MAPS	Synthetic	MN	Alum/microparticulate
V3-MAPS	Synthetic	15 strains/5 clades	Alum
V3-PPD	V3 peptide coupled to PPDC	MN	
V3-PPD	V3 peptide coupled to PPDC	5 strains	
V3-Toxin A	V3 peptide coupled to PPDC *Pseudomonas aeruginosa* toxin A	MN	None
V3 peptide coupled to *Mycobacterium* protein	Synthetic	MN	10K *Mycobacterium* protein
p24-V3 peptide (CLTB-36)	Synthetic chimeric	MN	Alum
C4-V3 peptides	Synthetic chimeric	MN, RF, CAN0, EV91	IFA
Recombinant V3 sequences in single peptide	*Escherichia coli*	Multiple Clade B	?
HGP-30	Synthetic p17 peptide	SF2	Alum
Lipopeptides	Synthetic (nef, gag, env)		± QS21
Particles			
p17/p24:Ty-VLP	Portion of p17/p24 + yeast transposon product	LAI	Alum/none
V3:Ty-VLP	V3-peptide + yeast transposon	LAI	Alum/none
Whole inactivated HIV-1, envelope depleted	Inactivated with betapropiolactone and γ-irradiation	HZ321	IFA

	Preparation	HIV strain	Adjuvant
Whole inactivated HIV-1, RNA depleted	Stabilized with formaldehyde		*Corynebacterium* extract Protein 40 and calcium phosphate
Recombinant viral vector			
Vaccinia-gp 160 (HIVAC-le)	Recombinant vaccinia	LAI	
Vaccinia-gp 160	Recombinant vaccinia	LAI	
Vaccinia-HIV-1 env, gag, pol (TBC-3B)	Recombinant vaccinia	LAI	
CP-gp 160 (vCP125)	Recombinant canarypox	MN	
CP-env, gag, protease (vCP205)	Recombinant canarypox	MN/LAI	
CP-env, gag, protease and other pol epitopes, nef epitopes (vCP300, vCP1433, vCP1452)	Recombinant canarypox	MN/LAI	
DNA			
gp 160 + revDNA	Plasmid	MN	Bupivacaine
gag + pol DNA	Plasmid	LAI	Bupivacaine
Retroviral vectors			
MoMLV-HIV-1 env, rev vector	Recombinant murine retrovirus	LAI	
Bacterial vectors			
S. typhi		LAI	

Abbreviations: CP = canarypox; LAI = group of closely related HIV isolates that include LAV, IIIB, BH10, and BRU; alum = aluminum hydroxide or aluminum phosphate; DOC = deoxycholate; IFA = incomplete Freund's adjuvant; MF59 = microfluidized oil-in-water emulsion; MoMLV = Moloney murine leukemia virus; MTP-PE = muramyl tripeptide-phosphatidylethanolamine; PPD = purified protein derivative of *Mycobacterium*; MAPS = multiple antigen presentation system; Ty = yeast retrotransposon; VLP = virus-like particle; SAF-M = Syntex adjuvant formulation; BCG = Bacillus Calmette-Guerin. Based on the Jordan Report. http://www.niaid.nih.gov/publications/pdf/jordan.pdf.

of human infants infected before or during birth, despite extensive exposure to infected secretions and blood, may point to a protective role for transplacentally acquired antibodies (116). Simian immunodeficiency virus, like primary HIV, is very difficult to neutralize; passive antibody is not very effective in preventing SIV infection of macaques. Current vaccine candidates, however, do not induce antibodies that neutralize a broad spectrum of circulating HIV candidates, and antibody titers wane within a few months to years. Therefore, the goal of complete protection by sterilizing, antibody-mediated immunity, seems unattainable at present.

An alternative and acceptable goal is to prevent the establishment of infection. This paradigm supposes that antibodies might reduce the infectious dose of virus, but that some cells will become infected. Then, cell-mediated immune responses or nonspecific effectors may limit HIV replication while cytotoxic cells search out and destroy infected cells. A rapid cell-mediated response to initial infection could conceivably eliminate HIV. Even if some HIV were to persist, neutralizing antibody and CTL might keep the virus in check. Thus, most scientists believe that a vaccine should induce the full range of immune functions, with a goal of eliminating virus replication, pathogenesis, and transmission.

The speed with which HIV replicates and changes to evade immune responses poses a severe challenge to the combined effect of cell-mediated immunity and antibodies. Whether T-cell responses could help tip the balance against HIV, especially during mucosal transmission, in which the chain of infectious events seems to be somewhat tenuous, is an intriguing possibility. Those who believe that exposed but uninfected individuals make protective responses against HIV look to hard-to-measure mucosal cellular responses as one possible mechanism of immunity.

Finally, great benefits might be conferred if vaccination could simply reduce HIV replication. Vaccine-induced immunity that can slow viral replication is likely to significantly extend the disease-free period. Individuals with a low viral burden are less likely to transmit the infection to their sexual partners or infants (117–118). The increased immune clearance of HIV and reduced viral burden might improve the effectiveness of antiretroviral therapy and delay the development of drug resistance. In short, vaccination before infection or, perhaps, immediately after infection if HIV replication was completely controlled by antiretroviral therapy, might prevent or postpone illness in infected people and reduce HIV transmission.

Regardless of the immune responses that are thought to be protective, two criteria can be applied to evaluation of vaccines. The immune responses must be durable, because the decades of sexual activity constitute a period of risk. The responses must prevent or limit infection by a wide range of genetic and antigenic variants of HIV-1, because the variability of HIV is enormous and continuously increasing.

II.   ASSESSING EFFICACY IN ANIMAL MODELS

Whether any vaccine "works" is determined by efficacy field trials and postmarketing surveillance to determine effectiveness in a public health setting. Because the first efficacy trials of HIV vaccine got under way in 1999, most vaccine approaches can currently be evaluated for efficacy only by experiments in nonhuman primates. Each animal model has its specific weaknesses: chimpanzees apparently suffer no illness as a result of infection with HIV-1 (except one strain) (119). In contrast, the disease caused in macaques by SIV is usually much more fulminant than HIV-1 in humans. Envelope structure and regulatory mechanisms of SIV differ in several respects from HIV-1. Recently created molecular chimeras between SIV and HIV-1, called SHIVs, infect macaques despite bearing components of HIV-1, usually envelope. Some of these are highly pathogenic. The env-bearing SHIVs allow the direct testing of HIV envelope vaccines in animal models (120–122).

In addition to efficacy in animal models, immunogenicity both in nonhuman primates and in humans can be used to evaluate various vaccine approaches. There is uncertainty in judging any vaccine by the immune responses it elicits, because the roles of specific immune responses in protection are not well understood. Nevertheless, the alternative is to make choices about moving vaccine candidates forward without the benefit of scientific judgment. Just as for other pathogens, the immune effector mechanisms against HIV are most likely quite complex, as are the responses to vaccines.

III.   VACCINE APPROACHES

In this section, studies that have tested the efficacy of various vaccine approaches in primate models are arranged by the type of vaccine. A comprehensive summary of the trials has been published (123). In addition, the immune responses measured in these in vivo primate studies, where possible, are compared with data from human clinical trials. Detailed descriptions of the clinical trials performed to date are presented in Table 1. Safety data and other aspects of human trials are discussed below. Only trials that have enrolled non–HIV-infected primates or humans are discussed.

A.   Live-Attenuated Retrovirus as a Vaccine

The first valid successes in protecting macaques against SIV employed live attenuated SIV. Attenuated vaccine strains make highly effective vaccines against viruses other than retroviruses (124). In AIDS, primate experiments have confirmed that these are the most effective vaccines against highly virulent, homologous SIV challenges (123). Successful protection against homologous virus by the rectal route also suggests that blocking mucosal transmission will not be a problem (98). However, protection is not as strong against heterologous challenges. Only 50% of macaques were protected against infection by a divergent SIV strain (109,125). In the chimpanzee, in which HIV acts essentially as an attenuated virus, one HIV strain has been used as a vaccine to protect against subsequent exposure to another. Within clade B, one strain appeared to be an effective vaccine against another B strain (126). However, prior infection with a clade B virus failed to prevent either infection with or persistence of a clade E virus (127), suggesting that the heterogeneity of HIV can be a problem, even for this vaccine approach.

Although proposals have been made to do limited trials of live attenuated HIV, no such vaccine is currently available for use, and many scientific, regulatory, and ethical hurdles would have to be overcome. Production of such a vaccine for human use could be difficult. Human immunodeficiency virus requires CD4-positive cells for efficient replication and large-scale production in uncharacterized PBMCs would not be practical. There are no acceptable human T-cell lines available for vaccine production, and growth in cultured cells selects variants that use different receptors than the commonly transmitted primary HIV strains. Virus variants would arise in each production lot. Utilizing an infectious DNA plasmid form of the attenuated strain might be the best approach for manufacturing. However, it is difficult to imagine how to predict the biological characteristics of a single cloned genome (as compared to the swarm of HIV variants from which it was selected).

Safety issues for an attenuated HIV vaccine are paramount. Attenuation may be less an intrinsic property of the virus than a reflection of its relationship with the host it infects. For example, an attenuated SIV construct that initially appeared safe in juvenile and adult macaques grew to high titer and could induce disease in neonatal macaques (128). There are rare cases of humans infected with spontaneously attenuated HIV (129–132). Recently, a decline in CD4 counts was noted in patients with HIV mutants lacking nef (132a). An attenuated SIV vaccine produced by the traditional empirical method of long-term culture appears to be safe (99,133), but it is not possible to develop a comparable HIV vaccine, because the genetic basis for the attenuation is not fully understood (133). The long-term risks of an attenuated human retrovirus as a vaccine could be assessed only in large and lengthy human trials. The impact of the epidemic has led some to advocate taking calculated risks (134), but safety testing of live attenuated HIV, given the current state of knowledge, would involve risks to human subjects that would be unacceptable to most physicians and scientists in the field.

B. Whole, Inactivated Virus and Virus-Like Particles

Traditionalists favor whole killed HIV, because vaccines of that type have worked well against other viral diseases. Such vaccines contain most HIV antigens. Design issues include the choice of strains upon which to base the vaccine and the choice of a method for inactivation that balances the need for reliable, complete inactivation with the presumption that viral structures should be preserved. The only support for effectiveness of whole killed retroviral vaccines in primates comes from the use of whole killed SIV as a boost after "priming" with live attenuated SIV in a model of mother-to-infant transfer of protective antibodies (135). Tests of killed virus vaccines as preventives in chimpanzees have not been encouraging from the standpoint of either envelope immunogenicity or protection from challenge (136,137). A series of successful protection experiments with whole killed vaccines in the SIV model (99,138–142) was, unfortunately, subsequently shown to depend not on the viral antigens but on cellular xenoantigens coming from the human cells that had been used to produce the vaccine (143,144).

A related approach is to create a pseudovirion, or genetically inactivated virus that already is replication incompetent (145,146). Such mutants would not require CD4$^+$ cells for production. They could be manufactured in cell lines, although developing a cell line acceptable for vaccine production might be difficult; however, chemical inactivation might still be required. Accessory proteins that might provide protective antigens, such as those encoded by nef, tat, or rev, would not be well represented in the vaccine. Such vaccines might have no special advantages for inducing cellular immune responses. Other virus-like particles have been studied (147–151), but their immunogenicity in nonhuman primates and humans has been modest to date.

If the native conformation of the envelope glycoprotein spikes in the virion could be maintained, thus providing the proper three-dimensional structure for inducing antibodies to recognize wild-type HIV, it could be the strongest advantage of a whole killed or pseudovirion vaccine. However, HIV easily sheds this surface glycoprotein. Producing virions or particles that retain a useful amount of glycoprotein, establishing an inactivation procedure that does not destroy the native conformation, and developing an acceptable tissue cell line for its production are significant obstacles. Testing for safety would be problematic. There is currently no good animal model for HIV pathogenicity, because HIV is usually innocuous for chimpanzees.

C. Recombinant Vectors

One potential solution to the apparent dichotomy between safety and vigor of immune responses is to incorporate some genetic material from HIV into a live or replication-competent viral or bacterial vector, and to induce a self-limited infection with the recombinant vector. This approach may have the advantage of authentic presentation of HIV antigens, often within lymphoid tissues, and stimulation by the vector of a vigorous immune response. Viral vectors code for antigens that will be synthesized by the human host's cells, whereas bacterial vectors yield antigens synthesized by prokaryotic systems that lack glycosylation and processing that would occur in a mammalian cell. Particularly if the vector is a known vaccine, safety and immunogenicity of the vector may be well understood. There are also disadvantages. Viral and bacterial pathogens may have evolved mechanisms for down-regulating or subverting human immune responses. In addition, safety of the vaccine may not be adequate for widespread use in an era when many people may harbor undiagnosed HIV infection, robbing them of their immune defenses against what would ordinarily be an innocuous infection by the vector. Design issues for recombinant vectors also include the identity and strain of the component HIV genes.

Properties of the vectors themselves may confer advantages or disadvantages. Vaccinia and vesicular stomatitis viruses infect many cell types and are generally eliminated by the immune system, whereas herpesviruses establish persistent infections. Vectors that naturally infect the oronasal mucosa (e.g., adenovirus, influenza, rhinovirus) or gut (*Salmonella typhi*, *Shigella*, poliovirus) might deliver their antigens and induce good mucosal immune responses as a consequence. An initial trial of a recombinant *S. typhi* vector (152) has been done in humans. Despite limited or absent replication capacity, these vectors can express the passenger antigens in the cells they infect and can induce immune responses. Whereas most vectors carry genes to direct endogenous synthesis of antigen by cells of the vaccine recipient, a few display vectors incorporate the HIV antigens as part of their structure (153).

Recombinant vectors must overcome the initial hurdle of prior immunity to the vector in the human population. Although such recombinant vectors cannot cause AIDS, there are nonetheless safety concerns. As with any live attenuated vaccine, genetic stability and transmissibility of the vaccine from person to person are important considerations. Such a vaccine would need to have extremely limited replication capacity, to avoid the possibility that some recipients could already be immunocompromised by HIV infection and unable to control infection by the vaccine vector. For this reason, the best developed vector, vaccinia, is generally excluded from consideration as an HIV vaccine carrier despite having been safe enough, in a pre-HIV era, to inoculate hundreds of millions of people as part of the successful worldwide campaign to eradicate smallpox.

Limited replication has been achieved in vectors under development for HIV vaccines in different ways. Replication is blocked when canarypox infects mammalian cells (154); multiple canarypox constructs bearing different combinations of HIV genes are being evaluated in human trials (155–156). One particular strain of vaccinia, through spontaneous deletion of 10% to 15% of its genes, has lost almost all replication capacity in mammalian cells. This modified virus (Modified Vaccinia, Ankara strain, or MVA) (157), is being tested preclinically, and human trials are planned, even though its future as a commercial product is uncertain because it is in the public domain. Another approach is to alter the packaged nucleic acid of the vector virus so that it can replicate only once in the host; this "replicon" technology is being evaluated in primate experiments for several vectors, including poliovirus (158), Semliki forest virus (159–161), and Venezuelan equine encephalitis virus (162,163).

Candidate vaccines have not induced strong, consistently measured CTL responses in humans and macaques, although this may relate to limitations in detection or in sampling, as discussed above. Proposals to improve CTL responses by adding specific cytokines such as interleukin (IL)-12 and interferon-gamma to the vaccine (164,165), or by targeting antigen to dendritic cells to improve cellular immune responses, are being evaluated in primates.

D. Plasmid Immunization

Immunization with DNA is a special case of vector presentation, wherein the vector organism is eliminated and just the encoding information is directly administered. Encouraging immunogenicity results in rodents have not translated well into primates for HIV vaccines (82,166), although a DNA form of a known successful hepatitis B vaccine was effective in the chimpanzee (167). These vaccines have been good at inducing CTLs in primates, but good neutralizing antibodies do not appear until after protein boosting (168,169). Early human trials of candidate DNA vaccines against HIV have begun.

Improvements in immunogenicity may depend on manipulating the antigen genes to optimize expression (170). Structures in the DNA itself, independent of the encoded information, appear to have self-adjuvanting properties (171,172), and the effects of such features may differ between rodents and primates. Inclusion of cytokine DNA along with the antigen DNA has improved responses in mice (173) and is beginning to be evaluated in primates. If antibody responses to nucleic acid immunization can be improved, this approach would the fastest way to compare multivalent envelope combinations to address the heterogeneity problem. An intriguing concept is immunization with DNA libraries prepared from the entire genome of the pathogen, bypassing the need to identify protective antigens in advance (174,175). Although this approach saves time, it requires that protective epitopes be confined to contiguous peptide sequences. Direct mucosal administration of nucleic acid is under study (175–179). Plasmid immunization has a number of significant manufacturing advantages, including stability, relatively low cost of production, and ease of purification.

E. Subunit Proteins and Peptides

Based on the model of the successful hepatitis B subunit vaccine, the first candidate HIV vaccines to be developed were envelope subunit proteins. Manufacture and purification of these large, heavily glycosylated, internally disulfide-bridged proteins in market quantities is technologically demanding. Until recently, these products were made exclusively from laboratory strains of HIV. The CTL responses have been minimal (180), although good proliferative responses are seen (181,182). Although better antibody responses were obtained with gp120 expressed in mammalian cells than from yeast or insect cell systems (24), responses to these subunits have been judged somewhat disappointing with respect to their breadth of neutralizing antibodies (although antibodies bind proteins from a wide variety of HIV strains) and their durability. The value of these neutralization responses against wild-type primary strains of HIV has been questioned (27,36,38). However, an objective way to set goals for protective antibody levels is lacking. These unknowns make for exciting science but contentious debate.

A pragmatic approach is to include multiple molecules and to search for a presentation that induces both cell-mediated and humoral responses. Human evaluations have begun with bivalent envelope vaccines that include gp120 from a primary isolate: clade E for Thailand and clade B for the United States (41). There is wide interest in using these subunit vaccines in combination with other modalities rather than as standalone vaccines.

Peptide vaccines focus even more precisely on linear B- and T-cell epitopes. Several human safety and immunogenicity trials have been conducted. Antibodies induced by peptide vaccines in humans have been disappointing (183–187). Synthesis of conformationally constrained synthetic peptides as immunogens (188,189) may increase the ability to induce antibodies against complex antibody-binding sites that depend on folded protein structure.

Several vaccines have been designed and tested for their ability to induce CTL responses to HIV peptides. Raising CTL responses to lipidated peptides has been successful in mice and macaques (190–192). Although there is intellectual appeal to including only the required CTL epitopes, mapping those epitopes so that the synthetic immunogen will be complete enough to cover MHC types in the recipient population would be a daunting task.

F. Combining Different Vaccines

There is an apparent dichotomy between the two main approaches tested in humans: protein subunits induce primarily antibodies (and T-helpers) whereas recombinant poxviruses induce primarily cell-mediated immunity, including CTL. This is consistent with immunological theory, but it is not the desired outcome. A possible solution is to combine two vaccines; this strategy has been called prime and boost, particularly where a recombinant poxvirus has been followed by a protein subunit. The practical and regulatory obstacles to obtaining licensure for a sequence of two different vaccines and effectively deploying such a combination will be substantial.

Live recombinant poxvirus vaccines generate cellular immune responses in humans, but they induce less antibody than multiple doses of adjuvanted preparations of envelope subunit vaccines. Conversely, human studies have shown virtu-ally no CTL induction by recombinant proteins (193). However, a single dose of envelope subunit administered after one or two priming doses of a live recombi-nant vector can yield the same levels of neutralization achieved after several doses of protein alone; CTL responses are the same or greater after the protein boost (155–155b,194,195). Combining the two approaches appears to preserve the best immune properties of each. Priming with a live vector for T-cell responses followed by protein boosting to optimize the B-cell response has become a common strategy. Recent efforts to use two different vaccines, a poxvirus vector and a subunit protein simultaneously, rather than sequentially, have shown encouraging results (194).

In animal studies, nucleic acid immunization behaves somewhat like a poxvirus vector, in that it primes for antibody responses which are brought out by the subsequent protein immunization (168,196). When used in combination with poxvirus vaccines, DNA is more effective as a prime than as a boost (196). Be-cause DNA and vectors are easier to produce and purify than proteins are, there may be some advantage to a vector/nucleic acid combination. DNA as a priming immunization followed by protein or poxvirus boosting has not yet been studied in human subjects.

IV. HIV VACCINE TRIALS

A. Safety of HIV Vaccine Candidates in Healthy Adults and Infants

More than 40 clinical trials of HIV vaccines have enrolled healthy adult volunteers not infected with HIV. In addition, two vaccines have been tested to date in trials enrolling newborn infants whose mothers are infected with HIV (most of these in-fants are not HIV-infected, but as a group they are at high risk of infection, rang-ing from approximately 25% to less than 5% if the mother and infant are treated with zidovudine and other antiretroviral drugs) (116,197,198). More than half of the trials have been supported by the National Institute of Allergy and Infectious Diseases (NIAID, NIH); some have been supported by other governments or by vaccine manufacturers, taking place in the United States, United Kingdom, France, Belgium, Switzerland, Israel, Thailand, Japan, China, Cuba, and Uganda, and em-ploying a variety of vaccine candidates (see Table 1). At the end of 1998, the first phase 3 efficacy trials of preventive HIV vaccine, bivalent gp120 (a laboratory strain and a regional primary isolate), were underway in the United States and Thai-land. Additional trials were being planned to take place in Africa and Asia, as well as in the United States and the Caribbean/Latin American region.

The overall safety of the HIV vaccines tested in NIH trials has been sum-marized. The parenterally administered vaccines have all caused some local reac-tions. Both alum and the oil-in-water emulsion MF59 have been generally well tolerated, but some more severe local reactions have been associated with the use of newer adjuvants. Systemic reactions, such as fever and malaise, have been uncommon, and there has been no evidence of harm based on laboratory tests such as blood counts, liver function tests, renal function tests, and urinalysis. Despite initial concerns that HIV envelope protein might cause immune dysfunction, autoimmunity, or other adverse health effects, no such pattern of serious adverse events has been observed and tests of immune function demonstrate no immunosuppression (199). None of the vaccines tested so far is capable of causing HIV infection.

Volunteers for most HIV vaccine trials are screened to exclude individuals at high risk for HIV infection because of unsafe sexual or needle-sharing practices. HIV risk may be episodic, and individuals who were originally at low risk may, over the course of the trial, engage in high-risk behavior. Phase 2 trials include individuals at higher risk of HIV exposure. A number of volunteers in AVEG trials (and a few in other trials) were known to have become infected with HIV, some during and some after completion of a vaccination series, as a result of high-risk exposures (200–203). Some of these individuals had received placebo preparations. There was no trend to indicate whether vaccinated individuals were at greater or lesser risk of HIV infection through sexual exposure or contaminated needles. The effect of vaccination on disease course cannot be evaluated in this small group (201).

B.   The Conduct of HIV Vaccine Trials: Special Safeguards

HIV vaccine trials must include safeguards for the volunteers against discrimination or harm coming from a mistaken belief that they are infected with HIV (204,205). At the same time, the ability to diagnose an authentic HIV infection in the face of vaccine-induced immune responses is critical for the medical care of the volunteer and for determining the endpoints in efficacy trials. Vaccination may induce antibodies that will be detected in diagnostic enzyme-linked immunosorbent assays (ELISA). In general, these have been transient, fading within 1 to 2 years, and they have been unusual among volunteers receiving only gp120 or peptide vaccines. Nevertheless, sensitive HIV tests may be employed for medical diagnosis or in conjunction with insurance applications or other situations, with or without a volunteer's knowledge, to screen for HIV infection. Anomalous Western blot patterns may not be recognized as vaccine-induced, particularly if there is a nonspecific band in the region of p24. More complex vaccines that include gag, pol, or regulatory proteins are much harder to distinguish from authentic infection. Use of a kit recognizing antibodies against antigens absent from the vaccine (e.g., the gp41 immunodominant region if only gp120 is included in the vaccine) may ameliorate these problems, or PCR can be used in an attempt to rule out infection (206). About one-fifth of volunteers report that they were tested for HIV infection, voluntarily or involuntarily, during trial participation (205). Voluntary disclosure of vaccine trial participation can lead to discrimination if friends, family, or employers misunderstand the trial and believe the volunteer to be infected with HIV. Physicians, nurses, and social workers associated with HIV vaccine trials can successfully assist volunteers to address these concerns.

C. Planning for Efficacy Trials

Conduct of efficacy trials for any vaccine is not simple. For HIV vaccine trials, some unique complications will arise (207,208). Human immunodeficiency virus transmission can be prevented by behavior change; however, education, counseling, and behavioral modification have not been completely successful. Nevertheless, the ethical conduct of HIV vaccine trials, or trials of other preventive interventions, requires trial organizers to educate, counsel, and provide protective devices such as condoms or clean needles and syringes to the extent that is feasible and legally permissible. The approximate incidence of HIV infection must be determined in the presence of such preventive measures in order to estimate needed sample size.

Volunteers must fully understand that the trial includes a placebo, that treatments are selected randomly, and that neither they nor the staff will know their treatment until the end of the trial. They must also understand that the vaccine, even if efficacious, may not protect every vaccinated individual, and they must be repeatedly counseled to avoid any increase in risky behavior based upon a false sense of security. Fortunately, vaccine preparedness research in the United States and other countries suggests that these goals are attainable (209,210).

Because of the difficulty surrounding evaluation of HIV vaccine candidates, some have proposed a smaller screening trial to estimate the approximate efficacy of one or more vaccine candidates before conducting a full-scale efficacy trial (208). Such a trial would not provide sufficient data for licensure, but it would efficiently screen out a vaccine candidate that is not efficacious. However, conducting a subsequent randomized, placebo-controlled definitive trial could be problematic if the preliminary estimate suggests the vaccine may be efficacious. Trials should be run in parallel in different regions of the world, and the data from these different trials, perhaps testing different regional variants of the vaccine, coordinated to allow efficient decision making.

V. THE FUTURE

Current HIV vaccine candidates do not induce immune responses as strong as those induced by HIV infection. It may be possible to induce stronger immune responses, and a variety of approaches are being pursued in the hope of improving neutralizing antibody, and/or T-cell responses, lytic or otherwise. These strategies are not mutually exclusive, and candidate vaccines often incorporate several ideas. Strategies to specifically improve mucosal responses are much less developed.

However, it may not be necessary to induce responses that match those in a chronically infected person. Immune effector mechanisms against HIV are not well understood and basic research on HIV biology, pathogenesis, and immunology may reveal the best line of attack or the best way of measuring vaccine-induced

Table 2 Rational Vaccine Design

 I. Hypothesis: induction of better neutralizing antibodies will improve the vaccine
    A. Modify antigen form
        env Based on macrophage-tropic strain
        "More native" structure
        Oligomeric envelope proteins
        Whole-killed virus
        gp120 Complexed to CD4
        Alter glycosylation of the env protein
        Specific epitopes
        Include envelope protein from several strains
    B. Improve "presentation"
        Improve adjuvants
        Coadminister cytokine as protein or DNA
        Optimize antigen expression by DNA vaccines
        Target dendritic antigen-presenting cells
        Combine vaccines of different types
 II. Hypothesis: making better CTL will improve the vaccine
    A. Include multiple antigens, including genes expressed early
    B. Improve endogenous "presentation"
        Lipidate peptides for CTL epitopes
        Optimize antigen expression by DNA
        GM-CSF to improve cellular responses
        Target dendritic antigen-presenting cells
III. Hypothesis: mucosal immunity will block sexual transmission
    A. Adjuvants specific for mucosal responses
    B. Target replicating vaccines to draining nodes
    C. Administer vaccines to mucosal sites
IV. Hypothesis: something other than neutralizing antibody or CTL is most important
    A. Coadminister cytokines to increase Th1 response
    B. Immunize with T-helper peptides only
    C. Immunize with tat
    D. Immunize with alloantigens
    E. Immunize with coreceptor peptides

---

immune responses. The extensive heterogeneity of the envelope protein, and the ability of HIV to persist in latent, integrated form to evade immune clearance from the body, pose the greatest problems for vaccine design. It is not clear which, if any, of the paths to rational vaccine design will lead to an effective HIV vaccine (Table 2).

A wide variety of vaccine candidates must be evaluated. Accumulating evidence from primate models about mechanisms of immunity to retrovirus challenge and evidence from epidemiological and clinical studies about mechanisms of HIV control can be integrated to develop hypotheses. Comparative immunogenicity testing in animals and humans is essential, but interpretation is limited by the absence of a well-defined correlate of protective immunity for HIV. Challenge studies in primates can be used not only to compare vaccine candidates but also to learn what immune responses are induced by effective vaccines. It is possible that no assay currently in use can measure a specific response that is predictive of protective efficacy in a field trial.

Systematic comparisons are beginning to be made, especially in the SHIV model, wherein vaccines with HIV env components can be evaluated by challenge in macaques (211). If vaccines are expected to reduce virus burden after challenge, it is essential that challenge studies employ viruses that have an immunodeficiency disease endpoint and whose replication and pathogenesis (e.g., plasma loads) in the test species are similar to that of HIV in humans (212). Although recent experiments in chimpanzees have generated much interest, use of the one known HIV strain that is pathogenic for chimpanzees as a challenge in vaccine trials is controversial (213).

Vaccine clinical trials will eventually identify one or more effective vaccines. Analysis of one or more successful or partially successful efficacy trials may show which immune responses predict or correlate with immunity to HIV.

REFERENCES

1. Barre-Sinoussi F, Chermann JC, Rey F, et al. Isolation of a T-lymphotropic retrovirus from a patient at risk for acquired immune deficiency syndrome (AIDS). Science 1983; 220:868–871.
2. Levy JA, Hoffman AD, Kramer SM, Landis JA, Shimabukuro JM, Oshiro LS. Isolation of lymphocytopathic retroviruses from San Francisco patients with AIDS. Science 1984; 225:840–842.
3. Gallo RC, Sarin PS, Gelmann EP, et al. Isolation of human T-cell leukemia virus in acquired immune deficiency syndrome (AIDS). Science 1983; 220:865–867.
4. Nathanson N, Gonzalez-Scarano F. Human immunodeficiency virus: an agent that defies vaccination. Adv Vet Sci Comp Med 1989; 33:397–412.
5. Ada GL. Prospects for HIV vaccines. J Acquir Immune Defic Syndr 1988; 1:295–303.

6. Ferdinand FJ, Dorner F, Kurth R. Perspectives of HIV vaccine developments. J Virol Methods 1987; 17:63–67.
7. Levy JA. Can an AIDS vaccine be developed? Transfus Med Rev 1988; 2:264–271.
8. Dalgleish AG, Chanh TC, Kennedy RC, Kanda P, Clapham PR, Weiss RA. Neutralization of diverse HIV-1 strains by monoclonal antibodies raised against a gp41 synthetic peptide. Virology 1988; 165:209–215.
9. Ho DD, Sarngadharan MG, Hirsch MS, et al. Human immunodeficiency virus neutralizing antibodies recognize several conserved domains on the envelope glycoproteins. J Virol 1987; 61:2024–2028.
10. Lyerly HK, Reed DL, Matthews TJ, et al. Anti-gp 120 antibodies from HIV seropositive individuals mediate broadly reactive anti-HIV ADCC. AIDS Res Hum Retroviruses 1987; 3:409–422.
11. Walker BD, Chakrabarti S, Moss B, et al. HIV-specific cytotoxic T lymphocytes in seropositive individuals. Nature 1987; 328:345–348.
12. Robey WG, Arthur LO, Matthews TJ, et al. Prospect for prevention of human immunodeficiency virus infection: purified 120-kDa envelope glycoprotein induces neutralizing antibody. Proc Natl Acad Sci U S A 1986; 83:7023–7027.
13. Buchbinder SP, Katz MH, Hessol NA, O'Malley PM, Holmberg SD. Long-term HIV-1 infection without immunologic progression [see comments]. AIDS 1994; 8:1123–1128.
14. Munoz A, Kirby AJ, He YD, et al. Long-term survivors with HIV-1 infection: incubation period and longitudinal patterns of CD4+ lymphocytes. J Acquir Immune Defic Syndr Hum Retrovirol 1995; 8:496–505.
15. Prince AM, Reesink H, Pascual D, et al. Prevention of HIV infection by passive immunization with HIV immunoglobulin. AIDS Res Hum Retroviruses 1991; 7:971–973.
16. Conley AJ, Kessler JA II, Boots LJ, et al. The consequence of passive administration of an anti-human immunodeficiency virus type 1 neutralizing monoclonal antibody before challenge of chimpanzees with a primary virus isolate. J Virol 1996; 70:6751–6758.
17. Shibata R, Igarashi T, Haigwood N, et al. Neutralizing antibody directed against the HIV-1 envelope glycoprotein can completely block HIV-1/SIV chimeric virus infections of macaque monkeys. Nat Med 1999; 5:204–210.
18. Burton DR. A vaccine for HIV type 1: the antibody perspective. Proc Natl Acad Sci U S A 1997; 94:10018–10023.
19. Burton DR, Montefiori DC. The antibody response in HIV-1 infection [see comments]. AIDS 1997; 11:S87–S98.
20. Wrin T, Loh TP, Vennari JC, Schuitemaker H, Nunberg JH. Adaptation to persistent growth in the H9 cell line renders a primary isolate of human immunodeficiency virus type 1 sensitive to neutralization by vaccine sera. J Virol 1995; 69:39–48.
21. Chanh TC, Dreesman GR, Kanda P, et al. Induction of anti-HIV neutralizing antibodies by synthetic peptides. EMBO J 1986; 5:3065–3071.
22. Zarling JM, Eichberg JW, Moran PA, McClure J, Pennathur S, Hu SL. Proliferative and cytotoxic T cells to AIDS virus glycoproteins in chimpanzees immunized with a recombinant vaccinia virus expressing AIDS virus envelope glycoproteins. J Immunol 1987; 139:988–990.

23. Nara PL, Robey WG, Pyle SW, et al. Purified envelope glycoproteins from human immunodeficiency virus type 1 variants induce individual, type-specific neutralizing antibodies. J Virol 1988; 62:2622–2628.

24. Graham BS. Serological responses to candidate AIDS vaccines. AIDS Res Hum Retroviruses 1994; 10:S145–S148.

25. Steimer KS, Scandella CJ, Skiles PV, Haigwood NL. Neutralization of divergent HIV-1 isolates by conformation-dependent human antibodies to gp120. Science 1991; 254:105–108.

26. Fast PE, Walker MC. Human trials of experimental AIDS vaccines. AIDS 1993; 7:S147–S159.

27. Dolin R. Human studies in the development of human immunodeficiency virus vaccines. J Infect Dis 1995; 172:1175–1183.

28. Graham BS, Wright PF. Candidate AIDS vaccines. N Engl J Med 1995; 333:1331–1339.

29. Belshe RB, Graham BS, Keefer MC, et al. Neutralizing antibodies to HIV-1 in seronegative volunteers immunized with recombinant gp120 from the MN strain of HIV-1. NIAID AIDS Vaccine Clinical Trials Network [see comments]. JAMA 1994; 272:475–480.

30. Cooney EL, Collier AC, Greenberg PD, et al. Safety of and immunological response to a recombinant vaccinia virus vaccine expressing HIV envelope glycoprotein [see comments]. Lancet 1991; 337:567–572.

31. Dolin R, Graham BS, Greenberg SB, et al. The safety and immunogenicity of a human immunodeficiency virus type 1 (HIV-1) recombinant gp160 candidate vaccine in humans. NIAID AIDS Vaccine Clinical Trials Network. Ann Intern Med 1991; 114:119–127.

32. Schwartz DH, Gorse G, Clements ML, et al. Induction of HIV-1-neutralising and syncytium-inhibiting antibodies in uninfected recipients of HIV-1IIIB rgp 120 subunit vaccine. Lancet 1993; 342:69–73.

33. Moore JP, Cao Y, Qing L, et al. Primary isolates of human immunodeficiency virus type 1 are relatively resistant to neutralization by monoclonal antibodies to gp120, and their neutralization is not predicted by studies with monomeric gp120. J Virol 1995; 69:101–109.

34. Zhang YJ, Fracasso C, Fiore JR, et al. Augmented serum neutralizing activity against primary human immunodeficiency virus type 1 (HIV-1) isolates in two groups of HIV-1-infected long-term nonprogressors. J Infect Dis 1997; 176:1180–1187.

35. Sattentau QJ, Moore JP. Human immunodeficiency virus type 1 neutralization is determined by epitope exposure on the gp120 oligomer. J Exp Med 1995; 182:185–196.

36. Mascola JR, Snyder SW, Weislow OS, et al. Immunization with envelope subunit vaccine products elicits neutralizing antibodies against laboratory-adapted but not primary isolates of human immunodeficiency virus type 1. The National Institute of Allergy and Infectious Disease AIDS Vaccine Evaluation Group. J Infect Dis 1996; 173:340–348.

37. VanCott TC, Bethke FR, Kalyanaraman V, Burke DS, Redfield RR, Birx DL. Preferential antibody recognition of structurally distinct HIV-1 gp120 molecules. J Acquir Immune Defic Syndr 1994; 7:1103–1115.

38. VanCott TC, Bethke FR, Burke DS, Redfield RR, Birx DL. Lack of induction of antibodies specific for conserved, discontinuous epitopes of HIV-1 envelope glycoprotein by candidate AIDS vaccines. J Immunol 1995; 155:4100–4110.

39. Zolla-Pazner S, Xu S, Burda S, Duliege AM, Excler JL, Clements-Mann ML. Neutralization of syncytium-inducing primary isolates by sera from human immunodeficiency virus (HIV)-uninfected recipients of candidate HIV vaccines. J Infect Dis 1998; 178:1502–1506.

40. Wrin T, Crawford L, Sawyer L, Weber P, Sheppard HW, Hanson CV. Neutralizing antibody responses to autologous and heterologous isolates of human immunodeficiency virus. J Acquir Immune Defic Syndr 1994; 7:211–219.

40a. Rübsamen-Waigmann H, von Briesen H, Holmes H, et al. Standard conditions of virus isolation reveal biological variability of HIV-1 in different regions of the world. AIDS Res Hum Retroviruses 1994; 10:1401–1409.

40b. De Wolf F, Hogervorst E, Goudsmit J, et al. Syncytium inducing (SI) and non-syncytium inducing (NSI) capacity of human immunodeficiency virus type 1 (HIV-1) subtypes other than B: phenotypic and genotypic characteristics. AIDS Res Hum Retroviruses 1994; 10:1387–1400.

40c. Osmanov S, Belsey EM, Heyward W, et al. HIV Type 1 variation in World Health Organization-sponsored vaccine evaluation sites: genetic screening, sequence analysis, and preliminary biological characterization of selected viral strains. AIDS Res Hum Retroviruses 1994; 10:1327–1343.

40d. Spaer EG, Lingenfelter P, Singal R, et al. Rapid genetic-characterization of HIV type-1 strains from 4 WHO-sponsored vaccine evaluation sites using a heteroduplex mobility assay. AIDS Res Hum Retroviruses 1994; 10:1345–1353.

40e. Gao F, Yue L, Craig S, et al. Genetic variation of HIV type 1 in 4; WHO-sponsored vaccine evaluation sites-generation of functional envelope (glycoprotein-160) clones representative of sequence subtype-A, subtype B, subtype C, and subtype E. AIDS Res Hum Retroviruses 1994; 10:1359–1368.

40f. Pau CP, Kai M, Hollomancadal DL, et al. Antigenic variation and serotyping of HIV type 1 from 4 WHO-sponsored HIV vaccine sites. AIDS Res Hum Retroviruses 1994; 10:1369–1377.

40g. Cheingsongpopov R, Lister S, Callow D, et al. Serotyping HIV type 1 by antibody-binding to the V3 loop-relationship to viral genotype. AIDS Res Hum Retroviruses 1994; 10:1379–1386.

41. First AIDS vaccine trial launched [news]. Science 1998; 280:1697.

42. Kwong PD, Wyatt R, Robinson J, Sweet RW, Sodroski J, Hendrickson WA. Structure of an HIV gp120 envelope glycoprotein in complex with the CD4 receptor and a neutralizing human antibody [see comments]. Nature 1998; 393:648–659.

43. Richardson TM Jr, Stryjewski BL, Broder CC, et al. Humoral response to oligomeric human immunodeficiency virus type 1 envelope protein. J Virol 1996; 70:753–762.

44. Luke W, Coulibaly C, Dittmer U, et al. Simian immunodeficiency virus (SIV) gp130 oligomers protect rhesus macaques (*Macaca mulatta*) against the infection with SIVmac32H grown on T-cells or derived ex vivo. Virology 1996; 216:444–450.

45. VanCott TC, Mascola JR, Kaminski RW, et al. Antibodies with specificity to native gp120 and neutralization activity against primary human immunodeficiency virus type 1 isolates elicited by immunization with oligomeric gp160. J Virol 1997; 71: 4319–4330.

46. LaCasse RA, Follis KE, Trahey M, Scarborough JD, Littman DR, Nunberg JH. Fusion-competent vaccines:broad neutralization of primary isolates of HIV [see comments]. Science 1999; 283:357–362.

47. Reitter JN, Means RE, Desrosiers RC. A role for carbohydrates in immune evasion in AIDS. Nat Med 1998; 4:679–684.

48. Wei X, Ghosh SK, Taylor ME, et al. Viral dynamics in human immunodeficiency virus type 1 infection [see comments]. Nature 1995; 373:117–122.

49. Ho DD, Neumann AU, Perelson AS, Chen W, Leonard JM, Markowitz M. Rapid turnover of plasma virions and CD4 lymphocytes in HIV-1 infection [see comments]. Nature 1995; 373:123–126.

50. Pantaleo G, Fauci AS. New concepts in the immunopathogenesis of HIV infection. Annu Rev Immunol 1995; 13:487–512.

51. Ahmad S, Lohman B, Marthas M, et al. Reduced virus load in rhesus macaques immunized with recombinant gp160 and challenged with simian immunodeficiency virus. AIDS Res Hum Retroviruses 1994; 10:195–204.

52. Hirsch VM, Goldstein S, Hynes NA, et al. Prolonged clinical latency and survival of macaques given a whole inactivated simian immunodeficiency virus vaccine. J Infect Dis 1994; 170:51–59.

52a. Hirsch VM, Fuerst TR, Sutter G, et al. Patterns of viral replication correlate with outcome in simian immunodeficiency virus (SIV)-infected macaques: effect of prior immunization with a trivalent SIV vaccine in modified vaccinia virus Ankara. J Virol 1996; 70:3741–3752.

53. Ourmanov I, Brown CR, Moss B, et al. Comparative efficacy of recombinant modified vaccinia virus ankara expressing simian immunodeficiency virus (SIV) gag-Pol and/or env in macaques challenged with pathogenic SIV. J Virol 2000; 74:2740–2751.

54. Lewis MG, Yalley-Ogunro J, Greenhouse JJ, et al. Limited protection from a pathogenic chimeric simian-human immunodeficiency virus challenge following immunization with attenuated simian immunodeficiency virus. J Virol 1999; 73:1262–1270.

55. Vogel TU, Fournier J, Sherring A. Presence of circulating CTL induced by infection with wild-type or attenuated SIV and their correlation with protection from pathogenic SHIV challenge. J Med Primatol 1998; 27:65–72.

56. Miller CJ, McGhee JR. Progress towards a vaccine to prevent sexual transmission of HIV. Nat Med 1996; 2:751–752.

57. Marx PA, Compans RW, Gettie A, et al. Protection against vaginal SIV transmission with microencapsulated vaccine. Science 1993; 260:1323–1327.

58. Girard M, Mahoney J, Wei Q, et al. Genital infection of female chimpanzees with human immunodeficiency virus type 1. AIDS Res Hum Retroviruses 1998; 14:1357–1367.

59. Clerici M, Giorgi JV, Chou CC, et al. Cell-mediated immune response to human immunodeficiency virus (HIV) type 1 in seronegative homosexual men with recent sexual exposure to HIV-1 [see comments]. J Infect Dis 1992; 165:1012–1019.

60. Fowke KR, Nagelkerke NJ, Kimani J, et al. Resistance to HIV-1 infection among persistently seronegative prostitutes in Nairobi, Kenya [see comments]. Lancet 1996; 348: 1347–1351.

61. Rowland-Jones SL, Nixon DF, Aldhous MC, et al. HIV-specific cytotoxic T-cell activity in an HIV-exposed but uninfected infant. Lancet 1993; 341:860–861.

62. Rowland-Jones S, Sutton J, Ariyoshi K, et al. HIV-specific cytotoxic T-cells in HIV-

exposed but uninfected Gambian women [published erratum appears in Nat Med 1995 Jun; 1(6):598]. Nat Med 1995; 1:59–64.

63. Beyrer C, Artenstein AW, Rugpao S, et al. Epidemiologic and biologic characterization of a cohort of human immunodeficiency virus type 1 highly exposed, persistently seronegative female sex workers in northern Thailand. Chiang Mai HEPS Working Group. J Infect Dis 1999; 179:59–67.

64. Schmitz JE, Kuroda MJ, Santra S, et al. Control of viremia in simian immunodeficiency virus infection by CD8+ lymphocytes. Science 1999; 283:857–860.

65. Jin X, Bauer DE, Tuttleton SE, et al. Dramatic rise in plasma viremia after CD8(+) T cell depletion in simian immunodeficiency virus-infected macaques. J Exp Med 1999; 189:991–998.

66. Matano T, Shibata R, Siemon C, Connors M, Lane HC, Martin MA. Administration of an anti-CD8 monoclonal antibody interferes with the clearance of chimeric simian/human immunodeficiency virus during primary infections of rhesus macaques. J Virol 1998; 72:164–169.

67. Borrow P, Lewicki H, Wei X, et al. Antiviral pressure exerted by HIV-1-specific cytotoxic T lymphocytes (CTLs) during primary infection demonstrated by rapid selection of CTL escape virus [see comments]. Nat Med 1997; 3:205–211.

68. Mortara L, Letourneur F, Gras-Masse H, Venet A, Guillet JG, Bourgault-Villada I. Selection of virus variants and emergence of virus escape mutants after immunization with an epitope vaccine. J Virol 1998; 72:1403–1410.

69. Haas G, Hosmalin A, Hadida F, Duntze J, Debre P, Autran B. Dynamics of HIV variants and specific cytotoxic T-cell recognition in nonprogressors and progressors. Immunol Lett 1997; 57:63–68.

70. Cao H, Kanki P, Sankale JL, et al. Cytotoxic T-lymphocyte cross-reactivity among different human immunodeficiency virus type 1 clades: implications for vaccine development. J Virol 1997; 71:8615–8623.

71. Betts MR, Krowka J, Santamaria C, et al. Cross-clade human immunodeficiency virus (HIV)-specific cytotoxic T-lymphocyte responses in HIV-infected Zambians. J Virol 1997; 7:8908–8911.

72. Durali D, Morvan J, Letourneur F, et al. Cross-reactions between the cytotoxic T-lymphocyte responses of human immunodeficiency virus-infected African and European patients. J Virol 1998; 72:3547–3553.

73. Ferrari G, Humphrey W, McElrath MJ, et al. Clade B-based HIV-1 vaccines elicit cross-clade cytotoxic T lymphocyte reactivities in uninfected volunteers. Proc Natl Acad Sci U S A 1997; 94:1396–1401.

74. Blazevic V, Ranki A, Krohn KJ. Helper and cytotoxic T cell responses of HIV type 1-infected individuals to synthetic peptides of HIV type 1 Rev. AIDS Res Hum Retroviruses 1995; 11:1335–1342.

75. Choppin J, Guillet JG, Levy JP. HLA class I binding regions of HIV-1 proteins. Crit Rev Immunol 1992; 12:1–16.

76. Hinkula J, Svanholm C, Schwartz S, et al. Recognition of prominent viral epitopes induced by immunization with human immunodeficiency virus type 1 regulatory genes. J Virol 1997; 71:5528–5539.

77. Koenig S, Conley AJ, Brewah YA, et al. Transfer of HIV-1-specific cytotoxic T lymphocytes to an AIDS patient leads to selection for mutant HIV variants and subsequent disease progression [see comments]. Nat Med 1995; 1:330–336.

78. Shankar P, Sprang H, Lieberman J. Effective lysis of HIV-1-infected primary CD4+ T cells by a cytotoxic T-lymphocyte clone directed against a novel A2-restricted reverse-transcriptase epitope. J Acquir Immune Defic Syndr Hum Retrovirol 1998; 19: 111–120.

79. Andersson S, Makitalo B, Thorstensson R, et al. Immunogenicity and protective efficacy of a human immunodeficiency virus type 2 recombinant canarypox (ALVAC) vaccine candidate in cynomolgus monkeys. J Infect Dis 1996; 174:977–985.

80. Daniel MD, Kirchhoff F, Czajak SC, Sehgal PK, Desrosiers RC. Protective effects of a live attenuated SIV vaccine with a deletion in the nef gene [see comments]. Science 1992; 258:1938–1941.

81. Daniel MD, Mazzara GP, Simon MA, et al. High-titer immune responses elicited by recombinant vaccinia virus priming and particle boosting are ineffective in preventing virulent SIV infection. AIDS Res Hum Retroviruses 1994; 10:839–851.

82. Lu S, Manson K, Wyand M, Robinson HL. SIV DNA vaccine trial in macaques: postchallenge necropsy in vaccine and control groups. Vaccine 1997; 15:920–923.

83. Yasutomi Y, Koenig S, Haun SS, et al. Immunization with recombinant BCG-SIV elicits SIV-specific cytotoxic T lymphocytes in rhesus monkeys. J Immunol 1993; 150:3101–3107.

84. Yasutomi Y, Koenig S, Woods RM, et al. A vaccine-elicited, single viral epitope-specific cytotoxic T lymphocyte response does not protect against intravenous, cell-free simian immunodeficiency virus challenge. J Virol 1995; 69:2279–2284.

85. Gallimore A, Cranage M, Cook N, et al. Early suppression of SIV replication by CD8+ nef-specific cytotoxic T cells in vaccinated macaques. Nat Med 1995; 1:1167–1173.

86. Kent SJ, Hu SL, Corey L, Morton WR, Greenberg PD. Detection of simian immunodeficiency virus (SIV)-specific CD8+ T cells in macaques protected from SIV challenge by prior SIV subunit vaccination. J Virol 1996; 70:4941–4947.

87. Walker CM, Moody DJ, Stites DP, Levy JA. CD8+ lymphocytes can control HIV infection in vitro by suppressing virus replication. Science 1986; 234:1563–1566.

88. Kannagi M, Chalifoux LV, Lord CI, Letvin NL. Suppression of simian immunodeficiency virus replication in vitro by CD8+ lymphocytes. J Immunol 1988; 140:2237–2242.

89. Yang OO, Kalams SA, Trocha A, et al. Suppression of human immunodeficiency virus type 1 replication by CD8+ cells: evidence for HLA class I-restricted triggering of cytolytic and noncytolytic mechanisms. J Virol 1997; 71:3120–3128.

90. Lehner T, Wang Y, Cranage M, et al. Protective mucosal immunity elicited by targeted iliac lymph node immunization with a subunit SIV envelope and core vaccine in macaques [see comments]. Nat Med 1996; 2:767–775.

91. Rosenberg ES, Billingsley JM, Caliendo AM, et al. Vigorous HIV-1-specific CD4+ T cell responses associated with control of viremia [see comments]. Science 1997; 278:1447–1450.

92. Keefer MC, Graham BS, Belshe RB, et al. Studies of high doses of a human immunodeficiency virus type 1 recombinant glycoprotein 160 candidate vaccine in HIV type 1-seronegative humans. The AIDS Vaccine Clinical Trials Network. AIDS Res Hum Retroviruses 1994; 10:1713–1723.

93. Kalams SA, Buchbinder SP, Rosenberg ES. Association between virus-specific cytotoxic T-lymphocyte and helper responses in human immunodeficiency virus type 1 infection. J Virol 1999; 73:6715–6720.

94. Walter EA, Greenberg PD, Gilbert MJ, et al. Reconstitution of cellular immunity against cytomegalovirus in recipients of allogeneic bone marrow by transfer of T-cell clones from the donor [see comments]. N Engl J Med 1995; 333:1038–1044.
95. Clerici M, Fusi ML, Ruzzante S, et al. Type 1 and type 2 cytokines in HIV infection—a possible role in apoptosis and disease progression [editorial]. Ann Med 1997; 29:185–188.
96. Romagnani S, Maggi E, Del Prete G. HIV can induce a TH1 to TH0 shift, and preferentially replicates in CD4+ T-cell clones producing TH2-type cytokines. Res Immunol 1994; 145:611–617; discussion 617–618.
97. Sabin AB. HIV vaccination dilemma [letter; comment]. Nature 1993; 362:212.
98. Cranage MP, Whatmore AM, Sharpe SA, et al. Macaques infected with live attenuated SIVmac are protected against superinfection via the rectal mucosa. Virology 1997; 229:143–154.
99. Marthas ML, Miller CJ, Sutjipto S, et al. Efficacy of live-attenuated and whole-inactivated simian immunodeficiency virus vaccines against vaginal challenge with virulent SIV. J Med Primatol 1992; 21:99–107.
100. Benson J, Chougnet C, Robert-Guroff M, et al. Recombinant vaccine-induced protection against the highly pathogenic simian immunodeficiency virus SIV(mac251): dependence on route of challenge exposure. J Virol 1998; 72:4170–4182.
101. Lehner T, Panagiotidi C, Bergmeier LA, et al. Genital-associated lymphoid tissue in female non-human primates. Adv Exp Med Biol 1995:357–365.
102. Lohman BL, Miller CJ, McChesney MB. Antiviral cytotoxic T lymphocytes in vaginal mucosa of simian immunodeficiency virus-infected rhesus macaques. J Immunol 1995; 155:5855–5860.
103. Murphey-Corb M, Wilson LA, Trichel AM, et al. Selective induction of protective MHC class I-restricted CTL in the intestinal lamina propria of rhesus monkeys by transient SIV infection of the colonic mucosa. J Immunol 1999; 162:540–549.
104. Trichel AM, Roberts ED, Wilson LA, Martin LN, Ruprecht RM, Murphey-Corb M. SIV/DeltaB670 transmission across oral, colonic, and vaginal mucosae in the macaque. J Med Primatol 1997; 26:3–10.
105. Lehner T, Wang Y, Cranage M, et al. Protective mucosal immunity elicited by targeted lymph node immunization with a subunit SIV envelope and core vaccine in macaques. Dev Biol Stand 1998; 92:225–235.
106. Burns JW, Siadat-Pajouh M, Krishnaney AA, Greenberg HB. Protective effect of rotavirus VP6-specific IgA monoclonal antibodies that lack neutralizing activity [see comments]. Science 1996; 272:104–107.
107. Mazanec MB, Kaetzel CS, Lamm ME, Fletcher D, Nedrud JG. Intracellular neutralization of virus by immunoglobulin A antibodies. Proc Natl Acad Sci U S A 1992; 89:6901–6905.
108. Joag SV, Liu ZQ, Stephens EB, et al. Oral immunization of macaques with attenuated vaccine virus induces protection against vaginally transmitted AIDS. J Virol 1998; 72:9069–9078.
109. Quesada-Rolander M, Makitalo B, Thorstensson R, et al. Protection against mucosal SIVsm challenge in macaques infected with a chimeric SIV that expresses HIV type 1 envelope. AIDS Res Hum Retroviruses 1996; 12:993–999.
110. Miller CJ, McChesney MB, Lu X, et al. Rhesus macaques previously infected with

simian/human immunodeficiency virus are protected from vaginal challenge with pathogenic SIVmac239. J Virol 1997; 71:1911–1921.

111. Artenstein AW, VanCott TC, Sitz KV, et al. Mucosal immune responses in four distinct compartments of women infected with human immunodeficiency virus type 1: a comparison by site and correlation with clinical information. J Infect Dis 1997; 175:265–271.

112. Haimovici F, Mayer KH, Anderson DJ. Quantitation of HIV-1-specific IgG, IgA, and IgM antibodies in human genital tract secretions. J Acquir Immune Defic Syndr Hum Retrovirol 1997; 15:185–191.

113. Belec L, Prazuck T, Payan C, et al. Cervicovaginal anti-HIV antibodies in index women from HIV-discordant, exclusively heterosexual, couples. Viral Immunol 1996; 9:155–158.

114. Gorse GJ, Rogers JH, Perry JE, et al. HIV-1 recombinant gp160 vaccine induced antibodies in serum and saliva. The NIAID AIDS Vaccine Clinical Trials Network. Vaccine 1995; 13:209–214.

115. Emini EA, Schleif WA, Nunberg JH, et al. Prevention of HIV-1 infection in chimpanzees by gp120 V3 domain-specific monoclonal antibody. Nature 1992; 355:728–730.

116. Ukwu HN, Graham BS, Lambert JS, Wright PF. Perinatal transmission of human immunodeficiency virus-1 infection and maternal immunization strategies for prevention. Obstet Gynecol 1992; 80:458–468.

117. Longini IM Jr, Datta S, Halloran ME. Measuring vaccine efficacy for both susceptibility to infection and reduction in infectiousness for prophylactic HIV-1 vaccines. J Acquir Immune Defic Syndr Hum Retrovirol 1996; 13:440–447.

117a. Quinn TC, Wawer MJ, Sewankambo N, et al. Viral load and heterosexual transmission of human immunodeficiency virus type 1. N Engl J Med 2000; 342:921–929.

118. Bryson YJ. Perinatal HIV-1 transmission: recent advances and therapeutic interventions. AIDS 1996; 10(Suppl 3):S33–S42.

119. Novembre FJ, Saucier M, Anderson DC, et al. Development of AIDS in a chimpanzee infected with human immunodeficiency virus type 1. J Virol 1997; 71:4086–4091.

120. Joag SV, Li Z, Foresman L, et al. Characterization of the pathogenic KU-SHIV model of acquired immunodeficiency syndrome in macaques. AIDS Res Hum Retroviruses 1997; 13:635–645.

121. Reimann KA, Li JT, Veazey R, et al. A chimeric simian/human immunodeficiency virus expressing a primary patient human immunodeficiency virus type 1 isolate env causes an AIDS-like disease after in vivo passage in rhesus monkeys. J Virol 1996; 70:6922–6928.

122. Shibata R, Kawamura M, Sakai H, Hayami M, Ishimoto A, Adachi A. Generation of a chimeric human and simian immunodeficiency virus infectious to monkey peripheral blood mononuclear cells. J Virol 1991; 65:3514–3520.

123. Warren JT, Levinson MA. Preclinical AIDS vaccine development: formal survey of global HIV, SIV, and SHIV in vivo challenge studies in vaccinated nonhuman primates. J Med Primatol 1997; 26:63–81.

124. Plotkin SA, Orenstein WA. Vaccines. Philadelphia: WB Saunders, 1999.

125. Putkonen P, Walther L, Zhang YJ, et al. Long-term protection against SIV-induced disease in macaques vaccinated with a live attenuated HIV-2 vaccine. Nat Med 1995; 1:914–918.

126. Shibata R, Seimon C, Cho MW, et al. Resistance of previously infected chimpanzees to successive challenges with a heterologous intraclade B strain of human immunodeficiency virus type 1. J Virol 1996; 70:4361–4369.

127. Girard M, Yue L, Barre-Sinoussi F, et al. Failure of a human immunodeficiency virus type 1 (HIV-1) subtype B-derived vaccine to prevent infection of chimpanzees by an HIV-1 subtype E strain. J Virol 1996; 70:8229–8233.

128. Baba TW, Jeong YS, Pennick D, Bronson R, Greene MF, Ruprecht RM. Pathogenicity of live, attenuated SIV after mucosal infection of neonatal macaques [see comments]. Science 1995; 267:1820–1825.

129. Deacon NJ, Tsykin A, Solomon A, et al. Genomic structure of an attenuated quasi species of HIV-1 from a blood transfusion donor and recipients [see comments]. Science 1995; 270:988–991.

130. Kirchhoff F, Greenough TC, Brettler DB, Sullivan JL, Desrosiers RD. Brief report: absence of intact nef sequences in a long-term survivor with nonprogressive HIV-1 infection [see comments]. N Engl J Med 1995; 332:228–232.

131. Learmont J, Cook L, Dunckley H, Sullivan JS. Update on long-term symptomless HIV type 1 infection in recipients of blood products from a single donor [letter]. AIDS Res Hum Retroviruses 1995; 11:1.

132. Greenough TC, Somasundaran M, Brettler DB, et al. Normal immune function and inability to isolate virus in culture in an individual with long-term human immunodeficiency virus type 1 infection. AIDS Res Hum Retroviruses 1994; 10:395–403.

132a. Learmont JC, Geczy AF, Mills J, et al. Immunologic and virologic status after 14 to 18 years of infection with an attenuated strain of HIV-1. A report from the Sydney Blood Bank Cohort. N Engl J Med 1999; 340:1715–1722.

133. Marthas ML, Ramos RA, Lohman BL, et al. Viral determinants of simian immunodeficiency virus (SIV) virulence in rhesus macaques assessed by using attenuated and pathogenic molecular clones of SIVmac. J Virol 1993; 67:6047–6055.

134. Desrosiers RC. Safety issues facing development of a live-attenuated, multiply deleted HIV-1 vaccine [letter]. AIDS Res Hum Retroviruses 1994; 10:331–332.

135. Van Rompay KK, Otsyula MG, Tarara RP, et al. Vaccination of pregnant macaques protects newborns against mucosal simian immunodeficiency virus infection. J Infect Dis 1996; 173:1327–1335.

136. Niedrig M, Gregersen JP, Fultz PN, Broker M, Mehdi S, Hilfenhaus J. Immune response of chimpanzees after immunization with the inactivated whole immunodeficiency virus (HIV-1), three different adjuvants and challenge. Vaccine 1993; 11:67–74.

137. Gibbs CJ Jr, Peters R, Gravell M, et al. Observations after human immunodeficiency virus immunization and challenge of human immunodeficiency virus seropositive and seronegative chimpanzees. Proc Natl Acad Sci U S A 1991; 88:3348–3352.

138. Johnson PR, Montefiori DC, Goldstein S, et al. Inactivated whole SIV vaccine in macaques: evaluation of protective efficacy against challenge with cell-free virus or infected cells. AIDS Res Hum Retroviruses 1992; 8:1501–1505.

139. Carlson JR, McGraw TP, Keddie E, et al. Vaccine protection of rhesus macaques against simian immunodeficiency virus infection. AIDS Res Hum Retroviruses 1990; 6:1239–1246.

140. Murphey-Corb M, Ohkawa S, Davison-Fairburn B, et al. A formalin-fixed whole SIV vaccine induces protective responses that are cross-protective and durable. AIDS Res Hum Retroviruses 1992; 8:1475–1478.

141. Mills KH, Page M, Chan WL, et al. Protection against SIV infection in macaques by immunization with inactivated virus from the BK28 molecular clone, but not with BK28-derived recombinant env and gag proteins. J Med Primatol 1992; 21:50–58.

142. Putkonen P, Thorstensson R, Cranage M, et al. A formalin inactivated whole SIV-mac vaccine in Ribi adjuvant protects against homologous and heterologous SIV challenge. J Med Primatol 1992; 21:108–112.

143. Le Grand R, Vogt G, Vaslin B, et al. Specific and non-specific immunity and protection of macaques against SIV infection. Vaccine 1992; 10:873–879.

144. Langlois AJ, Weinhold KJ, Matthews TJ, Greenberg ML, Bolognesi DP. Detection of anti-human cell antibodies in sera from macaques immunized with whole inactivated virus. AIDS Res Hum Retroviruses 1992; 8:1641–1652.

145. Haynes JR, Yao FL, Ma J, Cao SX, Klein MH. Strategy for developing a genetically-engineered whole-virus vaccine against HIV. Mol Immunol 1991; 28:231–234.

146. Rovinski B, Haynes JR, Cao SX, et al. Expression and characterization of genetically engineered human immunodeficiency virus-like particles containing modified envelope glycoproteins: implications for development of a cross-protective AIDS vaccine. J Virol 1992; 66:4003–4012.

147. Klavinskis LS, Bergmeier LA, Gao L, et al. Mucosal or targeted lymph node immunization of macaques with a particulate SIVp27 protein elicits virus-specific CTL in the genito-rectal mucosa and draining lymph nodes. J Immunol 1996; 157:2521–2527.

148. Martin SJ, Vyakarnam A, Cheingsong-Popov R, et al. Immunization of human HIV-seronegative volunteers with recombinant p17/p24:Ty virus-like particles elicits HIV-1 p24-specific cellular and humoral immune responses. AIDS 1993; 7:1315–1323.

149. Weber J, Cheingsong-Popov R, Callow D, et al. Immunogenicity of the yeast recombinant p17/p24:Ty virus-like particles (p24-VLP) in healthy volunteers. Vaccine 1995; 13:831–834.

150. Wagner R, Teeuwsen VJ, Deml L. Cytotoxic T cells and neutralizing antibodies induced in rhesus monkeys by virus-like particle HIV vaccines in the absence of protection from SHIV infection. Virology 1998; 245:65–74.

151. Grene E, Mezule G, Borisova G, Pumpens P, Bentwich Z, Arnon R. Relationship between antigenicity and immunogenicity of chimeric hepatitis B virus core particles carrying HIV type 1 epitopes. AIDS Res Hum Retroviruses 1997; 13:41–51.

152. Wu S, Pascual DW, Lewis GK, Hone DM. Induction of mucosal and systemic responses against human immunodeficiency virus type 1 glycoprotein 120 in mice after oral immunization with a single dose of a Salmonella-HIV vector. AIDS Res Hum Retroviruses 1997; 13:1187–1194.

153. Smith AD, Geisler SC, Chen AA, et al. Human rhinovirus type 14:human immunodeficiency virus type 1 (HIV-1) V3 loop chimeras from a combinatorial library induce potent neutralizing antibody responses against HIV-1. J Virol 1998; 72:651–659.

154. Limbach KJ, Paoletti E. Non-replicating expression vectors: applications in vaccine development and gene therapy. Epidemiol Infect 1996; 116:241–256.

155. Clements-Mann ML, Weinhold K, Matthews TJ, et al. Immune responses to human immunodeficiency virus (HIV) type 1 induced by canarypox expressing HIV-1MN gp120, HIV-1SF2 recombinant gp120, or both vaccines in seronegative adults. NIAID AIDS Vaccine Evaluation Group. J Infect Dis 1998; 177:1230–1246.

155a. Belshe RB, Gorse GJ, Mulligan MJ. Induction of immune responses to HIV-1 by canarypox virus (ALVAC) HIV-1 and gp120 SF-2 recombinant vaccines in uninfected volunteers. NIAID AIDS Vaccine Evalluation Group. AIDS 1998; 12:2407–2415.

155b. Clements-Mann ML, Weinhold K, Matthews TJ, et al. Immune responses to human immunodeficiency virus (HIV) type 1 induced by canarypox expressing HIV-1MN gp120, HIV-1SF2 recombinant gp120, or both vaccines in seronegative adults. NIAID AIDS Vaccine Evaluation Group. J Infect Dis 1998; 177:1230–1246.

156. Egan MA, Pavlat WA, Tartaglia J, et al. Induction of human immunodeficiency virus type 1 (HIV-1)-specific cytolytic T lymphocyte responses in seronegative adults by a nonreplicating, host-range-restricted canarypox vector (ALVAC) carrying the HIV-1MN env gene. J Infect Dis 1995; 171:1623–1627.

157. Sutter G, Moss B. Novel vaccinia vector derived from the host range restricted and highly attenuated MVA strain of vaccinia virus. Dev Biol Stand 1995; 84:195–200.

158. Anderson MJ, Porter DC, Moldoveanu Z, Fletcher TM 3rd, McPherson S, Morrow CD. Characterization of the expression and immunogenicity of poliovirus replicons that encode simian immunodeficiency virus SIVmac239 Gag or envelope SU proteins. AIDS Res Hum Retroviruses 1997; 13:53–62.

159. Berglund P, Quesada-Rolander M, Putkonen P, Biberfeld G, Thorstensson R, Liljestrom P. Outcome of immunization of cynomolgus monkeys with recombinant Semliki Forest virus encoding human immunodeficiency virus type 1 envelope protein and challenge with a high dose of SHIV-4 virus. AIDS Res Hum Retroviruses 1997; 13:1487–1495.

160. Brand D, Lemiale F, Turbica I, Buzelay L, Brunet S, Barin F. Comparative analysis of humoral immune responses to HIV type 1 envelope glycoproteins in mice immunized with a DNA vaccine, recombinant Semliki Forest virus RNA, or recombinant Semliki Forest virus particles. AIDS Res Hum Retroviruses 1998; 14:1369–1377.

161. Mossman SP, Bex F, Berglund P, et al. Protection against lethal simian immunodeficiency virus SIVsmmPBj14 disease by a recombinant Semliki Forest virus gp160 vaccine and by a gp120 subunit vaccine. J Virol 1996; 70:1953–1960.

162. Caley IJ, Betts MR, Irlbeck DM, et al. Humoral, mucosal, and cellular immunity in response to a human immunodeficiency virus type 1 immunogen expressed by a Venezuelan equine encephalitis virus vaccine vector. J Virol 1997; 71:3031–3038.

163. Pushko P, Parker M, Ludwig GV, Davis NL, Johnston RE, Smith JF. Replicon-helper systems from attenuated Venezuelan equine encephalitis virus: expression of heterologous genes in vitro and immunization against heterologous pathogens in vivo. Virology 1997; 239:389–401.

164. Kim JJ, Ayyavoo V, Bagarazzi ML, et al. Development of a multicomponent candidate vaccine for HIV-1. Vaccine 1997; 15:879–883.

165. Kim JH, Loveland JE, Sitz KV, et al. Expansion of restricted cellular immune responses to HIV-1 envelope by vaccination: IL-7 and IL-12 differentially augment cellular proliferative responses to HIV-1. Clin Exp Immunol 1997; 108:243–250.

166. Yasutomi Y, Robinson HL, Lu S, et al. Simian immunodeficiency virus-specific cytotoxic T-lymphocyte induction through DNA vaccination of rhesus monkeys. J Virol 1996; 70:678–681.

167. Davis HL. DNA-based immunization against hepatitis B: experience with animal models. Curr Top Microbiol Immunol 1998; 226:57–68.

168. Letvin NL, Montefiori DC, Yasutomi Y, et al. Potent, protective anti-HIV immune responses generated by bimodal HIV envelope DNA plus protein vaccination. Proc Natl Acad Sci U S A 1997; 94:9378–9383.

169. Shiver JW, Davies ME, Yasutomi Y, et al. Anti-HIV env immunities elicited by nucleic acid vaccines. Vaccine 1997; 15:884–887.

170. Andre S, Seed B, Eberle J, Schraut W, Bultmann A, Haas J. Increased immune response elicited by DNA vaccination with a synthetic gp120 sequence with optimized codon usage. J Virol 1998; 72:1497–1503.

171. Klinman DM, Yamshchikov G, Ishigatsubo Y. Contribution of CpG motifs to the immunogenicity of DNA vaccines. J Immunol 1997; 158:3635–3639.

172. Krieg AM, Yi AK, Schorr J, Davis HL. The role of CpG dinucleotides in DNA vaccines. Trends Microbiol 1998; 6:23–27.

173. Kim JJ, Weiner DB. DNA gene vaccination for HIV. Springer Semin Immunopathol 1997; 19:175–194.

174. Keller PM, Arnold BA, Shaw AR, et al. Identification of HIV vaccine candidate peptides by screening random phage epitope libraries. Virology 1993; 193:709–716.

175. Parren PW, Fisicaro P, Labrijn AF, et al. In vitro antigen challenge of human antibody libraries for vaccine evaluation: the human immunodeficiency virus type 1 envelope. J Virol 1996; 70:9046–9050.

176. Ishii N, Sugita Y, Nakajima H, Bukawa H, Asakura Y, Okuda K. Genetic control of immune responses to HIV-1 env DNA vaccine. Microbiol Immunol 1997; 41:421–425.

177. Klavinskis LS, Gao L, Barnfield C, Lehner T, Parker S. Mucosal immunization with DNA-liposome complexes. Vaccine 1997; 15:818–820.

178. Sasaki S, Sumino K, Hamajima K, et al. Induction of systemic and mucosal immune responses to human immunodeficiency virus type 1 by a DNA vaccine formulated with QS-21 saponin adjuvant via intramuscular and intranasal routes. J Virol 1998; 72:4931–4939.

179. Swain WF, Macklin MD, Neumann G, et al. Manipulation of immune responses via particle-mediated polynucleotide vaccines. Behring Inst Mitt 1997:73–78.

180. Stanhope PE, Clements ML, Siliciano RF. Human CD4+ cytolytic T lymphocyte responses to a human immunodeficiency virus type 1 gp160 subunit vaccine. J Infect Dis 1993; 168:92–100.

181. Picard O, Achour A, Bernard J, et al. A 2-year follow-up of an anti-HIV immune reaction in HIV-1 gp160-immunized healthy seronegative humans: evidence for persistent cell-mediated immunity. J Acquir Immune Defic Syndr 1992; 5:539–546.

182. Gorse GJ, McElrath MJ, Matthews TJ, et al. Modulation of immunologic responses to HIV-1MN recombinant gp160 vaccine by dose and schedule of administration. National Institute of Allergy and Infectious Diseases AIDS Vaccine Evaluation Group. Vaccine 1998; 16:493–506.

183. Kahn JO, Stites DP, Scillian J, et al. A phase I study of HGP-30, a 30 amino acid subunit of the human immunodeficiency virus (HIV) p17 synthetic peptide analogue sub-unit vaccine in seronegative subjects. AIDS Res Hum Retroviruses 1992; 8:1321–1325.

184. Rubinstein A, Goldstein H, Pettoello-Mantovani M, et al. Safety and immunogenicity of a V3 loop synthetic peptide conjugated to purified protein derivative in HIV-seronegative volunteers. AIDS 1995; 9:243–251.

185. Gorse GJ, Keefer MC, Belshe RB, et al. A dose-ranging study of a prototype synthetic HIV-1MN V3 branched peptide vaccine. The National Institute of Allergy and Infectious Diseases AIDS Vaccine Evaluation Group. J Infect Dis 1996; 173:330–339.

186. Kelleher AD, Emery S, Cunningham P, et al. Safety and immunogenicity of UBI HIV-1MN octameric V3 peptide vaccine administered by subcutaneous injection. AIDS Res Hum Retroviruses 1997; 13:29–32.

187. Phanuphak P, Teeratakulpixarn S, Sarangbin S, et al. International clinical trials of HIV vaccines: I. Phase I trial of an HIV-1 synthetic peptide vaccine in Bangkok, Thailand. Asian Pac J Allergy Immunol 1997; 15:41–48.

188. Robey FA, Harris-Kelson T, Robert-Guroff M, et al. A synthetic conformational epitope from the C4 domain of HIV Gp120 that binds CD4. J Biol Chem 1996; 271: 17990–17995.

189. Frey A, Neutra MR, Robey FA. Peptomer aluminum oxide nanoparticle conjugates as systemic and mucosal vaccine candidates: synthesis and characterization of a conjugate derived from the C4 domain of HIV-1MN gp120. Bioconjug Chem 1997; 8: 424–433.

190. Gahery-Segard H, Pialoux G, Charmeteau B, et al. Multiepitopic B- and T-cell responses induced in humans by a human immunodeficiency virus type 1 lipopeptide vaccine. J Virol 2000; 74:1694–1703.

191. Deprez B, Sauzet JP, Boutillon C, et al. Comparative efficiency of simple lipopeptide constructs for in vivo induction of virus-specific CTL. Vaccine 1996; 14:375–382.

192. Sauzet JP, Deprez B, Martinon F, Guillet JG, Gras- Masse H, Gomard E. Long-lasting anti-viral cytotoxic T lymphocytes induced in vivo with chimeric-multirestricted lipopeptides. Vaccine 1995; 13:1339–1345.

193. McElrath MJ, Corey L, Greenberg PD. Evaluation of cytotoxic T cell responses to candidate HIV-1 vaccines in HIV-1-uninfected individuals. AIDS Res Hum Retroviruses 1994; 10:S69–S72.

194. McElrath MJ, Corey L, Berger D, et al. Immune responses elicited by recombinant vaccinia-human immunodeficiency virus (HIV) envelope and HIV envelope protein: analysis of the durability of responses and effect of repeated boosting. J Infect Dis 1994; 169:41–47.

195. Graham BS, Gorse GJ, Schwartz DH, et al. Determinants of antibody response after recombinant gp160 boosting in vaccinia-naive volunteers primed with gp160-recombinant vaccinia virus. The National Institute of Allergy and Infectious Diseases AIDS Vaccine Clinical Trials Network. J Infect Dis 1994; 170:782–786.

196. Fuller DH, Corb MM, Barnett S, Steimer K, Haynes JR. Enhancement of immunodeficiency virus-specific immune responses in DNA-immunized rhesus macaques. Vaccine 1997; 15:924–926.

197. Dunn DT, Tess BH, Rodrigues LC, Ades AE. Mother-to-child transmission of HIV: implications of variation in maternal infectivity. AIDS 1998; 12:2211–2216.

198. Wara D, Luzuriaga K, Martin NL, Sullivan JL, Bryson YJ. Maternal transmission and diagnosis of human immunodeficiency virus during infancy. Ann N Y Acad Sci 1993; 693:14–19.

199. Keefer MC, Wolff M, Gorse GJ, et al. Safety profile of phase I and II preventive HIV type 1 envelope vaccination: experience of the NIAID AIDS Vaccine Evaluation Group. AIDS Res Hum Retroviruses 1997; 13:1163–1177.

200. Connor RI, Korber BT, Graham BS, et al. Immunological and virological analyses of persons infected by human immunodeficiency virus type 1 while participating in trials of recombinant gp120 subunit vaccines. J Virol 1998; 72:1552–1576.

201. Graham BS, McElrath MJ, Connor RI, et al. Analysis of intercurrent human immunodeficiency virus type 1 infections in phase I and II trials of candidate AIDS vaccines. AIDS Vaccine Evaluation Group and the Correlates of HIV Immune Protection Group. J Infect Dis 1998; 177:310–319.

202. Kahn JO, Steimer KS, Baenziger J, et al. Clinical, immunologic, and virologic observations related to human immunodeficiency virus (HIV) type 1 infection in a volunteer in an HIV-1 vaccine clinical trial [see comments]. J Infect Dis 1995; 171:1343–1347.

203. McElrath MJ, Corey L, Greenberg PD, et al. Human immunodeficiency virus type 1 infection despite prior immunization with a recombinant envelope vaccine regimen. Proc Natl Acad Sci U S A 1996; 93:3972–3977.

204. Fast PE, Sawyer LA, Wescott SL. Clinical considerations in vaccine trials with special reference to candidate HIV vaccines. Pharmacol Biotechnol 1995; 6:97–134.

205. Sheon AR, Wagner L, McElrath MJ, et al. Preventing discrimination against volunteers in prophylactic HIV vaccine trials: lessons from a phase II trial. J Acquir Immune Defic Syndr Hum Retrovirol 1998; 19:519–526.

206. Belshe RB, Clements ML, Keefer MC, et al. Interpreting HIV serodiagnostic test results in the 1990s: social risks of HIV vaccine studies in uninfected volunteers. NIAID AIDS Vaccine Clinical Trials Group. Ann Intern Med 1994; 121:584–589.

207. Rida WN, Lawrence DN. Some statistical issues in HIV vaccine trials. Stat Med 1994; 13:2155–2177.

208. Rida W, Fast P, Hoff R, Fleming T. Intermediate-size trials for the evaluation of HIV vaccine candidates: a workshop summary. J Acquir Immune Defic Syndr Hum Retrovirol 1997; 16:195–203.

209. Koblin BA, Taylor PE, Avrett S, Stevens CE. The feasibility of HIV-1 vaccine efficacy trials among gay/bisexual men in New York City: Project ACHIEVE. AIDS Community Health Initiative Enroute to the Vaccine Effort. AIDS 1996; 10:1555–1561.

210. McKirnan DJ, Doetsch J, Vanable P, Buchbinder S, Douglas JM, Judson F. Preparations for AIDS vaccine trials. Developing brief valid screening instruments for HIV-related sexual risk behavior among gay and bisexual men. AIDS Res Hum Retroviruses 1994; 10:S285–S288.

211. Lu Y, Salvato MS, Pauza CD, et al. Utility of SHIV for testing HIV-1 vaccine candidates in macaques. J Acquir Immune Defic Syndr Hum Retrovirol 1996; 12:99–106.

212. Mellors JW, Munoz A, Giorgi JV, et al. Plasma viral load and CD4+ lymphocytes as prognostic markers of HIV-1 infection [see comments]. Ann Intern Med 1997; 126:946–954.

213. Prince AM, Allan J, Andrus L, et al. Virulent HIV strains, chimpanzees, and trial vaccines [letter] [see comments]. Science 1999; 283:1117–1118.

7
Gene Therapy of HIV Infection

Stefan A. Klein, Christian Klebba, and Dieter Hoelzer
Johann Wolfgang Goethe-Universität, Frankfurt am Main, Germany

Manuel Grez
Georg-Speyer Haus, Frankfurt am Main, Germany

I. INTRODUCTION

The introduction of combination antiretroviral therapy resulted in a remarkable improvement of the life expectancy and the acquired immunodeficiency syndrome (AIDS)-free survival of individuals infected with human immunodeficiency virus (HIV). Despite this progress, HIV infection is still not a curable disease. Furthermore, the problems of drug therapy such as its toxicity and, above all, the emergence of resistance clearly show the need for alternative therapeutic approaches.

Retroviral infection with HIV results in the stable integration of a proviral DNA in the genome of the target cell. This provirus becomes a hereditary part of the genetic information of the host cell. The HIV can be therefore considered as a kind of acquired genetic disease. Thus, the modulation of HIV replication by the gene therapeutic expression of antiviral genes may be a therapeutic option for HIV infection. The concept of gene therapy as an intracellular immunization against HIV was suggested for the first time in 1988 by Baltimore (1). Recently, a large number of different anti-HIV gene therapy approaches have been developed and brought into clinical trials. The gene therapy strategies can be divided into two main categories: (a) genetic modification of HIV target cells or their progenies in order to inhibit HIV replication and (b) genetic modification of cells in order to generate an immune response against HIV or HIV-infected cells. The second category can be described as a gene therapy–based immunotherapy. This field involves two major principles: (a) the generation of immune cells, such as cytotoxic T cells against HIV-infected cells and (b) the gene therapeutic application of genetic information encoding for HIV proteins in order to generate or to enhance a humoral or cellular response against the virus. Such vaccination approaches are not discussed in this chapter; rather, this chapter focuses mainly on the first category. It involves the transfer of genetic material into HIV target cells or their progenitor cells (CD4$^+$ T cells, hematopoietic stem cells) in order to inhibit intracellularly HIV gene expression and HIV replication. A typical approach for gene therapy of HIV infection is schematically depicted in Figure 1. As potential anti-HIV genes, several different protein and nucleic acid–based antiviral principles have been developed. Simultaneously, different efficient, reliable, and secure methods for ex vivo manipulation and gene transfer of potential HIV target cells have been established. This chapter addresses the different antiviral strategies, the transfer of the genetic material encoding for these antivirals into the target cells, and the first steps of clinical application of gene therapy for HIV infection.

II. ANTIVIRAL STRATEGIES

Intracellular immunization by the expression of anti-HIV genes utilizes either nucleic acids, primarily RNA molecules, or proteins with an antiviral activity. Antisense oligonucleotides, ribozymes, and decoys fall into the first group. The HIV inhibitory proteins are intracellularly acting antibody fragments, single-chain variable fragments (sFV), or transdominant negative HIV or cellular proteins. Most of these approaches target viral RNA or proteins. In addition, cellular factors, which are prerequisites for HIV infection and replication or which at least have important influence on HIV replication, are potential targets for anti-HIV gene therapy. The viral and cellular targets for the different anti-HIV genes are listed in Table 1.

A. RNA-Based Strategies

1. Antisense

Antisense strategies have been widely used to inhibit gene expression, especially to suppress the expression of viral genes as a therapeutic approach. Antisense RNA molecules act by hybridization to the target RNA molecules, leading to the degradation of the duplexed RNA. Additionally, antisense molecules inhibit mRNA transport and translation. Antisense sequences have been utilized as chemically synthesized phosphorothioate-labeled RNA strains (52), or they have been expressed after gene transfer by the target cell itself (53). Antisense molecules can theoretically be targeted against each sequence within the HIV genome and they are able to act during each active step of the HIV replication cycle. Therefore, antisense sequences have already been directed against almost all parts of the HIV genome. Sequences encoding for both structural as well as for regulatory elements

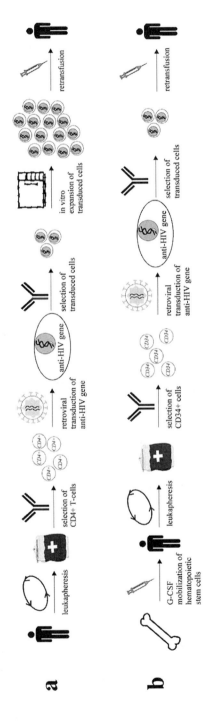

Figure 1 Schematic illustration of gene therapy strategies in clinical trials involving retroviral ex vivo gene transfer into CD4+ T cells (a) or CD34+ hematopoietic stem cells (b).

Table 1 Viral and Cellular Targets and Their Corresponding Anti-HIV Genes

Target	Antiviral strategy
Gag	Antisense (2,3), Ribozymes, transdominant gag mutants (4)
Pol	Ribozymes (5–7), anti RT Ab fragments (8), anti integrase sFV (9), transdominant neg. protease (10)
Env	Anti gp120 single chain variable fragments (11), intracellular soluble CD4 (12,13), ribozymes (14,15), transdominant rev mutants (16)
Tat/TAR	Transdominant neg. tat (17,18), TAR decoy (19,20), antisense oligonucleotides against TAR and tat (21), ribozymes against tat (22,23), anti tat sFV (24)
Rev/RRE	Transdominant neg. rev (25–28), RRE decoy (29,30), antisense oligonucleotides against RRE (31), ribozymes against rev (15,22), anti rev single chain variable fragments (32), transdominant neg. EIF-5A (33)
Nef	Ribozymes (34)
5′ leader sequence (U5)	Ribozymes (35–38)
Chemokine receptors	Antisense oligonucleotides, ribozymes against chemokine receptor mRNA (39), RANTES intrakine (40–42), transdominant CCR-5 mutant (43)
NFκB	IκB (44), transdominant IκB mutant (45–47)
eIF-5A	Transdominant eukaryotic initiation factor 5A mutants (33)
RNA binding protein$_{9-27}$	IFN-β gene expression (48–51)

have been targeted (2,3,22,31,54–59). Antisense molecules against regulatory components of HIV, such as TAR (54) and Tat (56), as well as against RRE (31) and Rev (22) have been demonstrated to be very effective. Chatterjee et al. showed a greater than 99% reduction of infectious virus production by an adeno-associated virus (AAV)-expressed antisense, including the TAR sequence. To make the generation of resistant mutants against antisense molecules less likely, large subgenomic antisense sequences have been developed. These antisense molecules are thousands of bases long and cover simultaneously several genes of the HIV genome (53). Several clinical trials of anti-HIV antisense molecules expressed retrovirally in hematopoietic stem cells and CD4+ T cells are in preparation or have already started (NIH##9503-103, 9806-261, and 9812-277).

2. Ribozymes

Ribozymes are small antisense molecules with a catalytic activity (60). They are able to specifically cleave a target RNA sequence. Among the large number of different ribozyme types, those with hammerhead or hairpin structures have been applied as antivirals. Both ribozyme types are originally small cis-cleaving motives isolated from plant virusoids such as the tobacco ringspot virus (60–62). By in vitro mutagenesis, trans-cleaving molecules were created (60). Hairpin and hammerhead ribozymes are relatively small molecules with about 40 to 60 nucleotides. The catalytic core of most of the ribozyme types is directed against GUC triplets. Alternatively, some ribozymes are directed against GAU (63), GUU (64), or AUC (65) triplets. The binding of a ribozyme is mediated by way of the antisense sequence of the ribozyme, which should have a minimal length of 8 to 12 nucleotides to guarantee a specific cleavage. Similar to antisense molecules, ribozymes can be targeted against virtually any HIV sequence (if it possesses an appropriate target triplet). However, ribozymes have several advantages in comparison to antisense molecules. Usually they are smaller. Thus, they are expressed more easily and efficiently, and multiple ribozyme sequences can be expressed by a single vector. The main advantage of ribozymes are, at least in theory, their capability of multiple turnovers and regeneration after each catalytic interaction.

Ribozymes against several sequences of the HIV genome have been designed and expressed retrovirally in hematopoietic stem cells (66,67), T-cell lines, and primary $CD4^+$ T cells (36,65,68). Human immunodeficiency virus replication (p24 antigen level in culture supernatants) was reduced by 1 to 4 orders of magnitude (log 10) by some of the anti-HIV ribozymes. Effective ribozymes were targeted against, for example, the second GUC triplet of the 5′ LTR (5′ leader sequence/U5) (35,69), the first GUC triplet in the tat gene (21,65), a GUA triplet in the tat sequence (70,71), and the second GUC in the pol gene (5). Some of these ribozymes have already been introduced into clinical trials (NIH## 9309-057, 9508-117, and 9604-153) (72).

A different type of ribozyme that could be used for gene therapeutic HIV inhibition is the group I intron from *Tetrahymena thermophilia*. This originally cis-splicing intron was modified to a trans-cleaving and -splicing ribozyme. In addition to the cleavage reaction, the tetrahymena group I ribozyme can specifically transfer an RNA sequence downstream from the cleavage site (73). Utilizing such a specific splicing tool, suicide genes could be added into HIV transcripts (74). Such an approach should specifically result in the death of HIV-infected cells.

3. Decoys

Decoys are RNA molecules that mimic binding motives for virus-specific regulatory proteins. These binding motives are the Rev responsive element (RRE) for the Rev protein and the transactivation response element (TAR) for the Tat protein. Highly expressed decoys lead to competitive inhibition of the binding of the virus RNA to the regulatory proteins. RRE decoys suppress the Rev-mediated HIV RNA transport and TAR decoys inhibit the transactivation of HIV replication conferred by Tat (19,20,29,30,75,76). Especially, retrovirally expressed RRE decoys have been demonstrated as efficient inhibitors of HIV replication in cell lines, primary $CD4^+$ T cells and hematopoietic stem cell–derived monocytes (29,30). A phase I clinical trial of hematopoietic stem cell gene therapy in HIV-1 infected children with retrovirally expressed RRE decoys was initiated in 1997 (NIH# 9602-147) (77,78).

B. Protein-Based Strategies

1. Transdominant HIV Proteins

In general, transdominant proteins are mutated viral proteins that have lost at least a part of their function but still compete with the wild-type protein. Transdominant mutants have been generated to interfere with structural proteins such as Gag (4,79) and Env (16,80) and to compete with regulatory factors such as Tat (17,18,81–83) and Rev (25,26,84). The most favored transdominant HIV protein is a mutant Rev designated as RevM10. While it still binds the RRE, its binding site for exportin 1, a cellular nuclear export factor, is mutated. Therefore, the Rev-mediated transport of unspliced or single spliced HIV transcripts is inhibited competitively by RevM10. Although its antiviral capacity is relatively low in comparison to antisense sequences or ribozymes, RevM10 is the anti-HIV gene therapeutic approach with the most ongoing clinical trials. Both CD4$^+$ T cells and hematopoietic stem cells are targeted by retrovirally expressed RevM10 in these trials (NIH## 9306-048,9503-103, 9806-261, and 9812-277) (59,85).

2. Intrabodies, Single-Chain Variable Fragments (sFv)

Intrabodies are intracellularly expressed genetically engineered antibody fragments. They are single-chain antibodies in which the variable domain of the heavy chain is joined to the light chain through a peptide linker, preserving the affinity of the original antibody (86). Such single-chain variable fragments (SFv) have been targeted against structural and regulatory HIV proteins such as Env, Gag, Tat, and Rev (24,86–91). Clinical trials on anti-HIV intrabodies have already been initiated (NIH## 9506-112 and 9512-141) (92).

3. Suicide Genes

Suicide genes under the control of a Tat-dependent HIV promoter have been demonstrated to kill cells after infection with HIV and to inhibit HIV spread in vitro (93). Suicide genes that have already been used in vitro studies for HIV gene therapy are genes encoding for the herpes simplex virus thymidine kinase (93,94), for the herpes simplex virus host shutoff protein (95), for cytosindeaminase, or for bacterial toxins such as the diphtheria toxin A (181). A major problem of the gene therapeutic application of HIV promoter driven suicide genes is that this promoter can be activated not only by Tat but also by a variety of cellular and other viral transcription factors leading to an unspecific destruction of HIV-negative cells. Alternatively, suicide genes can be employed for specific killing of HIV-infected cells by the tetrahymena group I intron–mediated ligation of the suicide gene to HIV transcripts (74).

The expression of suicide genes as well as of other protein-based anti-HIV genes, such as intrabodies or mutant HIV proteins, involves the problem of expressing foreign nonhuman proteins that are potentially immunogenic. For the thymidine kinase (96) and RevM10 (97), immune responses against the expressed gene products have been already demonstrated in animal models.

C. Combination of Antiviral Strategies

Similar to the conventional antiretroviral drug therapy, gene therapy with anti-HIV genes is faced with the problem of the emergence of resistance. Therefore, the expression of multiple anti-HIV genes within a target cell would certainly be of benefit. In theory, all the aforementioned antiviral strategies can be combined. Several combinations of anti-HIV genes expressed by a single vector have been already tested in vitro (Table 2). Furthermore, clinical trials on combination strategies have already started (NIH## 9806-261 and 9812-277). Some of the combinations con-

Table 2 Combined Expression of Anti-HIV Genes

Combination	Targets
Decoy with decoy	RRE decoy + TAR decoy (104)
Ribozyme with ribozyme	Multitarget ribozymes against 9 sites with the Env gene (14,98)
	Dimer minizymes (maxizyme) directed against 2 cleavage sites within the tat mRNA (99,105)
	Shotgun ribozymes, release of multiple independent ribozymes by cis cleavage (100–102)
Antisense with antisense	Antisense against Tat + antisense against Rev (106)
Combination of transdominant mutants	Transdominant Tat mutant + transdominant Rev mutant (107,108)
Decoy with ribozyme	RRE decoy + ribozyme against the 5' leader sequence (109)
	RRE decoy + ribozymes against the 5' leader sequence and the Env gene (110)
	TAR decoy + gag specific ribozyme (111)
Decoy with antisense	TAR decoy + gag specific antisense (112)
Decoy with transdominant mutant	Transdominant Tat mutant + RRE decoy (108)
	Transdominant Gag mutant + TAR decoy (112)
SFv with ribozyme	Anti Rev single chain variable fragment (SFv) + RRE specific ribozyme (113)
SFv with decoy	Anti Rev single chain variable fragment (SFv) + RRE decoy (114)
Transdominant mutant with suicide gene	Transdominant Gag mutant + eosinophil derived neurotoxin (115)

ferred an additive antiviral effect, whereas others even displayed synergism. The expression of multiple proteins by one vector is problematic. More than two or three different proteins can hardly be expressed even by a bicistronic or tricistronic vector system. Therefore, RNA-based strategies appear to be superior for antiviral combination therapy. Particularly short sequences such as decoys and ribozymes can be used in multitarget approaches. Chen et al. developed a multitarget ribozyme construct simultaneously targeting up to nine sites in the Env gene (14,98).

Kuwabara et al. developed shortened mutants of hammerhead ribozymes (minizymes) that form very active dimers designated as maxizymes. Heterodimeric maxizymes have been utilized as a combination antiviral approach to express ribozymes to cleave HIV-1 tat RNA at two sites simultaneously (99).

A further modification of multitarget ribozymes is the recently described principle of "shotgun" ribozymes: Multiple differently targeted ribozymes are released by a cis-acting ribozyme, resulting in multiple independently cleaving ribozymes (100–102). Currently, this promising approach is not usable in retroviral vector, because cis-acting ribozymes would destroy their own vector system. Alternatively, AAV vectors could be used (103).

D. Gene Therapeutic Immunotherapy

The genetic immunotherapy approach deals with the enhancement of the activity of cytotoxic T lymphocytes. Walker and colleagues developed a chimeric receptor protein composed of the gp120 binding domain from the CD4 molecule and the T-cell receptor CD3ζ chain (116). In CD8[+] T-cells expressing the chimeric receptor, binding of the CD4 domain to gp120 on the surface of HIV-infected cells result in a CD3ζ chain–mediated cell activation, which should immediately initiate a cytotoxic response. In vitro, such gene-modified CD8[+] T cells demonstrated a strong cytolytic activity against cells expressing gp120. Several clinical phase I/II studies with autologous and syngeneic gene-modified cytotoxic T lymphocytes against HIV-1 infected cells have been initiated (NIH## 9403-068, 9510-131, 9703-181, 9709-213, and 9805-253) (116,117).

III. DELIVERY OF ANTIVIRAL GENES

Several different methods are available to transfer genetic material into human cells. Nonviral (e.g., particle bombardment and liposome/DNA complexes) and viral (adenoviral, adeno-associated, retroviral, herpes simplex virus) delivery systems have been developed for clinical application. For gene therapy of HIV infection by intracellular immunization, some prerequisites have to be considered. The expression of the transferred gene must be stable and the genetic information should be inherited to daughter cells. Furthermore, the transfection efficiency has to be high and the biological characteristics of the modified cells should not be altered. Above all, the transfer system has to be safe: Side effects for the treated patient should be minimized and there must not be any danger for other individuals.

Although nonviral delivery systems such as liposome/DNA complexes or particle bombardment are very safe and easily manufactured, they currently play almost no role in the field of applied gene therapy. Their transfection efficiency is low, the majority of the targeted cells are destroyed during the transfection process, and stable integration of the transferred genetic material is rather rare. Totally synthetic gene delivery systems might be the preferred choice in the future to avoid the danger of producing recombinant virus or other toxic effects engendered by biologically active viral particles (118).

Adenoviral vectors and herpes simplex virus–based vectors do not stably integrate into the genome of the target cells and, consequently, vector expression decreases as the transduced cells proliferate (119). Currently, only viral vectors that integrate into the host genome of targeted cells provide stable gene transfer and expression. Therefore, the integrating retroviral and adeno-associated virus vectors are the most widely used gene transfer modalities for HIV gene therapy (120).

A. Retroviral Vectors

Within the group of Retroviridae, two subgroups, Oncoviridae (murine leukemia viruses) and Lentiviridae (HIV-1 and -2), are utilized to generate vectors for gene transfer. Moloney murine leukemia virus (MMLV)–based vectors have been selected in the earliest days of work on somatic gene therapy as the most promising gene transfer system (121). Currently, approximately 60% of all clinical gene transfer protocols use such retroviral vectors (118). For HIV gene therapy, wherein long-term expression of antiviral genes is required, almost all current protocols employ murine leukemia virus–based vectors.

1. Murine Leukemia Virus–Based Vectors

In principle, murine leukemia viruses have the same genome structure as all retroviruses. To serve as a gene delivery system, all viral genes (Gag, Pol, and Env) have been removed. The vectors only retain the viral long terminal repeats and the RNA packaging signal (ψ). The removal of all viral genes results in the important safety characteristic of replication incompetence. Retroviral vectors provide room for up to 8 kb of exogenous DNA. The genetic information that has to be transferred can be inserted downstream of the packaging signal. Alternatively, the genetic information is cloned into the LTR. Because of the doubling of the LTR during the reverse transcription, this architecture results in a double copy vector (19,122,123). The transcription of the inserted gene can be driven by the viral LTR promoter or by its own promoter. In addition to the inserted gene (e.g., an anti-HIV gene), a reporter gene has to be cloned into the vector. The reporter gene gives the opportunity to detect and to select cells that express the transferred gene. The most commonly used reporter gene is the neomycin resistance gene. Recently, the gene for the low-affinity nerve growth factor-receptor (LNGF-R) has become a very attractive selectable marker (124–126).

To infect the gene therapy target cells, recombinant vectors are generated by transfection of the vector DNA into packaging cell lines (127). Packaging cells are transfected with the viral genes that have been deleted in the vector genome in order to provide the structural proteins for virus production. To prevent the formation of replication-competent retroviruses, the viral genes are expressed without the packaging signal (ψ). In second and third generation packaging cells, the viral genes are transfected separately to make a packaging by chance even more unlikely (128–133). The Moloney murine leukemia virus targets the amphotropic receptor, which is expressed by almost all human cell types. Unfortunately, some cell types (e.g., hematopoietic stem cells) express the amphotropic receptor weakly. Therefore, pseudotyped vectors bearing the envelope from the gibbon ape leukemia virus (GALV) have been generated (134). Pseudotyping is an attractive method to generate more efficient or cell type–specific vectors. Because of the fragility of the envelope, Moloney envelope–bearing vectors cannot be ultracentrifuged. The G-protein of vesicular stomatitis virus was therefore applied to generate vector particles that can be concentrated, resulting in a higher multiplicity of infection (MOI) for transduction (135). For CD4[+] cell–specific transduction, HIV-1-env or SIV-env pseudotyped Moloney vectors have been designed (136,137). In comparison to the current ex vivo HIV gene therapy approaches, the potential for targeting HIV-1-env pseudotyped MMLV–based vectors to CD4[+] T cells by direct injection into the patient would greatly advance HIV gene therapy strategies (120).

The main risks involved in the application of MMLV–based vectors are the problems of possible insertional mutagenesis and the production of replication-competent virus (138–140). The major disadvantage of MMLV–based gene transfer is the problem that nondividing cells, such as hematopoietic stem cells or noncycling T cells, are hardly transducable. Therefore, cell cycle independent lentiviral vectors have been developed.

2. Lentiviral Vectors

"Similia similibus curantur," Samuel Hahnemann, the founder of homeopathy, established in the late 18th century a system of therapeutics based on the theory that "like cures like." Currently, HIV-based vectors are suggested as gene delivery systems for gene therapy of HIV infection.

The main target cells of anti-HIV gene transfer are hematopoietic stem cells and CD4[+] T cells. Without prior mitogenic stimulation, which may alter the normal characteristics of these cells, they are not transducable via MMLV-based vectors.

For transduction of nonmitotic cells, such as hematopoietic stem cells, neurons, or muscle cells, lentiviral (HIV-1 or -2 based) vectors have been developed

(141–152). For HIV gene therapy, lentivirus-based vectors would provide several advantages

1. Lentivirus-based vectors allow the ability to transduce nondividing cells. Using a lentiviral vector, Corbeau et al. were able to transduce terminally differentiated macrophages (149). More relevant, lentiviral vectors can transduce nonproliferating primitive ($CD34^+$, $CD38^-$) hemotopoietic stem cells (153). The ability to transduce quiescent cells provides the opportunity to transduce cells without prior stimulation. Thus, stem cells might be transduced without affecting their characteristics of self-renewal and differentiation into all lymphatic and myeloid progenitors. Likewise, $CD4^+$ T cells could be transduced without prior mitogenic stimulation preventing the occurrence of activation-induced apoptotic cell death.

2. HIV-based vectors allow specific transduction of $CD4^+$ cell populations. Like HIV-Env pseudotyped MMLV vectors, lentiviral vectors can specifically transduce $CD4^+$ cells in vitro without prior cell sorting, and they might be used for in vivo gene delivery by direct injection of the viral vector into the patient.

3. A rescue of the vector by wild-type HIV would result in spread and delivery of the anti-HIV genes to additional $CD4^+$ cells. Although this feature is fascinating, one has to consider the risks of such an uncontrolled vector replication. Donahue et al. have demonstrated the occurrence of lymphomas in 3 among 10 rhesus monkeys challenged by an uncontrolled spread of replication-competent murine leukemia virus (154). Furthermore, the spread of the viral vector could result in an unintentional infection of a second individual. Finally, recombination of vector and wild-type HIV could result in the generation of a new pathogenic virus.

B. Adeno-Associated Viral Vectors

Adeno-associated virus (AAV) is a nonpathogenic virus that is widespread in the human population. The wild-type AAV is the only known mammalian virus that preferentially integrates into a specific locus in the genome (short arm of human chromosome 19) (155,156). Because AAV is nonpathogenic and integrates in a site-specific manner, it would be the ideal candidate for a safe gene therapy. Unfortunately, integration of the current recombinant AAV vectors appears not to be strictly specific (157,158). A further major disadvantage of AAV vector is its small genome, which only provides space for about 4 to 5 kb of additional genetic information. However, AAV appears to be capable of infecting and integrating into nondividing cells, such as hematopoietic stem cells (159,160). Therefore, AAV is a promising vector system for stem cell–based gene therapy of HIV infection.

IV. TARGET CELLS

The HIV host cells have to be the targets of a gene therapeutic approach for HIV infection. Thus, $CD4^+$ T cells and their progenies, monocytic progenitors, monocytes, and all cells belonging to the mononuclear phagocyte system, such as tissue macrophages, microglial cells, or dendritic cells, must be protected by intracellular immunization. All these immune cells are derived from hematopoietic stem cells. Therefore, this cell type is the most attractive target for HIV gene therapy. Alternatively, mature peripheral blood CD4$^+$ T cells are a second important target. Both cell types have several advantages and inherent problems. However, both cellular approaches are meanwhile subject of clinical trials on gene therapy of HIV infection.

A. Hematopoietic Stem Cells

Hematopoietic stem cells expressing a potent anti-HIV gene should confer antiviral protection to all lymphohematopoietic cell lineages. Theoretically, such modified stem cells could provide a lifelong inhibition of HIV replication in all potential HIV host cells, resulting in complete reconstitution of immune function.

Besides potent anti-HIV genes, the prerequisites for a stem cell–based gene therapy of HIV infection are (a) the mobilization, collection, and separation of hematopoietic stem cells, (b) the efficient gene delivery into the stem cells without affecting their stem cell properties, (c) the engraftment of the modified stem cells after retransfusion, and (d) the in vivo development of protected mature HIV target cells.

Mobilization of peripheral blood hematopoietic stem cells by G-CSF (granulocyte-colony stimulating factor), collection of the stem cells by way of leukocyte apheresis, and selection of CD34$^+$ stem cells by immunoabsorption methods are routinely used for autologous and allogeneic stem cell transplantation. For isolation of hematopoietic stem cells from HIV-infected individuals, these methods have been employed successfully (161). The most critical point of stem cell–based gene therapy is to deliver genes into hematopoietic stem cells without destroying their potential for long-term engraftment in the bone marrow (162). In recent years, methods for highly efficient retroviral gene transfer into hematopoietic stem cells have been developed (7,152,153,163–165). Furthermore, in animal models, transduction of pluripotent long-term repopulating stem cells has been demonstrated (150,166,167). The ongoing clinical trials on hematopoietic stem cell–based gene therapy will elucidate whether human pluripotent stem cells can be successfully transduced in a clinical gene therapy setting. The next important issue is the ability of transduced hematopoietic stem cells to engraft in patients without prior cytoreductive or myeloablative conditioning (168). It has been shown in recent studies that transduced stem cells were detectable in unconditioned patients several months after receiving a stem cell graft (169,170). However, in the majority of gene therapy trials, the frequency of genetically modified cells is very low or even undetectable. Further clinical studies have to evaluate the importance of cytoreductive conditioning. Particularly in immune-compromised HIV-infected individuals, a cytoreductive chemotherapy has to be considered carefully. Finally, immunocompetent T lymphocytes have to be generated by thymic education. In HIV-infected individuals, the thymic as well as the lymph node stroma are significantly impaired (171,172). Thus, the capacity of HIV-infected individuals to provide sufficient conditions for maturation of T lymphocytes derived from genetically modified stem cell has to be investigated. In conclusion, hematopoietic stem cells are the most attractive target cells for gene therapy of HIV infection. However, there are still several fundamental questions that must be answered prior to a successful transduction and engraftment of hematopoietic stem cells transduced with an anti-HIV gene.

B. CD4+ T Lymphocytes

To date, most of the clinical studies dealing with HIV gene therapy involve the ex vivo transfer of anti-HIV genes, subsequent in vitro expansion of the genetically modified cells, and finally their reinfusion. The genetic modification of mature CD4+ T cells with anti-HIV genes is based on the rationale that the antiviral activity confers a selective survival advantage. Because of the high turnover of CD4+ T cells in HIV-1–infected individuals, such a selective advantage should result in an increasing ratio of protected cells by in vivo selection.

Mature CD4+ T cells have several characteristics that make them attractive targets for HIV gene therapy. First, they are the most important target cells of HIV. Thus, protection of the CD4+ T cell compartment would be of benefit. Second, they are easily obtained in large numbers from the peripheral blood of the patient by leukapheresis. Furthermore, CD4+ T cells can be isolated and expanded under very well-characterized conditions. Finally, in past years, very efficient protocols for retroviral transduction of T-cells have been developed (135,173,174).

A disadvantage of a T-lymphocyte–based HIV gene therapy is that this cell type represents only one of the cell types susceptible to HIV infection. Inhibition of HIV replication in CD4+ T cells would be therefore not able to stop virus spread, for example, in monocytes and tissue macrophages. Moreover, mature CD4+ lymphocytes are terminally differentiated. Thus, the in vivo growth potential and lifespan of genetically modified cells might be limited. Nevertheless, Walker et al. were able to demonstrate a long-term engraftment of syngeneic neomycin phosphotransferase transduced T-cells in HIV-infected individuals (175). The concept to apply CD4+ T cells for transfer of anti-HIV genes has been supported even more by the data of Nabel's group who were able to demonstrate a selective survival advantage for RevM10 expressing CD4+ T cells in vivo (28,176).

V. CLINICAL PROTOCOLS

Based on the aforementioned gene therapeutic concepts, several clinical trials have been initiated. In Table 3, the clinical protocols are listed that have been reviewed

Table 3 NIH Reviewed Protocols on Gene Therapy and Gene Marking in HIV Infection (Last Updated 5/18/99)

Principal investigator, institution	Transduction NIH #	Title	Initial NIH review Final NIH approval	Reference
S. R. Riddel University of Washington, Seattle	ex vivo 9202-017	Phase 1 study of cellular adoptive immunotherapy using genetically modified CD8+ HIV-specific T cells for HIV seropositive patients undergoing allogeneic bone marrow transplant	11/21/91 4/17/92	178
R. E. Walker NIH, Bethesda	ex vivo 9209-026	A study of the safety and survival of the adoptive transfer of genetically marked syngeneic lymphocytes in HIV-infected identical twins	9/14/92 9/3/93	177
J. E. Galpin University of Southern California, Los Angeles	ex vivo 9306-048	A Phase I clinical trial to evaluate the safety and biological activity of HIV-IT (TAF) (HIV-1IIIB env-transduced, autologous fibroblasts) in asymptomatic HIV-1 infected patients	6/7/93 9/3/93	179
G. J. Nabel University of Michigan, Ann Arbor	ex vivo 9306-048	A molecular genetic intervention for AIDS— effects of a transdominant negative form of Rev	6/7/93 9/3/93	85
F. Wong-Staal University of California, San Diego	ex vivo 9309-057	A controlled, phase 1 clinical trial to evaluate the safety and effects of HIV-1 infected humans of autologous lymphocytes transduced with a ribozyme that cleaves HIV-1 RNA	9/10/93 10/25/94	72
R. Haubrich University of California, San Diego	in vivo 9312-062	An open label, phase I/II clinical trial to evaluate the safety and biological activity of HIV-IT (V) (HIV-1IIIB env/rev retroviral vector) in HIV-1-infected subjects	12/3/93 4/19/94	180

Investigator/Institution	Type/Protocol	Description	Dates	Ref
R. Walker NIH, Bethesda Sponsor: NIH/Cell Genesys, Inc.	ex vivo 9403-068	A phase I/II pilot study of the safety of the adoptive transfer of syngeneic gene-modified cytotoxic T lymphocytes in HIV-infected identical twins	3/3/94 8/23/94	116
R. Morgan NIH, Bethesda	ex vivo 9503-103	Gene therapy for AIDS using retroviral mediated gene transfer to deliver HIV-1 antisense TAR and transdominant Rev protein genes to syngeneic lymphocytes in HIV-1 infected identical twins	3/7/95 4/1/95	59
D. Parenti George Washington University, Washington, DC	in vivo 9503-105	A repeat dose safety an efficacy study of HIV-IT(V) in HIV-1 infected subjects with greater than 100 CD4+ T cells and no AIDS defining symptoms	3/11/95 3/11/95 11/30/94 (FDA approval)	
W. A. Marasco Dana Farber Cancer Institute, Boston	ex vivo 9506-112	Intracellular antibodies against HIV-1 envelope protein for AIDS gene therapy	6/10/95 7/27/95	92
M. Conant Conant Medical Group and ViRx Inc., San Francisco	in vivo 9504-113	A randomized, double blinded phase I/II dosing study to evaluate the safety and optimal CTL inducing dose of HIV-1 infected subjects	5/6/94 (FDA approved)	
J. D. Rosenblatt University of California, Los Angeles	ex vivo 9508-117	A phase I trial of autologous CD34+ hematopoietic progenitor cells transduced with anti-HIV-1 ribozyme	8/7/95 (sole FDA review recommended by NIH/ORDA)	
S. R. Riddel Fred Hutchinson Cancer Center, Seattle Sponsor: Targeted Genetics Corp.	ex vivo 9508-119	Phase I study to evaluate the safety of cellular adoptive immunotherapy using autologous unmodified and genetically modified CD8+ HIV specific	8/7/95 (sole FDA review recommended by NIH/ORDA)	

Table 3 Continued

Principal investigator, institution	Transduction NIH #	Title	Initial NIH review Final NIH approval	Reference
E. Connick University of Colorado, Denver Sponsor: Cell Genesys, Inc.	ex vivo 9510-131	A randomized, controlled, phase II study of the activity and safety of autologous CD4-Zeta gene modified T cells in HIV-infected patients	10/17/95 (sole FDA review recommended by NIH/ORDA)	
P. D. Greenberg Fred Hutchinson Cancer Center, Seattle	ex vivo 9511-134	Phase I study to evaluate the safety and in vivo persistence of adoptively transferred autologous CD4+ T cells genetically modified to resist HIV replication	11/1/95 (sole FDA review recommended by NIH/ORDA)	
R. J. Pomerantz Jefferson Medical University, Philadelphia	ex vivo 9512-141	Intracellular immunization against HIV-1 infection using anti-Rev single chain variable fragments (SFv)	12/13/95 (sole FDA review recommended by NIH/ORDA)	
D. B. Kohn Childrens Hospital, Los Angeles	ex vivo 9602-147	Transduction of CD34+ cells from bone marrow of HIV-1 infected children: Comparative marking by a RRE decoy	2/8/96 (sole FDA review recommended by NIH/ORDA)	78
D. B. Kohn Childrens Hospital, Los Angeles	ex vivo 9604-153	Transduction of CD34+ autologous peripheral blood progenitor cells from HIV-1 infected persons: a phase I study of comparative marking using a ribozyme gene and a neutral gene	4/24/96 (sole FDA review recommended by NIH/ORDA)	
E. Connick University of Colorado, Denver Sponsor: Cell Genesys, Inc.	ex vivo 9703-181	A phase II study of the activity and safety of autologous CD4-zeta gene modified T cells with or without exogenous IL-2 in HIV infected patients	4/18/97 (sole FDA review recommended by NIH/ORDA)	

S. G. Deeks University of California, San Francisco Sponsor: Cell Genesys, Inc.	ex vivo 9709-213	A phase II study of autologous CD4-zeta gene modified T cells in HIV infected patients with undetectable plasma viraemia on combination antiretroviral drug therapy	10/10/97 (sole FDA review recommended by NIH/ORDA)
D. T. Scadden Massachusetts General Hospital Cancer Center, Boston Sponsor: Cell Genesys, Inc.	ex vivo 9805-253	A phase I study of the activity and safety of autologous CD4-zeta gene modified T cells in HIV infected patients with undetectable plasma viraemia and highly active anti-retroviral drug therapy	6/3/98 (sole FDA review recommended by NIH/ORDA)
R. G. Amado University of California, Los Angeles Sponsor: Systemix, Inc.	ex vivo 9806-261	A phase I/II study of the feasibility of RevM10 or RevM10/Antisense Pol 1 transduced hematopoietic stem cells (HSC) in HIV-1 related non-Hodgkin's lymphoma treated with high dose chemotherapy and peripheral blood stem cell support	7/20/98 (sole FDA review recommended by NIH/ORDA)
S. R. Riddel Fred Hutchinson Cancer Center, Seattle	ex vivo 9812-273	The safety and antiviral efficacy of cellular adotive immunotherapy with autologous CD8+ HIV specific cytotoxic T cells combined with interleukin-2 for HIV seropositive individuals	1/5/99 (sole FDA review recommended by NIH/ORDA)
R. G. Amado University of California, Los Angeles Sponsor: Systemix, Inc.	ex vivo 9812-277	A Phase I/II study in HIV-1 infected patients infused with CD34+ Thy1+ hematopoietic stem cells (HCS) from G-CSF mobilized peripheral blood retrovirally transduced with RevM10 or RevM10/Antisense Pol 1	1/19/99 (sole FDA review recommended by NIH/ORDA)

by the NIH Recombinant DNA Advisory Committee (RAC). Most of the ongoing or planned HIV gene therapy trials are classified as phase I or phase I/II. Thus, the intention of these trials is at first the assessment of safety and toxicity. The antiviral activity of the transferred anti-HIV genes and their potential clinical benefit is not the primary aim of the studies. Only a few investigators have published results of the clinical trials. A very important issue of T-cell based gene therapy was addressed by Walker et al. (175,177).

Studying syngeneic twin pairs discordant for HIV infection, the investigators were able to demonstrate the persistence of genetically marked cells from the HIV-negative donor in the circulation of the HIV-positive recipient for 4 to 18 weeks after transfer. After approximately 6 months, marked cells were detectable in lymphoid tissues in proportions comparable to those found in peripheral blood. This study clearly indicated that mature T cells can engraft and persist in an HIV-infected individual after genetic modification. For a successful application of CD4$^+$ T cells expressing an anti-HIV gene, a selective survival advantage would be pivotal. In 1996, Woffendin et al. published data on autologous CD4$^+$ T cells transfected by particle bombardment with the RevM10 gene. For those cells expressing the antiviral gene, a prolonged T-cell survival resulting in a selective advantage could be demonstrated (28). Ranga et al. repeated the experiments with retrovirally transduced CD4$^+$ T cells. Again, a significant difference in survival was determined: RevM10-transduced cells were detected after retransfusion for an average of 6 months compared to less than 3 weeks for cells expressing a Rev mutant without antiviral activity (176). These clinical results are a "proof of principle" for a CD4$^+$ T lymphocyte–based gene therapy. So far, from most of the other trials, only preliminary results have been reported but not published. First data on genetically modified autologous hematopoietic stem cells indicate an engraftment in HIV-infected individuals. One year after transfusion of RRE decoy-expressing autologous CD34$^+$ cells, gene-containing leukocytes in peripheral blood samples were still detectable (78).

The most important result of all clinical trials has been that no severe side effects occurred in the past years, indicating that the infusion of genetically modified autologous or syngeneic cells is a safe method for therapy of HIV-1 infection.

VI. CONCLUSIONS AND PERSPECTIVES

Although several critical issues still remain, there is reason for optimism that gene therapy can be established as a successful therapy approach in HIV infection. Especially, the current in vitro and in vivo data on CD4$^+$ T cell–based anti-HIV gene transfer encourage establishing in the near future a gene therapeutic antiretroviral therapy, not as an alternative but as an additive concept together with drug antiretroviral therapy.

Antiretroviral drug therapy became successful after the application of several different potent antivirals in an antiretroviral combination therapy. Therefore, it can be assumed that vector systems that are able to strongly express multiple anti-HIV genes would confer a long-term inhibition of HIV replication by preventing early emergence of resistance.

Infection with HIV is still an incurable disease. Neither combination drug therapy nor gene therapeutic approaches have been able to provide optimism that a therapy capable of curing the disease by total clearance of the virus will be feasible. All available therapeutic principles only inhibit productive infection without affecting the integrated HIV provirus. Thus, the main challenge for research on HIV gene therapy should be to find methods to eliminate the integrated provirus in already infected cells.

REFERENCES

1. Baltimore D. Gene therapy. Intracellular immunization [news]. Nature 1988; 335: 395–396.
2. Sczakiel G, Pawlita M, Kleinheinz A. Specific inhibition of human immunodeficiency virus type 1 replication by RNA transcribed in sense and antisense orientation from the 5´-leader/gag region. Biochem Biophys Res Commun 1990; 169:643–651.
3. Sczakiel G, Pawlita M. Inhibition of human immunodeficiency virus type 1 replication in human T cells stably expressing antisense RNA. J Virol 1991; 65:468–472.
4. Trono D, Feinberg MB, Baltimore D. HIV-1 Gag mutants can dominantly interfere with the replication of the wild-type virus. Cell 1989; 59:113–120.
5. Yu M, Poeschla E, Yamada O, et al. In vitro and in vivo characterization of a second functional hairpin ribozyme against HIV-1. Virology 1995; 206:381–386.
6. Sioud M, Drlica K. Prevention of human immunodeficiency virus type 1 integrase expression in Escherichia coli by a ribozyme. Proc Natl Acad Sci U S A 1991; 88: 7303–7307.
7. Gervaix A, Schwarz L, Law P, et al. Gene therapy targeting peripheral blood CD34+ hematopoietic stem cells of HIV-infected individuals. Hum Gene Ther 1997; 8:2229–2238.
8. Maciejewski JP, Weichold FF, Young NS, et al. Intracellular expression of antibody fragments directed against HIV reverse transcriptase prevents HIV infection in vitro. Nat Med 1995; 1:667–673.
9. Kitamura Y, Ishikawa T, Okui N, et al. Inhibition of replication of HIV-1 at both early and late stages of the viral life cycle by single-chain antibody against viral integrase. J Acquir Immune Defic Syndr Hum Retrovirol 1999; 20:105–114.
10. Junker U, Escaich S, Plavec I, et al. Intracellular expression of human immunodeficiency virus type 1 (HIV-1) protease variants inhibits replication of wild-type and protease inhibitor-resistant HIV-1 strains in human T-cell lines. J Virol 1996; 70: 7765–7772.

11. Marasco WA, Haseltine WA, Chen SY. Design, intracellular expression, and activity of a human anti-human immunodeficiency virus type 1 gp120 single-chain antibody. Proc Natl Acad Sci U S A 1993; 90:7889–7893.

12. Buonocore L, Rose JK. Blockade of human immunodeficiency virus type 1 production in CD4+ T cells by an intracellular CD4 expressed under control of the viral long terminal repeat. Proc Natl Acad Sci U S A 1993; 90:2695–2699.

13. Buonocore L, Rose JK. Prevention of HIV-1 glycoprotein transport by soluble CD4 retained in the endoplasmic reticulum. Nature 1990; 345:625–628.

14. Chen CJ, Banerjea AC, Harmison GG, Haglund K, Schubert M. Multitarget-ribozyme directed to cleave at up to nine highly conserved HIV-1 env RNA regions inhibits HIV-1 replication—potential effectiveness against most presently sequenced HIV-1 isolates. Nucleic Acids Res 1992; 20:4581–4589.

15. Yamada O, Kraus G, Leavitt MC, Yu M, Wong-Staal F. Activity and cleavage site specificity of an anti-HIV-1 hairpin ribozyme in human T cells. Virology 1994; 205: 121–126.

16. Buchschacher GL Jr, Freed EO, Panganiban AT. Cells induced to express a human immunodeficiency virus type 1 envelope gene mutant inhibit the spread of wild-type virus. Hum Gene Ther 1992; 3:391–397.

17. Green M, Ishino M, Loewenstein PM. Mutational analysis of HIV-1 Tat minimal domain peptides: identification of trans-dominant mutants that suppress HIV-LTR-driven gene expression. Cell 1989; 58:215–223.

18. Rossi C, Balboni PG, Betti M, et al. Inhibition of HIV-1 replication by a Tat trans-dominant negative mutant in human peripheral blood lymphocytes from healthy donors and HIV-1-infected patients. Gene Ther 1997; 4:1261–1269.

19. Sullenger BA, Gallardo HF, Ungers GE, Gilboa E. Overexpression of TAR sequences renders cells resistant to human immunodeficiency virus replication. Cell 1990; 63: 601–608.

20. Lee SW, Gallardo HF, Gaspar O, Smith C, Gilboa E. Inhibition of HIV-1 in CEM cells by a potent TAR decoy. Gene Ther 1995; 2:377–384.

21. Lo KM, Biasolo MA, Dehni G, Palu G, Haseltine WA. Inhibition of replication of HIV-1 by retroviral vectors expressing tat-antisense and anti-tat ribozyme RNA. Virology 1992; 190:176–183.

22. Sczakiel G, Oppenlander M, Rittner k, Pawlita M. Tat- and Rev-directed antisense RNA expression inhibits and abolishes replication of human immunodeficiency virus type 1: a temporal analysis. J Virol 1992; 66:5576–5581.

23. Sun LQ, Wang L, Gerlach WL, Symonds G. Target sequence-specific inhibition of HIV-1 replication by ribozymes directed to tat RNA. Nucleic Acids Res 1995; 23: 2909–2913.

24. Mhashilkar AM, LaVecchio J, Eberhardt B, et al. Inhibition of human immunodeficiency virus type 1 replication in vitro in acutely and persistently infected human CD4+ mononuclear cells expressing murine and humanized anti-human immunodeficiency virus type 1 Tat single-chain variable fragment intrabodies. Hum Gene Ther 1999; 10:1453–1467.

25. Malim MH, Bohnlein S, Hauber J, Cullen BR. Functional dissection of the HIV-1 Rev Trans-activator—derivation of a trans-dominant repressor of Rev function. Cell 1989; 58:205–214.

26. Malim MH, Freimuth WW, Liu J, et al. Stable expression of transdominant Rev protein in human T cells inhibits human immunodeficiency virus replication. J Exp Med 1992; 176:1197–1201.

27. Escaich S, Kalfoglou C, Plavec I, Kaushal S, Mosca JD, Bohnlein E. RevM10-mediated inhibition of HIV-1 replication in chronically infected T cells. Hum Gene Ther 1995; 6:625–634.

28. Woffendin C, Ranga U, Yang Z, Xu L, Nabel GJ. Expression of a protective gene-prolongs survival of T cells in human immunodeficiency virus-infected patients. Proc Natl Acad Sci U S A 1996; 93:2889–2894.

29. Bahner I, Kearns K, Hao QL, Smogorzewska EM, Kohn DB. Transduction of human CD34+ hematopoietic progenitor cells by a retroviral vector expressing an RRE decoy inhibits human immunodeficiency virus type 1 replication in myelomonocytic cells produced in long-term culture. J Virol 1996; 70:4352–4360.

30. Lee SW, Gallardo HF, Gilboa E, Smith C. Inhibition of human immunodeficiency virus type 1 in human T cells by a potent Rev response element decoy consisting of the 13-nucleotide minimal Rev-binding domain. J Virol 1994; 68:8254–8264.

31. Li G, Lisziewicz J, Sun D, et al. Inhibition of Rev activity and human immunodeficiency virus type 1 replication by antisense oligodeoxynucleotide phosphorothioate analogs directed against the Rev-responsive element. J Virol 1993; 67:6882–6888.

32. Duan L, Zhu M, Bagasra O, Pomerantz RJ. Intracellular immunization against HIV-1 infection of human T lymphocytes: utility of anti-rev single-chain variable fragments [published erratum appears in Hum Gene Ther 1998 Mar 20;9(5):765]. Hum Gene Ther 1995; 6:1561–1573.

33. Junker U, Bevec D, Barske C, et al. Intracellular expression of cellular eIF-5A mutants inhibits HIV-1 replication in human T cells: a feasibility study. Hum Gene Ther 1996; 7:1861–1869.

34. Larsson S, Hotchkiss G, Su J, et al. A novel ribozyme target site located in the HIV-1 nef open reading frame. Virology 1996; 219:161–169.

35. Ojwang JO, Hampel A, Looney DJ, Wong-Staal F, Rappaport J. Inhibition of human immunodeficiency virus type 1 expression by a hairpin ribozyme. Proc Natl Acad Sci U S A 1992; 89:10802–10806.

36. Yamada O, Yu M, Yee JK, Kraus G, Looney D, Wong-Staal F. Intracellular immunization of human T cells with a hairpin ribozyme against human immunodeficiency virus type 1. Gene Ther 1994; 1:38–45.

37. Yu M, Ojwang J, Yamada O, et al. A hairpin ribozyme inhibits expression of diverse strains of human immunodeficiency virus type 1 [published erratum appears in Proc Natl Acad Sci U S A 1993 Sep 1;90(17):8303]. Proc Natl Acad Sci U S A 1993; 90: 6340–6344.

38. Leavitt MC, Yu M, Yamada O, et al. Transfer of an anti-HIV-1 ribozyme gene into primary human lymphocytes. Hum Gene Ther 1994; 5:1115–1120.

39. Gonzalez MA, Serrano F, Llorente M, Abad JL, Garcia-Ortiz MJ, Bernad A. A hammerhead ribozyme targeted to the human chemokine receptor CCR5. Biochem Biophys Res Commun 1998; 251:592–596.

40. Yang AG, Zhang X, Torti F, Chen SY. Anti-HIV type 1 activity of wild-type and functional defective RANTES intrakine in primary human lymphocytes. Hum Gene Ther 1998; 9:2005–2018.

41. Yang AG, Bai X, Huang XF, Yao C, Chen S. Phenotypic knockout of HIV type 1 chemokine coreceptor CCR-5 by intrakines as potential therapeutic approach for HIV-1 infection. Proc Natl Acad Sci U S A 1997; 94:11567–11572.

42. Bai X, Chen JD, Yang AG, Torti F, Chen SY. Genetic co-inactivation of macrophage- and T-tropic HIV-1 chemokine coreceptors CCR-5 and CXCR-4 by intrakines. Gene Ther 1998; 5:984–994.

43. Benkirane M, Jin DY, Chun RF, Koup RA, Jeang KT. Mechanism of transdominant inhibition of CCR5-mediated HIV-1 infection by ccr5delta32. J Biol Chem 1997; 272:30603–30606.

44. Wu BY, Woffendin C, Duckett CS, Ohno T, Nabel GJ. Regulation of human retroviral latency by the NF-kappa B/I kappa B family: inhibition of human immunodeficiency virus replication by I kappa B through a Rev-dependent mechanism. Proc Natl Acad Sci U S A 1995; 92:1480–1484.

45. Beauparlant P, Kwon H, Clarke M, et al. Transdominant mutants of I kappa B alpha block Tat-tumor necrosis factor synergistic activation of human immunodeficiency virus type 1 gene expression and virus multiplication. J Virol 1996; 70:5777–5785.

46. Kwon H, Pelletier N, DeLuca C, et al. Inducible expression of IkappaBalpha repressor mutants interferes with NF-kappaB activity and HIV-1 replication in Jurkat T cells. J Biol Chem 1998; 273:7431–7440.

47. Hiscott J, Beauparlant P, Crepieux P, et al. Cellular and viral protein interactions regulating I kappa B alpha activity during human retrovirus infection. J Leukoc Biol 1997; 62:82–92.

48. Vieillard V, Lauret E, Rousseau V, De Maeyer E. Blocking of retroviral infection at a step prior to reverse transcription in cells transformed to constitutively express interferon beta. Proc Natl Acad Sci U S A 1994; 91:2689–2693.

49. Viellard V, Lauret E, Maguer V, et al. Autocrine interferon-beta synthesis for gene therapy of HIV infection: increased resistance to HIV-1 in lymphocytes from healthy and HIV-infected individuals. AIDS 1995; 9:1221–1228.

50. Vieillard V, Cremer I, Lauret E, et al. Interferon beta transduction of peripheral blood lymphocytes from HIV-infected donors increases Th1-type cytokine production and improves the proliferative response to recall antigens. Proc Natl Acad Sci U S A 1997; 94:11595–11600.

51. Matheux F, Le Grand R, Rousseau V, De Maeyer E, Dormont D, Lauret E. Macaque lymphocytes transduced by a constitutively expressed interferon beta gene display an enhanced resistance to SIVmac251 infection. Hum Gene Ther 1999; 10:429–440.

52. Weichold FF, Lisziewicz J, Zeman RA, et al. Antisense phosphorothioate oligodeoxynucleotides alter HIV type 1 replication in cultured human macrophages and peripheral blood mononuclear cells. AIDS Res Hum Retroviruses 1995; 11:863–867.

53. Kretschmer A, Antonicek HP, Baumgarten J, et al. Expressionsvektoren für HIV resistente Zellen. Le A 28 518. USA: Patent US S583035.

54. Chatterjee S, Johnson PR, Wong KK Jr. Dual-target inhibition of HIV-1 in vitro by means of an adeno-associated virus antisense vector. Science 1992; 258:1485–1488.

55. Veres G, Escaich S, Baker J, et al. Intracellular expression of RNA transcripts complementary to the human immunodeficiency virus type 1 gag gene inhibits viral replication in human CD4+ lymphocytes. J Virol 1996; 70:8792–8800.

56. Biasolo MA, Radaelli A, Del Pup L, Franchin E, De Giuli-Morghen C, Palu G. A

new antisense tRNA construct for the genetic treatment of human immunodeficiency virus type 1 infection. J Virol 1996; 70:2154–2161.

57. Veres G, Junker U, Baker J, et al. Comparative analyses of intracellularly expressed antisense RNAs as inhibitors of human immunodeficiency virus type 1 replication. J Virol 1998; 72:1894–1901.

58. Sczakiel G. The design of antisense RNA. Antisense Nucleic Acid Dug Dev 1997; 7:439–444.

59. Morgan RA, Walker R. Gene therapy for AIDS using retroviral mediated gene transfer to deliver HIV-1 antisense TAR and transdominant Rev protein genes to syngeneic lymphocytes in HIV-1 infected identical twins. Hum Gene Ther 1996; 7:1281–1306.

60. Haseloff J, Gerlach WL. Simple RNA enzymes with new and highly specific endoribonuclease activities. Nature 1988; 334:585–589.

61. Kikuchi Y, Sasaki N. Site-specific cleavage of natural mRNA sequences by newly designed hairpin catalytic RNAs. Nucleic Acids Res 1991; 19:6751–6755.

62. Sarver N, Cantin EM, Chang PS, et al. Ribozymes as potential anti-HIV-1 therapeutic agents. Science 1990; 247:1222–1225.

63. Weerasinghe M, Liem SE, Asad S, Read SE, Joshi S. Resistance to human immunodeficiency virus type 1 (HIV-1) infection in human CD4+ lymphocyte-derived cell lines conferred by using retroviral vectors expressing an HIV-1 RNA-specific ribozyme. J Virol 1991; 65:5531–5534.

64. Ohkawa J, Yuyama N, Takebe Y, Nishikawa S, Taira K. Importance of independence in ribozyme reactions: kinetic behavior of trimmed and of simply connected multiple ribozymes with potential activity against human immunodeficiency virus. Proc Natl Acad Sci U S A 1993; 90:11302–11306.

65. Zhou C, Bahner IC, Larson GP, Zaia JA, Rossi JJ, Kohn EB. Inhibition of HIV-1 in human T-lymphocytes by retrovirally transduced anti-tat and rev hammerhead ribozymes. Gene 1994; 149:33–39.

66. Bauer G,. Valdez P, Kearns K, et al. Inhibition of human immunodeficiency virus-1 (HIV-1) replication after transduction of granulocyte colony-stimulating factor-mobilized CD34+ cells from HIV-1-infected donors using retroviral vectors containing anti-HIV-1 genes. Blood 1997; 89:2259–2267.

67. Yu M, Leavitt MC, Maruyama M, et al. Intracellular immunization of human fetal cord blood stem/progenitor cells with a ribozyme against human immunodeficiency virus type 1. Proc Natl Acad Sci U S A 1995; 92:699–703.

68. Leavitt MC, Yu M, Wong-Staal F, Looney DJ. Ex vivo transduction and expansion of CD4+ lymphocytes from HIV+ donors: prelude to a ribozyme gene therapy trial. Gene Ther 1996; 3:599–606.

69. Heidenreich O, Eckstein F. Hammerhead ribozyme-mediated cleavage of the long terminal repeat RNA of human immunodeficiency virus type 1. J Biol Chem 1992; 267:1904–1909.

70. Ramezani A, Joshi S. Comparative analysis of five highly conserved target sites within the HIV-1 RNA for their susceptibility to hammerhead ribozyme-mediated cleavage in vitro and in vivo. Antisense Nucleic Acid Drug Dev 1996; 6:229–235.

71. Wang L, Witterington C, King A, et al. Preclinical characterization of an anti-tat ribozyme for therapeutic application. Hum Gene Ther 1998; 9:1283–1291.

72. Wong-Staal F, Poeschla EM, Looney DJ. A controlled, Phase 1 clinical trial to eval-

uate the safety and effects in HIV-1 infected humans of autologous lymphocytes transduced with a ribozyme that cleaves HIV-1 RNA. Hum Gene Ther 1998; 9:2407–2425.

73. Sullenger BA, Cech TR. Ribozyme-mediated repair of defective mRNA by targeted, trans-splicing. Nature 1994; 371:619–622.

74. Lee SW, Sullenger BA. Trans splicing ribozymes as potential HIV gene inhibitors. In: Smith C, ed. Gene therapy for HIV infection: Springer-Verlag, 1998:49–58.

75. Smith C, Lee SW, Wong E, et al. Transcient protection of human T-cells from human immunodeficiency virus type 1 infection by transduction with adeno-associated viral vectors which express RNA decoys. Antiviral Res 1996; 32:99–115.

76. Browning CM, Cagnon L, Good PD, Rossi J, Engelke DR, Markovitz DM. Potent inhibition of human immunodeficiency virus type 1 (HIV-1) gene expression and virus production by an HIV-2 tat activation-response RNA decoy. J Virol 1999; 73: 5191–5195.

77. Bauer B, Valdez P, Rice CR, et al. Clinical trial of stem cell gene therapy in HIV-1 infected children. First Annual Meeting of the American Society of Gene Therapy, Seattle, 1998.

78. Kohn DB, Bauer G, Rice CR, et al. A clinical trial of retroviral-mediated transfer of a rev-responsive element decoy gene into CD34(+) cells from the bone marrow of human immunodeficiency virus-1-infected children. Blood 1999; 94:368–371.

79. Smythe JA, Sun D, Thomson M, et al. A Rev-inducible mutant gag gene stably transferred into T lymphocytes: an approach to ene therapy against human immunodeficiency virus type 1 infection. Proc Natl Acad Sci U S A 1994; 91:3657–3661.

80. Steffy KR, Wong-Staal F. Transdominant inhibition of wild-type human immunodeficiency virus type 2 replication by an envelope deletion mutant. J Virol 1993; 67: 1854–1859.

81. Pearson L, Garcia J, Wu F, Modesti N, Nelson J, Gaynor R. A transdominant tat mutant that inhibits tat-induced gene expression from the human immunodeficiency virus long terminal repeat. Proc Natl Acad Sci U S A 1990; 87:5079–5083.

82. Orsini MJ, Debouck CM. Inhibition of human immunodeficiency virus type 1 and type 2 Tat function by transdominant Tat protein localized to both the nucleus and cytoplasm. J Virol 1996; 70:8055–8063.

83. Caputo A, Grossi MP, Bozzini R, et al. Inhibition of HIV-1 replication and reactivation from latency by tat transdominant negative mutants in the cysteine rich region. Gene Ther 1996; 3:235–245.

84. Bahner I, Zhou C, Yu XJ, Hao QL, Guatelli JC, Kohn DB. Comparison of trans-dominant inhibitory mutant human immunodeficiency virus type 1 genes expressed by retroviral vectors in human T lymphocytes. J Virol 1993; 67:3199–3207.

85. Nabel GJ, Fox BA, Post L, Thompson CB, Woffendin C. A molecular genetic intervention for AIDS—effects of a transdominant negative form of Rev. Hum Gene Ther 1994; 5:79–92.

86. Isaac J, Rondon IJ, Marasco WA. Intracellular antibodies (intrabodies) for gene therapy of infectious diseases. Annu Rev Microbiol 1997; 51;275–283.

87. Mhashilkar AM, Biswas DK, LaVecchio J, Pardee AB, Marasco WA. Inhibition of human immunodeficiency virus type 1 replication in vitro by a novel combination of anti-Tat single-chain intrabodies and NF-kappa B antagonists. J Virol 1997; 71:6486–6494.

88. Mhashilkar AM, Bagley J, Chen SY, Szilvay AM, Helland DG, Marasco WA. Inhibition of HIV-1 Tat-mediated LTR transactivation and HIV-1 infection by anti-Tat single chain intrabodies. Embo J 1995; 14:1542–1551.

89. Chen SY, Bagley J, Marasco WA. Intracellular antibodies as a new class of therapeutic molecules for gene therapy. Hum Gene Ther 1994; 5:595–601.

90. Levin R, Mhashilkar AM, Dorfman T, et al. Inhibition of early and late events of the HIV-1 replication cycle by cytoplasmic Fab intrabodies against the matrix protein, p17. Mol Med 1997; 3:96–110.

91. Marasco WA. Intracellular antibodies (intrabodies) as research reagents and therapeutic molecules for gene therapy. Immunotechnology 1995; 1:1–19.

92. Marasco WA, Chen S, Richardson JH, Ramstedt U, Jones SD. Intracellular antibodies against HIV-1 envelope protein for AIDS gene therapy. Hum Gene Ther 1998; 9:1627–1642.

93. Caruso M, Klatzmann D. Selective killing of CD4+ cells harboring a human immunodeficiency virus-inducible suicide gene prevents viral spread in an infected cell population. Proc Natl Acad Sci U S A 1992; 89:182–186.

94. Caruso M, Bank A. Efficient retroviral gene transfer of a Tat-regulated herpes simplex virus thymidine kinase gene for HIV gene therapy. Virus Res 1997; 52:133–143.

95. Hamouda T, McPhee R, Hsia SC, Read GS, Holland TC, King SR. Inhibition of human immunodeficiency virus replication by the herpes simplex virus virion host shutoff protein. J Virol 1997; 71:5521–5527.

96. Jung D, Jaeger E, Cayeux S, et al. Strong immunogenic potential of a B7 retroviral expression vector: generation of HLA-B7-restricted CTL response against selectable marker genes. Hum Gene Ther 1998; 9:53–62.

97. Chan SY, Louie MC, Piccotti JR, et al. Genetic vaccination-induced immune responses to the human immunodeficiency virus protein Rev: emergence of the interleukin 2-producing helper T lymphocyte. Hum Gene Ther 1998; 9:2187–2196.

98. Chen CJ, Banerjea AC, Haglund K, Harmison GG, Schubert M. Inhibition of HIV-1 replication by novel multitarget ribozymes. Ann N Y Acad Sci 1992; 660:271–273.

99. Kuwabara T, Warashina M, Nakayama A, Ohkawa J, Taira K. tRnaval-heterodimeric maxizymes with high potential as geneinactivating agents: simultaneous cleavage at two sites in Hiv-1 Tat mRna in cultured cells. Proc Natl Acad Sci U S A 1999; 96: 1886–1891.

100. Ohkawa J, Yuyama N, Taira K. Activities of HIV-RNA targeted ribozymes transcribed from a "shot-gun" type ribozyme-trimming plasmid. Nucleic Acids Symp Ser 1992:15–16.

101. Ohkawa J, Yuyama N, Takebe Y, et al. Multiple site-specific cleavage of HIV RNA by transcribed ribozymes from shotgun-type trimming plasmid. Nucleic Acids Symp Ser 1993:121–122.

102. Yuyama N, Ohkawa J, Koguma T, Shirai M, Taira K. A multifunctional expression vector for an anti-HIV-1 ribozyme that produces a 5´- and 3´-trimmed trans-acting ribozyme, targeted against HIV-1 RNA, and cis-acting ribozymes that are designed to bind to and thereby sequester trans-activator proteins such as Tat and Rev. Nucleic Acids Res 1994; 22:5060–5067.

103. Gottfredsson M. Gene therapy strategies for inhibition of HIV. In: Smith C, ed. Gene Therapy for HIV Infection. New York: Springer, 1998:13–47.

104. Fraisier C, Irvine A, Wrighton C, Craig R, Dzierzak E. High level inhibition of HIV replication with combination RNA decoys expressed from an HIV-Tat inducible vector. Gene Ther 1998; 5:1665–1676.

105. Kuwabara T, Amontov SV, Warashina M, Ohkawa J, Taira K. Characterization of several kinds of dimer minizyme: simultaneous cleavage at two sites in HIV-1 tat mRNA by dimer minizymes. Nucleic Acids Res 1996; 24:2302–2310.

106. Liu D, Donegan J, Nuovo G, Mitra D, Laurence J. Stable human immunodeficiency virus type 1 (HIV-1) resistance in transformed CD4+ monocytic cells treated with multitargeting HIV-1 antisense sequences incorporated into U1 snRNA. J Virol 1997; 71:4079–4085.

107. Ulich C, Harrich D, Estes P, Gaynor RB. Inhibition of human immunodeficiency virus type 1 replication is enhanced by a combination of transdominant Tat and Rev proteins. J Virol 1996; 70:4871–4876.

108. Caputo A, Rossi C, Bozzini R, et al. Studies on the effect of the combined expression of anti-tat and anti-rev genes on HIV-1 replication. Gene Ther 1997; 4:288–295.

109. Yamada O, Kraus G, Luznik L, Yu M, Wong-Staal F. A chimeric human immunodeficiency virus type 1 (HIV-1) minimal Rev response element-ribozyme molecule exhibits dual antiviral function and inhibits cell-cell transmission of HIV-1. J Virol 1996; 70:1596–1601.

110. Gervaix A, Li X, Kraus G, Wong-Staal F. Multigene antiviral vectors inhibit diverse human immunodeficiency virus type 1 clades. J Virol 1997; 71:3048–3053.

111. Lisziewicz J, Sun D, Smythe J, et al. Inhibition of human immunodeficiency virus type 1 replication by regulated expression of a polymeric Tat activation response RNA decoy as a strategy for gene therapy in AIDS. Proc Natl Acad Sci U S A 1993; 90:8000–8004.

112. Lori F, Lisziewicz J, Smythe J, et al. Rapid protection against human immunodeficiency virus type 1 (HIV-1) replication mediated by high efficiency non-retroviral delivery of genes interfering with HIV-1 tat and gag. Gene Ther 1994; 1:27–31.

113. Duan L, Zhu M, Ozaki I, Zhang H, Wei DL, Pomerantz RJ. Intracellular inhibition of HIV-1 replication using a dual protein- and RNA-based strategy. Gene Ther 1997; 4:533–543.

114. Inouye RT, Du B, Boldt-Houle D, et al. Potent inhibition of human immunodeficiency virus type 1 in primary T cells and alveolar macrophages by a combination anti-Rev strategy delivered in an adeno-associated virus vector [published erratum appears in J Virol 1998 Apr;72(4):3506]. J Virol 1997; 71:4071–4078.

115. Cara A, Rybak SM, Newton DL, et al. Inhibition of HIV-1 replication by combined expression of gag dominant negative mutant and a human ribonuclease in a tightly controlled HIV-1 inducible vector. Gene Ther 1998; 5:65–75.

116. Walker RE. A phase I/II pilot study of the safety of the adoptive transfer of syngeneic gene-modified cytotoxic T lymphocytes in HIV-infected identical twins. Hum Gene Ther 1996; 7:367–400.

117. Bitton N, Gorochov G, Debre P, Eshhar Z. Gene therapy approaches to HIV-infection: immunological strategies: use of T bodies and universal receptors to redirect cytolytic T-cells. Front Biosci 1999; 4:D386–D393.

118. Anderson WF. Human gene therapy. Nature 1998; 392:25–30.

119. Kass-Eisler A, Falck-Pedersen E, Elfenbein DH, Alvira M, Buttrick PM, Leinwand

LA. The impact of developmental stage, route of administration and the immune system on adenovirus-mediated gene transfer. Gene Ther 1994; 1:395–401.

120. Phillips KL. Viral vectors for HIV gene therapy. In: Smith C, ed. Gene Therapy for HIV Infection. New York: Springer, 1998:59–75.

121. Anderson WF. Prospects for human gene therapy. Science 1984; 226:401–409.

122. Junker U, Bohnlein E, Veres G. Genetic instability of a MoMLV-based antisense double-copy retroviral vector designed for HIV-1 gene therapy. Gene Ther 1995; 2:639–646.

123. Ilves H, Barske C, Junker U, Bohnlein E, Veres G. Retroviral vectors designed for targeted expression of RNA polymerase III-driven transcripts: a comparative study. Gene 1996; 171:203–208.

124. Mavilio F, Ferrari G, Rossini S, et al. Peripheral blood lymphocytes as target cells of retroviral vector-mediated gene transfer. Blood 1994; 83:1988–1997.

125. Rudoll T, Phillips K, Lee SW, et al. High-efficiency retroviral vector mediated gene transfer into human peripheral blood CD4+ T lymphocytes. Gene Ther 1996; 3:695–705.

126. Phillips K, Gentry T, McCowage G, Gilboa E, Smith C. Cell-surface markers for assessing gene transfer into human hematopoietic cells. Nat Med 1996; 2:1154–1156.

127. Mann R, Mulligan RC, Baltimore D. Construction of a retrovirus packaging mutant and its use to produce helper-free defective retrovirus. Cell 1983; 33:153–159.

128. Miller AD, Buttimore C. Redesign of retrovirus packaging cell lines to avoid recombination leading to helper virus production. Mol Cell Biol 1986; 6:2895–2902.

129. Danos O, Mulligan RC. Safe and efficient generation of recombinant retroviruses with amphotropic and ecotropic host ranges. Proc Natl Acad Sci U S A 1988; 85: 6460–6464.

130. Markowitz D, Goff S, Bank A. A safe packaging line for gene transfer: separating viral genes on two different plasmids. J Virol 1988; 62:1120–1124.

131. Markowitz D, Goff S, Bank A. Construction and use of a safe and efficient amphotropic packaging cell line. Virology 1988; 167:400–406.

132. Pear WS, Nolan GP, Scott ML, Baltimore D. Production of high-titer helper-free retroviruses by transient transfection. Proc Natl Acad Sci U S A 1993; 90:8392–8396.

133. Finer MH, Dull TJ, Qin L, Farson D, Roberts MR. kat: A high-efficiency retroviral transduction system for primary human T lymphocytes. Blood 1994; 83:43–50.

134. Bauer TR Jr, Miller AD, Hickstein DD. Improved transfer of the leukocyte integrin CD18 subunit into hematopoietic cell lines by using retroviral vectors having a gibbon ape leukemia virus envelope. Blood 1995; 86:2379–2387.

135. Sharma S, Cantwell M, Kipps TJ, Friedmann T. Efficient infection of a human T-cell line and of human primary peripheral blood leukocytes with a psuedotyped retrovirus vector. Proc Natl Acad Sci U S A 1996; 93:11842–11847.

136. Mammano F, Salvatori F, Indraccolo S, De Rossi A, Chieco-Bianchi L, Gottlinger HG. Truncation of the human immunodeficiency virus type 1 envelope glycoprotein allows efficient pseudotyping of Moloney murine leukemia virus particles and gene transfer into CD4+ cells. J Virol 1997; 71:3341–3345.

137. Indraccolo S, Minuzzo S, Feroli F, et al. Pseudotyping of Moloney leukemia virus-based retroviral vectors with simian immunodeficiency virus envelope leads to targeted infection of human CD4+ lymphoid cells. Gene Ther 1998; 5:209–217.

138. Vanin EF, Kaloss M, Broscius C, Nienhuis AW. Characterization of replication-competent retroviruses from nonhuman primates with virus-induced T-cell lymphomas and observations regarding the mechanism of oncogenesis. J Virol 1994; 68:4241–4250.

139. Dunbar CE, Emmons RV. Gene transfer into hematopoietic progenitor and stem cells: progress and problems. Stem Cells (Dayt) 1994; 12:563–576.

140. Grosovsky AJ, Skandalis A, Hasegawa L, Walter BN. Insertional inactivation of the tk locus in a human B lymphoblastoid cell line by a retroviral shuttle vector. Mutant Res 1993; 289:297–308.

141. Parolin C, Sodroski J. A defective HIV-1 vector for gene transfer to human lymphocytes. J Mol Med 1995; 73:279–288.

142. Naldini L, Blomer U, Gallay P, et al. In vivo gene delivery and stable transduction of nondividing cells by a lentiviral vector. Science 1996; 272:263–267.

143. Zufferey R, Nagy D, Mandel RJ, Naldini L, Trono D. Multiply attenuated lentiviral vector achieves efficient gene delivery in vivo. Nat Biotechnol 1997; 15:871–875.

144. Kafri T, van Praag H, Ouyang L, Gage FH, Verma IM. A packaging cell line for lentivirus vectors. J Virol 1999; 73:576–584.

145. Dull T, Zufferey R, Kelly M, et al. A third-generation lentivirus vector with a conditional packaging system. J Virol 1998; 72:8463–8471.

146. Poeschla E, Corbeau P, Wong-Staal F. Development of HIV vectors for anti-HIV gene therapy. Proc Natl Acad Sci U S A 1996; 93:11395–11399.

147. Corbeau P, Kraus G, Wong-Staal F. Efficient gene transfer by a human immunodeficiency virus type 1 (HIV-1)-derived vector utilizing a stable HIV packaging cell line. Proc Natl Acad Sci U S A 1996; 93:14070–14075.

148. Corbeau P, Wong-Staal F. Anti-HIV effects of HIV vectors. Virology 1998; 243:268–274.

149. Corbeau P, Kraus G, Wong-Staal F. Transduction of human macrophages using a stable HIV-1/HIV-2-derived gene delivery system. Gene Ther 1998; 5:99–104.

150. Miyoshi H, Smith KA, Mosier DE, Verma IM, Torbett BE. Transduction of human CD34+ cells that mediate long-term engraftment of NOD/SCID mice by HIV vectors. Science 1999; 283:682–686.

151. White SM, Renda M, Nam NY, et al. Lentivirus vectors using human and simian immunodeficiency virus elements. J Virol 1999; 73:2832–2840.

152. Douglas J, Kelly P, Evans JT, Garcia JV. Efficient transduction of human lymphocytes and CD34+ cells via human immunodeficiency virus-based gene transfer vectors. Hum Gene Ther 1999; 10:935–945.

153. Case SS, Price MA, Jordan CT, et al. Stable transduction of quiescent CD34(+)CD38(-) human hematopoietic cells by HIV-1-based lentiviral vectors. Proc Natl Acad Sci U S A 1999; 96:2988–2993.

154. Donahue RE, Kessler SW, Bodine D, et al. Helper virus induced T cell lymphoma in nonhuman primates after retroviral mediated gene transfer. J Exp Med 1992; 176:1125–1135.

155. Linden RM, Berns KI. Site-specific integration by adeno-associated virus: a basis for a potential gene therapy vector [editorial]. Gene Ther 1997; 4:4–5.

156. Linden RM, Ward P, Giraud C, Winocour E, Berns KI. Site-specific integration by adeno-associated virus. Proc Natl Acad Sci U S A 1996; 93:11288–11294.

157. Ponnazhagan S, Erikson D, Kearns WG, et al. Lack of site-specific integration of the recombinant adeno-associated virus 2 genomes in human cells. Hum Gene Ther 1997; 8:275–284.

158. Kearns WG, Afione SA, Fulmer SB, et al. Recombinant adeno-associated virus (AAV-CFTR) vectors do not integrate in a site-specific fashion in an immortalized epithelial cell line. Gene Ther 1996; 3:748–755.

159. Fisher-Adams G, Wong KK, Jr, Podsakoff G, Forman SJ, Chatterjee S. Integration of adeno-associated virus vectors in CD34+ human hematopoietic progenitor cells after transduction. Blood 1996; 88:492–504.

160. Podsakoff G, Wong KK Jr, Chatterjee S. Efficient gene transfer into nondividing cells by adeno-associated virus-based vectors. J Virol 1994; 68:5656–5666.

161. Law P, Lane TA, Gervaix A, et al. Mobilization of peripheral blood progenitor cells for human immunodeficiency virus-infected individuals. Exp Hematol 1999; 27:147–154.

162. Storms R. Stem cell based gene therapies in the treatment of AIDS. In: Smith C, ed. Gene Therapy for HIV Infection. New York: Springer 1998:95–117.

163. Su L, Lee R, Bonyhadi M, et al. Hematopoietic stem cell-based gene therapy for acquired immunodeficiency syndrome: efficient transduction and expression of RevM10 in myeloid cells in vivo and in vitro. Blood 1997; 89:2283–2290.

164. Glimm H, Flugge K, Mobest D, et al. Efficient serum-free retroviral gene transfer into primitive human hematopoietic progenitor cells by a defined, high-titer, non-concentrated vector-containing medium. Hum Gene Ther 1998; 9:771–778.

165. Schilz AJ, Brouns G, Knoss H, et al. High efficiency gene transfer to human hematopoietic SCID-repopulating cells under serum-free conditions. Blood 1998; 92:3163–3171.

166. Keim HP, Darovsky B, von Kalle C, et al. Retrovirus-mediated gene transduction into canine peripheral blood repopulation cells. Blood 1994; 83:1467–1473.

167. Van Beusechem VW, Valerio D. Gene transfer into hematopoietic stem cells of non-human primates. Hum Gene Ther 1996; 7:1649–1668.

168. Zaia JA, Cairns JS, Sarver N. Genetic modification and transplantation of hematopoietic cells for treatment of Human Immunodeficiency Virus infection. In: Donnall ET, Blume KG, Forman SJ, eds. Hematopoietic Cell Transplantation: Malden, MA: Blackwell Science, 1998: 1105–1116.

169. Malech HL, Maples PB, Whiting-Theobald N, et al. Prolonged production of NADPH oxidase-corrected granulocytes after gene therapy of chronic granulomatous disease. Proc Natl Acad Sci U S A 1997; 94:12133–12138.

170. Dunbar CE, Kohn DB, Schiffmann R, et al. Retroviral transfer of the glucocerebrosidase gene into CD34+ cells from patients with Gaucher disease: in vivo detection of transduced cells without myeloablation. Hum Gene Ther 1998; 9:2629–2640.

171. Maroder M, Scarpa S, Screpanti I, et al. Human immunodeficiency virus type 1 tat protein modulates fibronectin expression in thymic epithelial cells and impairs in vitro thymocyte development. Cell Immunol 1996; 168:49–58.

172. Racz P, Tenner-Racz K, van Vloten F, et al. Lymphatic tissue changes in AIDS and other retrovirus infections: tools and insights. Lymphology 1990; 23:85–91.

173. Bunnell BA, Muul LM, Donahue RE, Blaese RM, Morgan RA. High-efficiency retroviral-mediated gene transfer into human and nonhuman primate peripheral blood lymphocytes. Proc Natl Acad Sci U S A 1995; 92:7739–7743.

174. Pollok KE, Hanenberg H, Noblitt TW, et al. High-efficiency gene transfer into normal and adenosine deaminase-deficient T lymphocytes is mediated by transduction on recombinant fibronectin fragments. J Virol 1998; 72:4882–4892.

175. Walker RE, Carter CS, Muul L, et al. Peripheral expansion of pre-existing mature T cells is an important means of CD4+ T-cell regeneration HIV-infected adults. Nat Med 1998; 4:852–856.

175. Ranga U, Woffendin C, Verma S, et al. Enhanced T cell engraftment after retroviral delivery of an antiviral gene in HIV-infected individuals. Proc Natl Acad Sci U S A 1998; 95:1201–1206.

177. Walker R, Blaese RM, Carter CS, et al. A study of the safety and survival of the adoptive transfer of genetically marked syngeneic lymphocytes in HIV-infected identical twins. Hum Gene Ther 1993; 4:659–680.

178. Riddell SR, Greenberg PD, Overell RW, et al. Phase I study of cellular adoptive immunotherapy using genetically modified CD8+ HIV-specific T cells for HIV seropositive patients undergoing allogeneic bone marrow transplant. Hum Gene Ther 1992; 3:319–338.

179. Galpin JE, Casciato DA, Richards SB. A phase I clinical trial to evaluate the safety and biological activity of HIV-IT (TAF) (HIV-1IIIBenv-transduced, autologous fibroblasts) in asymptomatic HIV-1 infected subjects. Hum Gene Ther 1994; 5:997–1017.

180. Haubrich R, McCutchan JA, Holdredge R, Heiner L, Merritt J, Merchant B. An open label, phase I/II clinical trial to evaluate the safety and biological activity of HIV-IT (V) (HIV-1IIIBenv/rev retroviral vector) in HIV-1-infected subjects. Hum Gene Ther 1995; 6:941–955.

181. Ragheb JA, Couture L, Mullen C, Ridgway A, Morgan RA. Inhibition of human immunodeficiency virus type 1 by Tat/Rev-regulated expression of cytosine deaminase, interferon alpha2, or diphtheria toxin compared with inhibition by transdominant Rev. Hum Gene Ther 1999; 10:103–112.

8
Antagonism of Chemokine Receptors in Preventing Infection by HIV

Amanda E. I. Proudfoot and Timothy N. C. Wells
Serono Pharmaceutical Research Institute S.A., Geneva, Switzerland

Alexandra Trkola
University Hospital Zurich, Zurich, Switzerland

I. INTRODUCTION

The human immunodeficiency virus (HIV) has to interact with two essential proteins on the host cell surface in order to bind, fuse, and subsequently infect the cell. These two proteins are the glycoprotein CD4, identified more than a decade ago, and a second receptor, which proved to be elusive until members of the chemokine receptor family were discovered to function as HIV-coreceptors in mid-1996. The virus binds to its two receptors by a recognition complex referred to as virus envelope, which consists of trimers built by two subunits, gp120 and gp41, products of the viral *env* gene.

Chemokines and their receptors mediate leukocyte trafficking. Specific cellular recruitment is essential for embryonic development and routine immunosurveillance in the adult, but it also plays a major role in inflammation. Chemokine receptors belong to the seven-transmembrane G-protein–coupled receptor superfamily. Initial research on these receptors had focused principally on their role in inflammation. Their identification as HIV coreceptors has broadened the scenario. The first chemokine receptor identified to function as an HIV-coreceptor, CXCR4, is the main coreceptor for T-cell line adapted (TCLA) strains of HIV, whereas the second to be identified, CCR5, allows entry of macrophage tropic strains of HIV.

The identification of the chemokine receptors as HIV coreceptors and the characterization of the interaction between these receptors and the viral envelope proteins opened the possibility of developing new types of anti-HIV drugs that target the host cell. Many of the pharmaceutical agents currently on the market are the result of a focused attempt to obtain small molecules that act via these G-protein–coupled receptors. This chapter discusses the progress in understanding the mechanism of the HIV–chemokine receptor interaction and the approaches taken to block infection.

II. CHEMOKINES AND THEIR RECEPTORS

Chemokine biology has blossomed over the past decade, resulting in a vast wealth of data from numerous laboratories, both academic as well as industrial. The aim of this chapter is not to review the background to the field in great detail; refer to recent reviews on the subject for more information (1–3). The discovery of a subfamily of cytokines, through their properties of selective cellular recruitment, gave rise to the name chemokines, a contraction of "*chemo*attractant cyto*kines*". The first to be identified was the neutrophil attractant, initially named NAP-1 (neutrophil activating peptide-1) and then renamed IL-8 in the tradition of the emerging interleukin immune modulating family. Shortly after, the monocyte chemoattractant chemokines were identified, namely MCP-1 and MIP-1α and β. These proteins are all small, approximately 8 kD, and shared a common four-cysteine motif. The overall level of sequence identity within the family can be less than 20%. The amino terminal sequence of these proteins showed a significant difference in the cysteine motif. The IL-8 has a single residue between the first two cysteines, whereas in MCP-1 and the two MIP-1 proteins, the first two cysteines are adjacent. This led to the division of the family into two subclasses: the CXC, or α subclass, and the CC, or β subclass. Two proteins have been found which fall outside of the CC and the CXC subclasses: the C chemokine, lymphotactin, which lacks a disulfide pair and is postulated to be an evolutionary ancestral form, and the CX₃C chemokine fractalkine, or neurotactin. The latter two groups show a deviation from the classic four-cysteine motif; however, only one member exists to date for each.

Initially, chemokines were identified in classic purifications from cell culture media or directly from tissue samples. Later cDNA cloning by homology was used. The real explosion in the chemokine field has come from the identification of new chemokine ligands from EST (expressed sequence tag) databases (4). Thus, the number of ligands is currently between 40 and 50 for the human system.

After their identificaiton, chemokines were initially principally associated with inflammatory disease, where they were found at elevated levels in biological fluids or tissues both from patients and from animal models of inflammation. However, more recently, chemokines have been classified into two groups. Some are constitutively expressed and play a role in development; others are inducible and play a major role in inflammation. There may be a certain overlap between these two broad categories. However, this division is particularly relevant in light of the prevention of HIV infection by interfering with the chemokine system. Deletion of the CXCR4 ligand, SDF-1α, in mice resulted in embryonic lethality (5), but there is no evidence to date that blocking the activity of this chemokine in the adult will be deleterious.

Another feature of chemokines that differentiated them from other cytokines and interleukins was the fact that they activate members of the superfamily of seven-transmembrane spanning (7TM), G-protein–coupled receptors. This family has been one of the most fruitful classes of targets for the pharmaceutical industry because the receptors very often have small ligands. As recently as 6 years ago, only three chemokine receptors had been identified: the two IL-8 receptors CXCR1 and CXCR2, and CCR1, initially known as the shared RANTES/MIP-1α receptor, which made the targets for therapeutic intervention for inflammation to appear simple. By 1996, the year that the chemokine receptors were identified as HIV coreceptors, the list had grown to nine; currently, the list has 16 members (Fig. 1).

Initial research focused on the expression levels of the chemokine ligands, but the principal player is probably the receptor itself, particularly in immune modulation and inflammation. Newcomers to the chemokine field are often perplexed by the complexity and apparent lack of specificity seen in the chemokine system, in which few receptors bind only one ligand and certain chemokines bind to more than one receptor as shown in Fig. 1. However, emerging data show that there is a tight level of control of receptor expression. For example, CD4$^+$ T cells have recently been extensively studied in regard to their receptor profiles, providing insights as to which subsets are susceptible to infection by HIV strains with different tropisms. T cells were shown to express almost all of the chemokine receptors, at least at the mRNA level. However, resting T cells principally express CXCR4 and not CCR5, whereas activated T cells predominantly express CCR5 and CXCR3, the expression of the former being dependable on the mode of activation, and CXCR4 is also expressed. Furthermore, T-cell subsets have been described as preferentially expressing certain chemokine receptors: the Th1 phenotype expresses CCR5 (6), whereas the Th2 phenotype expresses CCR3 and CCR4 (7,8). A second example is the dendritic cell—again, mRNA for many chemokine receptors has been found in dendritic cells, but while undergoing activation and maturation, receptor expression has been shown to follow distinctive patterns (9). Similarly, as monocytes acquire the macrophage phenotype as they become adherent, the level of CCR5 increases dramatically.

With antibodies becoming available for many chemokine receptors recently, many laboratories have been able to focus on the receptors that are up-regulated in pathological situations. Before antibodies became available, workers in the field

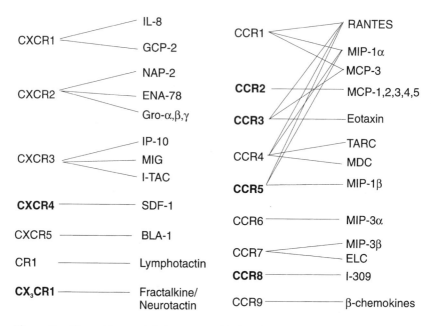

Figure 1 Chemokines and their receptors. To date, five CXC and nine CC chemokine receptors have been identified, as well as the receptors for the C and CX$_3$C chemokines. There are few receptors that only bind one ligand, and in addition, certain chemokines bind to more than one receptor. The chemokine receptors that have been shown to act as coreceptors, at least in vitro, are shown in bold. As discussed in the text, in vivo, the most important are CCR5 and CXCR4.

were restricted to analyses at the mRNA level, and, even though these studies were useful in identifying the genes in question, there is no doubt that correlation of these results by direct measurements of protein levels are preferable. Recent publications have shown the importance of CXCR3 and CCR5 on activated T cells in a number of disease states (10), and presentations from relevant meetings have disclosed that many more will soon be reported.

III.   HIV ENTRY THROUGH THE CD4 AND CHEMOKINE RECEPTOR COMPLEX

The HIV particles enter host cells by means of their envelope glycoprotein subunits gp120 and gp41, which are covalently associated, and assemble to trimers on the HIV viral membrane. Viral entry is achieved by fusion on the cell surface as a result of conformational changes in the envelope glycoproteins upon binding to the CD4 molecule (11–13). It was shown more than a decade ago that expression of CD4 on otherwise resistant human cells renders them susceptible for infection with at least one type of HIV-1 strain, the T-cell line adapted (TCLA) strains, but failed to induce the same in nonhuman cells (11,12). It was therefore concluded that HIV-1, in addition to CD4, utilizes additional surface molecules on human cells to succeed in efficient entry.

A second line of evidence that not one but at least two different second receptor molecules are involved in HIV-1 entry, that HIV isolates have a distinct cellular tropism, was an observation made by several groups over the past years. When studying HIV tropism, one has to distinguish between primary strains, unselected by passage in transformed T-cell lines, and T-cell line adapted strains, which have been cultured in vitro. Certain primary HIV-1 isolates only replicate in macrophages or activated primary CD4$^+$ T cells and were hence referred to as macrophage tropic (M-tropic) isolates. M-tropic isolates are unable to replicate in transformed T-cell lines, despite the presence of CD4 on these cells. Another group of isolates replicates very efficiently on these cell lines and are referred to as T-tropic isolates. Upon infection, the latter viruses induce large multicell fusion bodies called syncitia and are therefore referred to as syncitium-inducing (SI) isolates. T-tropic isolates distinguish themselves further from M-tropic isolates—which cannot form syncitia in cell lines and so are referred to as non–syncitium-inducing (NSI) isolates—by their lack of replication in macrophages. A third group of isolates, referred to as dual-tropic isolates, harbors the ability to replicate in all three cell types: macrophages, primary T cells, and T-cell lines. These viruses fall into the class of SI isolates. The differences in tropism between isolates have been mapped to regions on the gp120 molecule. Changes in gp120 that conferred change of tropism were often found in the V3 loop region of gp120, but changes in other regions on gp120 were also shown to be of importance (13a).

The nomenclature based on tropism is not completely accurate, because the different groups overlap (for more details see Ref. 14). Classification based on chemokine receptor usage adds an extra dimension to the nomenclature, which may help to simplify the picture (24).

IV. THE IDENTIFICATION OF THE CHEMOKINE RECEPTORS AS THE HIV CORECEPTOR

The initial observation by Cocchi et al. that the CC chemokines MIP-1α, MIP-1β, and RANTES can block infection by NSI isolates (15), was followed by the identification of a seven-transmembrane G-protein–coupled orphan receptor to be the missing cofactor for T-tropic isolates (16). After several name changes and identification of its chemokine ligand, the receptor was finally defined as the CXC chemokine receptor CXCR4 (17,18). The discovery of CCR5 as the coreceptor for macrophage tropic HIV strains by several laboratories followed shortly afterward (19–21). Several other chemokine and related orphan receptors have since been shown to function as HIV coreceptors for at least some isolates (22). The chemokine receptors that have been shown to function as coreceptors, at least in vitro, are shown in bold in Fig. 1. However, CCR5 and CXCR4 remain the dominant coreceptors and all isolates identified to date use at least one of these two receptors (23). Recently, a standardized nomenclature has been adopted that is based on coreceptor usage (24). M-tropic or NSI viruses were shown to use CCR5 for entry and are hence referred to as R5 viruses. T-tropic viruses use CXCR4 and are referred to as X4 isolates. Dual tropic isolates, which interact with both CCR5 and CXCR4, are called R5X4 viruses.

V. THE LINK BETWEEN HIV TROPISM, PATHOGENESIS, AND CHEMOKINE RECEPTORS

Much of the underlying biology of HIV-1 is linked to differential coreceptor usage. The HIV virus tropism is closely associated with transmission and pathogenesis. It had been shown early on that sexually transmitted isolates are preferentially R5 (NSI) viruses and stay prevalent early on in infection (25,26). The importance of CCR5 in viral transmission was further underlined by the discovery of a variant in the CCR5 gene, which prevents the formation of a functional receptor molecule, and the finding that individuals that are homozygote for this deletion are highly resistant to HIV-1 infection (27–29). This observation strengthened the hypothesis that the cell compartments involved in the initial infection might predominantly express CCR5, in that macrophages and dendritic cells, which are present in the mucosal sites of infection during sexual transmission, express CCR5. As time progresses after infection, X4 viruses emerge and their appearance is closely linked with progression of disease, although this is not observed in all individuals studied. What drives this phenotypic switch and which factors suppress the emergence of the highly pathogenic X4 isolates in the earlier years of infection are still unclear. Differential expression of chemokine receptors in tissues and on the peripheral CD4$^+$ T cells during progression might be partially responsible. In addition, local overexpression of chemokines might suppress replication of certain groups of viruses.

VI. INTERACTION OF VIRUS ENVELOPE AND THE CHEMOKINE RECEPTOR

The initial interaction between CD4 and the viral envelope drives a conformational change in gp120, which exposes the binding site to allow interaction with the chemokine receptor (30,31). The precise regions of gp120 that interact with the coreceptors are not yet completely identified, but studies with monoclonal antibodies against gp120 epitopes have suggested the gp120/CCR5 interaction site (30,31,31a). A molecular complex of soluble gp120, membrane associated CD4, and CXCR4 can be immunoprecipitated, proving the close association of these three players (32).

Fusion of the viral and cell membrane is then thought to be induced by the conformational change in the gp41/gp120/CD4 complex driving the glycoprotein gp41 into the host membrane. The hypothesis is that this interaction is driven by the hydrophobic amino terminus of gp41 and the model is based on the mechanism of membrane fusion for the influenza virus (33). Chemokine receptors may mediate the conformational change of the HIV envelope proteins required for the insertion of gp41 into the host membrane. The signaling activities of the chemokine receptors mediated by G proteins or receptor internalization are not required for the chemokine receptor to function as an HIV coreceptor. Infection is not abolished by pertussis toxin (15,34) and mutant receptors that are unable to internalize still support viral entry (35).

Mapping the binding region of the viral envelope protein on the chemokine coreceptors is an area of active research. For R5 viruses, the N-terminus of CCR5 has been shown to be crucial for recognition and coreceptor activity (36,37). Chimeric CCR2b/CCR5 receptors containing only the CCR5 N-terminus are active for R5/NSI virus infection (28). The N-terminal region of CCR5 has three tyrosine residues, which are conserved in the orphan receptors BONZO and BOB. Despite the low identity of these orphans with the chemokine receptors, they still act as coreceptors for HIV, which suggests that these tyrosines are important recognition elements (39). In addition, several negatively charged residues at the N-terminus are crucial for CCR5 coreceptor activity. Mutations of aspartic acid residues at positions 2 and 11, as well as a glutamic acid at position 18, impair CCR5 coreceptor activity (37). yet, monoclonal antibodies that recognize the second extracellular loop (E2) of CCR5 efficiently blocked HIV-1 infection, whereas those specific for the N-terminus were weaker inhibitors (40), suggesting that this loop might not have a specific function in interaction with the envelope but that it nevertheless plays an important role in the fusion process.

For X4 strains, the regions on their coreceptor, CXCR4, that are recognized by the envelope are different. Their key site is the E2 loop of CXCR4. It was shown that a chimeric receptor containing the N-terminus of CCR5 and E2 of CXCR4 functions for a range of R5 and X4 viruses (36). Truncation of N-terminal sequences of CXCR4 showed that some X4 viruses required a full length N-terminus, whereas others were unaffected by removal of most or all N-terminal sequences (41). This different pattern of receptor binding sites between R5 and X4 strains may play an important role in the switch that occurs when the virus mutates form R5 to X4 during the later stages of infection.

VII. CHEMOKINE RECEPTOR LIGANDS CAN SUPPRESS VIRAL INFECTIVITY

The chemokine ligands also play a key role in the HIV infection process: CCR5 ligands—MIP-Iα, MIP-Iβ, and RANTES—were identified as components secreted by $CD8^+$ T cells that block infection of human cells by R5 strains at nanomolar concentration (15). Their efficiency of inhibition generally parallels their affinity for CCR5, with RANTES being the highest affinity ligand and the most potent blocker (42). Similarly, the CXCR4 ligand SDF-1 can block infection of the TCLA or X4 strains, although higher concentrations are required to achieve the effect (18,43).

The ligands for the other chemokine receptors, which function as coreceptors, are also able to inhibit their coreceptor function. Thus, eotaxin inhibits CCR3 using strains (44), and I-309 inhibits infection of diverse HIV-1 strains through CCR8 (45), but so far there are no reports of MCP-1 inhibition of R2b strains. Poxviruses and herpes viruses have been recently shown to encode a large number of chemokines (46). HHV8, the virus associated with Karposi's sarcoma, encodes three such molecules, which have been called vMIP-I, vMIP-II, and BCK/vMIP-III. vMIP-II is the best studied of these molecules (47,48). It is unique among the chemokines in that it can bind to members of the CXC and CC chemokine receptors: CXCR4, CCR5 CCR3, as well as the cytomegalovirus-encoded open reading frame US28. The vMIP-II protein is thus able to block infection by both R5 and X4 strains of HIV-1, as well as dual tropic strains known to utilize CCR3. The molecular basis of this selectivity is not yet fully understood. However, it points to the fact that these receptors have been selected for in the evolution of the HHV8 chemokines. The role of these chemokines in sarcoma production (the control of cell recruitment and angiogenesis) is clear, but their effect on HIV-1 infection in vivo has not been well studied yet.

VIII. CHEMOKINE RECEPTOR ANTAGONISTS

Alterations in the amino termini of certain chemokines have been shown to result in profound changes on their activity. Chemokines are thought to interact with their receptors according to a two-site model: The main body of the chemokine first reacts with an extracellular domain of the receptor, which is thus defined as site 1. Site 1 has been identified for certain receptors, CCR2 and CCR5, as being the second extracellular loop. The binding to the receptor has been suggested to induce a conformational change, which allows the amino terminal region to interact with a second site, site 2. This model is based on the one proposed for another small chemoattractant protein, C5a, in which this protein triggers site 2 through its C-terminal region (49). Alanine spanning mutagenesis of RANTES and the analysis of the affinities for the mutants for CCR1, CCR3, and CCR5 have lent evidence in favor of this model (50).

Amino terminal truncation of chemokines or modifications of the amino terminal region can result in proteins that have lost their capacity to activate their receptors through site 2, although they retain the ability to bind to the receptors through site 1. In this manner, receptor antagonists can be generated because they will compete for the binding of the natural ligand. The first example of this phenomenon was demonstrated with IL-8, which was shown to have a three amino acid motif: Glu-Leu-Arg (ELR) preceding the CXC motif, which was required for optimal binding (51). Removal of the first five amino acid residues while retaining the Arg produced a protein that was still able to bind to the receptor and could antagonize the actions of IL-8 (52). Similar modifications of other members of the CXC family have since been shown to produce antagonists (53).

CC chemokines can also be modified in this way. RANTES, MCP-1, and MCP-3 have been produced as amino terminally truncated proteins, and these variants antagonize the effects of their parent ligands in vitro. Furthermore, removal of the first eight residues from the amino terminal of RANTES changed its specificity and the truncated protein was able to bind to CCR2, which the full-length protein does not normally do (54). Similarly, removal of eight residues from the amino terminal region of MCP-1 forms an antagonist protein (55). But the most potent chemokine receptor antagonists have been produced by extending the amino terminal. The retention of the initiating methionine (Met-RANTES) in the bacterial *Escherichia coli* expression system produces a protein that inhibits both RANTES and MIP-1α induced monocyte and T-cell chemotaxis in vitro at nanomolar concentrations (56).

Met-RANTES can also significantly reduce inflammation in several murine models of inflammation. When administered to mice that have been sensitized with collagen which provokes symptoms resembling rheumatoid arthritis in humans, the onset and severity of the arthritic symptoms are reduced in a dose-related manner, if the antagonist is administered before disease onset (57). Met-RANTES administration to mice, in which crescentic glomerulonephritis is induced by nephrotoxic sheep serum results in a reduction of both T-cell and macrophage accumulation in the renal tissues (58). The inflammation involved in organ transplant rejection in a rat model of kidney transplant was significantly abrogated by Met-RANTES treatment (58a). Lastly, in the ovalbumin-sensitized murine model of airways inflammation, which has symptoms of human asthma, the efficacy of chemokine receptor antagonism by Met-RANTES administration was compared to blocking the action of chemokines that had been previously identified to be overexpressed (58b). The inhibition of eosinophil recruitment to the airways observed by the administration of Met-RANTES was greater than that observed by the blocking of individual chemokine ligands by neutralizing antibodies, demonstrating that blocking the receptor is more efficient than blocking ligands.

Extension of the amino terminal of RANTES by the chemical coupling of a five-carbon alkyl chain to the oxidized N-terminal serine residue produces a modified RANTES protein called amino-oxy pentane RANTES (AOP-RANTES). This protein was found to have an increased affinity over RANTES and Met-RANTES for CCR5 (59) and, furthermore, to have a greater affinity for CCR1 and CCR3. However, even though neither Met-RANTES nor AOP-RANTES induced chemotaxis or calcium mobilization using freshly isolated peripheral blood mononuclear cells (PBMCs), both were capable of calcium mobilization in CHO cells, which had been transfected to express high levels of CCR5 receptors (60). Thus, modifications of the N-terminus of RANTES result in partial agonists on certain receptors, and their ability to induce cellular responses depends on the number of receptors expressed at the cell surface.

IX. CHEMOKINE-MEDIATED INHIBITION OF HIV INFECTION

Both the chemokine receptor ligands and modified RANTES proteins are able to inhibit infection by HIV-1 strains. As discussed, infection by X4 strains can be blocked by SDF-1, R3 using strains can be blocked by eotaxin, R8 by I-309, and R5 strains by RANTES, MIP-1α, and MIP-1β. Three functional chemokine receptor antagonists, (9-68)RANTES (61), Met-RANTES, and AOP-RANTES (59) have all been shown to inhibit PBMC infection by R5 strains of HIV-1. However, both (9-68)RANTES and Met-RANTES are less potent than RANTES itself, whereas AOP-RANTES is significantly more potent than RANTES. Although the inhibition by RANTES of R5 strains of both fusion and infection in recombinant cell lines expressing CD4 and CCR5 as well as that of PBMCs has been widely reported by many different groups, the inhibition of macrophages by RANTES is still controversial. In fact, enhancement of infection of macrophages in the presence of RANTES has been reported (62). However, Simmons et al. were able to show that AOP-RANTES was very efficient in inhibiting the infection of macrophages by four R5 strains, whereas RANTES showed inhibition of only one of the strains tested, and Met-RANTES showed no inhibition at all (59). To date, AOP-RANTES remains the most potent inhibitor of R5 strains. However, recent studies have shown that high concentrations, greater than 1 μg/ml, of RANTES cause enhancement of infection of several types of virus, independent of receptor usage, and of the mechanism of viral fusion and entry in vitro (63). Whereas AOP-RANTES inhibited HIV-1 infection mediated through CCR5, it was similarly shown to enhance infection of X4 strains, as well as other viruses. These observations were made at concentrations that are superphysiological in vivo, and the mechanism of this enhancement remains to be elucidated.

X. MECHANISMS OF BLOCKING THE HIV/CHEMOKINE RECEPTOR INTERACTION

Once the chemokine receptors had been identified as coreceptors and it was shown that it is possible to block infection using chemokines, the immediate question was whether cellular activation by an agonist was required for this effect. Upon activation, chemokine receptors, in a manner that is common to all 7TMs, are internalized from the cell surface. This is a possible mechanism for chemokine ligands to block viral infection. However, a second hypothesis could be proposed, that is, simply, there is steric hindrance where the binding of the chemokine to the receptor prevents access to the binding site of the HIV virus to the coreceptor. These two hypotheses, depicted in Fig. 2, do not exclude the possibility that other mechanisms may exist that depend on signaling mechanisms that have not yet been elucidated for chemokine receptors. The observation by several groups that the natural ligands of the coreceptors could block HIV infection does not distinguish between the mechanisms.

As discussed, it has been established that signaling is not an absolute requirement because pertussis toxin treatment, which inhibits G_i mediated signaling, does not prevent infection (15). In addition, mutant receptors that do not signal still

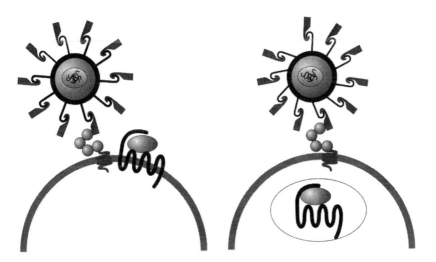

Figure 2 Two hypotheses for the mechanism of inhibition of HIV infectivity by chemokines. *Left*, The binding of the chemokine to its receptor may sterically hinder the interaction of the viral glycoproteins with the coreceptor. *Right*, The chemokine induces the signaling events that trigger the endocytosis of the receptor, thereby removing it from the surface and preventing it from functioning as a coreceptor.

function as coreceptors (34). Neither is internalization of the chemokine receptor a requisite for infection because carboxy terminal truncated CXCR4 receptors, which are unable to internalize upon ligand binding, also still function as coreceptors (35). The observation that modified RANTES proteins, which are unable to induce calcium mobilization and chemotaxis of certain primary cells such as monocytes, are capable of inhibiting HIV-1 infection, the mechanism of steric hindrance, appeared to be most likely. However, these modified proteins are all capable of receptor activation and should thus be defined as partial agonists, which does not exclude that receptor activation may play a role.

Whereas (9-68)RANTES has been reported to be unable to mobilize calcium and induce chemotaxis, it is able to induce CCR5 internalization. Down-regulation of 7TM receptors is known to be an agonist-mediated event, which requires phosphorylation mediated by the GRK family of serine/threonine kinases of the carboxy terminal region of the receptor. This is followed by interaction with β-arrestins before sequestration into clathrin-coated pits (64,65). Both (9-68)RANTES and AOP-RANTES efficiently down-regulate CCR5 in stably transfected CHO cells as well as PBMCs (35,60). Met-RANTES, on the other hand, has been shown to be unable to mediate CCR1 down-regulation (66) and is very poor in inducing CCR5 down-regulation (60). The ability of chemokines to remove cell surface receptors has been suggested to contribute to their anti-infectivity properties, both for X4 strains because SDF-1 causes receptor internalization and for R5 strains since the modified RANTES proteins (9-68)RANTES and AOP-RANTES cause internalization of CCR5. In the case of AOP-RANTES, the receptor down-regulation was, in fact, greater than that induced by RANTES, possibly explaining its superior potency as an inhibitor of HIV infection.

Furthermore, AOP-RANTES has identified a novel mechanism that may be important in the inhibition of HIV infection. After down-regulation and trafficking into early endosomes, 7TM receptors may undergo one of two fates. They are either targeted to late endosomes and then lysosomes where they are degraded, or they are targeted to a recycling compartment where, following dissociation of the ligand, the receptor is dephosphorylated and then recycled to the cell surface. Although the fate of chemokine receptors following internalization has not yet been studied extensively, examples of both pathways have been demonstrated. CCR2b has been shown to follow the degradative pathway through the lysosomal compartment, whereas CXCR4 (67) and CCR5 (60) recycle to the cell surface. Removal of RANTES from the culture medium after down-regulation of CCR5 allows the internalized receptors to recycle, but, surprisingly, removal of AOP-RANTES significantly abrogates receptor recycling (60). Under these circumstances, cell surface expression of the receptor is prevented and HIV infection becomes impossible. This conclusion is further supported by the infection of cells with the cDNA coding for CCR5 ligands, including the KDEL motif. This amino acid sequence targets proteins to the endoplasmic reticulum (ER), and it is believed that ligands expressed with this amino acid sequence, named intrakines, trap the nascent chemokine receptors in the ER and thus prevent cell surface expression (68). Cells transfected with these cDNA sequences were effectively unable to be infected by HIV-1 viruses.

XI. ORALLY ACTIVE ANTI-HIV THERAPEUTICS?

The observations that HIV infection can be inhibited both by the natural ligands as well as the modified chemokines suggests chemokine receptors as good targets for therapeutic intervention. The question remains as to what the negative effect of blocking a receptor involved in the maintenance of a fully competent immune system would be. The effect may not be dramatic: In the 1% of the Caucasian population which are homozygous for the ΔCCR5 mutation, there are no apparent immune defects, but a high level of resistance to HIV infection. Whereas CXCR4 appears essential for fetal development, there is no evidence that blocking this receptor in the adult is deleterious. Pharmaceutical companies are therefore putting great efforts into screening the coreceptors for small molecules that block the coreceptors. Such small molecules could be useful therapeutic adjuncts to the combined therapies currently used in clinic. The current therapies target essential proteins produced by the virus itself and which are required for the viral replication life cycle, in contrast to the chemokine receptor target molecules that are host proteins.

This screening effort is beginning to pay off. Because seven-transmembrane receptors have an exceptionally good track record for being susceptible to low molecular weight therapeutic drugs that can be taken orally, once the worry of crucial interference with the immune system was diminished, these receptors appeared an ideal target. However, the majority of these receptors have small ligands, of which, histamine, adrenalin, serotonin, and dopamine are representative examples. The interaction of chemokines and their receptors involves a larger protein ligand, of about 8 kDa, which may explain why small molecule inhibitors were not found rapidly. However, the outlook is hopeful because reports of such compounds are appearing in the patent and scientific literature, and have recently been well documented in a specialized review (69). Whereas no compounds have yet been reported for CCR5, three classes of compounds were recently described that were identified by their ability to block infection of PBMCs by T-tropic HIV-1 strains. These compounds have all been shown to be CXCR4 receptor antagonists in that they block binding of its ligand, SDF-1, as well as inhibiting SDF-1–induced receptor activation. The most potent class of compounds is the bicyclam series, in which the prototype AMD3100 is 10 to 50-fold more potent in inhibiting HIV infection than SDF-1 itself (70,71). The second type of antagonist is a cyclic 18-mer peptide containing two disulfides that was isolated from *Limulus ployphemus*, and the third is pseudo 9-mer peptide. However, only the bicyclam family may be small enough to allow their development into an orally available compound.

Thus, even though the development of modified chemokines as therapeutic agents appears to be the most advanced, the discovery of low molecular weight inhibitors is following closely on its heels. The observation that RANTES and AOP-RANTES, at least in vitro, cause enhancement of viral infection, albeit at concentrations that are most likely not physiological, suggests that the relevant control experiments must be carried out before envisaging the use of these proteins as therapeutics. However, the modified chemokine AOP-RANTES has opened up a new potential mechanism of inhibition of receptor recycling, which could suggest a novel target area. Taken together, it is clear that blocking the ability of chemokine receptors to function as coreceptors in HIV cell entry may soon become feasible and could add another component to the successful strategy of combined therapies that block different processes essential to the productive infection of cells by HIV.

REFERENCES

1. Baggiolini M. Chemokines and leukocyte traffic. Nature 1998; 392:565–568.
2. Luster AD. Chemokines—chemotactic cytokines that mediate inflammation. N Engl J Med 1998; 338:436–445.
3. Wells TNC, Power CA, Proudfoot AEI. Definition, function and pathophysiological significance of chemokine receptors. Trends Pharmacol Sci 1998; 19:376–380.
4. Wells TNC, Peitsch MC. The chemokine information source: identification and characterization of novel chemokines using the WorldWideWeb and expressed sequence tag databases. J Leukoc Biol 1997; 61:545–550.
5. Nagasawa T, Hirota S, Tachibana K, Takakura N, Nishikawa S, Kitamura Y, Yoshida N, Kikutani H, Kishimoto T. Defects of B-cell lymphopoiesis and bone-marrow myelopoiesis in mice lacking the CXC chemokine PBSF/SDF-1. Nature 1998; 382:635–638.
6. Loetscher P, Uguccioni M, Bordoli L, Baggiolini M, Moser B, Chizzolini C, Dayer JM. CCR5 is characteristic of Th1 lymphocytes. Nature 1998; 391:344–345.
7. Sallusto F, Mackay CR, Lanzavecchia A. Selective expression of the eotaxin receptor CCR3 by human T helper 2 cells. Science 1997; 277:2005–2007.
8. Bonecchi R, Bianchi G, Pordignon PP, Dambrosio D, Lang R, Borsatti A, Sozzani S, Allavena P, Gray PA, Mantovani A, Sinigaglia F. Differential expression of chemokine receptors and chemotactic responsiveness of type 1 T helper cells (Th1s and Th2s). J Exp Med 1998; 187:129–134.
9. Desaintvis B, Fugiervivier I, Massacrier C, Gaillard C, Vanbervliet BA, Banchereau J, Liu YJ, Lebecque S, Caux C. The cytokine profile expressed by human dendritic cells is dependent on cell subtype and mode of activation. J Immunol 160:1666–1676.
10. Qin S, Rottman JB, Myers P, Kassam N, Weinblatt M, Loetscher M, Koch AE, Moser B, Mackay CR. The chemokine receptors CXCR3 and CCR5 mark subsets of T cells associated with certain inflammatory reactions. J Clin Invest 1998; 101:746–754.
11. Dalgleish AG, Beverley PC, Clapham PR, Crawford DH, Greaves MF, Weiss RA. The CD4 (T4) antigen is an essential component of the receptor for the AIDS retrovirus. Nature 1984; 312:763–767.
12. Maddon PJ, Dalgleish AG, McDougal JS, Clapham PR, Weiss RA, Axel R. The T4 gene encodes the AIDS virus receptor and is expressed in the immune system and the brain. Cell 1986; 47:333–348.

13. Chesebro B, Buller R, Portis J, Wehrly K. Failure of human immunodeficiency virus entry and infection in CD4-positive human brain and skin cells. J Virol 1990; 64:215–221.

13a. Chesebro B, Wehrly K, Nishio J, Perryman S. Mapping of independent V3 envelope determinants of human immunodeficiency virus type 1 macrophage tropism and syncytium formation in lymphocytes. J Virol 1996; 70(12):9055–9059.

14. Clapham P, McKnight A, Simmons G, Weiss R. Is CD4 sufficient for HIV entry? Cell surface molecules involved in HIV infection. Philos Trans R Soc Lond Series B: Biol Sci 1993; 342:67–73.

15. Cocchi F, DeVico AL, Garzino-Demo A, Arya SK, Gallo RC, Lusso P. Identification of RANTES, MIP-1 alpha and MIP-1 beta as the major HIV-suppressive factors produced by CD8+ T cells. Science 1995; 270:1811–1815.

16. Feng Y, Broder CC, Kennedy PE, Berger EA. HIV-1 entry cofactor: functional cDNA cloning of a seven-transmembrane, G protein-coupled receptor. Science 1996; 272:872–877.

17. Bleul CC, Farzan M, Choe H, Parolin C, Clarklewis I, Sodroski J, Springer TA. The lymphocyte chemoattractant SDF-1 is a ligand for LESTR/FUSIN and blocks HIV-1 entry. Nature 1996; 382:829–833.

18. Oberlin E, Amara A, Bachelerie F, Bessia C, Virelizier JL, Arenzana-Seisdedos F, Schwartz O, Heard JM, Clark-Lewis I, Legler DF, Loetscher M, Baggiolini M, Moser B. The CXC chemokine SDF-1 is the ligand for LESTR/fusin and prevents infection by T-cell-line-adapted HIV-1. Nature 1996; 382:833–835.

19. Dragic T, Litwin V, Allaway GP, Martin SR, Huang Y, Nagashima KA, Cayanan C, Maddon PJ, Koup RA, Moore JP, Paxton WA. HIV-1 entry into CD4+ cells is mediated by the chemokine receptor CC-CKR-5. Nature 381:667–673.

20. Alkhatib G, Combadiere C, Broder CC, Feng Y, Kennedy PE, Murphy PM, Berger EA. CC CKR5: a RANTES, MIP-1alpha, MIP-1beta receptor as a fusion cofactor for macrophage-tropic HIV-1. Science 1996; 272:1955–1958.

21. Deng H, Liu R, Ellmeier W, Choe S, Unutmaz D, Burkhart M, DiMarzio P, Marmon S, Sutton RE, Hill CM, Davis CB, Peiper SC, Schall TJ, Littman DR, Landau NR. Identification of a major coreceptor for primary isolates of HIV-1. Nature 1996; 381:661–666.

22. Clapham PR. HIV and chemokines: Ligands sharing cell-surface receptors. Trends Cell Biol 1997; 7:264–268.

23. Doms RW, Moore JP. HIV-1 Coreceptor Use: A Molecular Window into Viral Tropism. Human Retroviruses and AIDS 1997: A Compilation and Analysis of Nucleic Acid and Amino Acid Sequences 1997.

24. Berger EA, Doms RW, Fenyo EM, Korber BT, Littman DR, Moore JP, Sattentau QJ, Schuitemaker H, Sodroski J, Weiss RA. A new classification for HIV-1. Nature 1998; 391:240.

25. Connor RI, Ho DD. Transmission and pathogenesis of human immunodeficiency virus type 1. AIDS Res Hum Retroviruses 1994; 10:321–323.

26. Schuitemaker H, Koot M, Kootstra NA, Dercksen MW, de Goede RE, van Steenwijk RP, Lange JM, Schattenkerk JK, Miedema F, Tersmette M. Biological phenotype of human immunodeficiency virus type 1 clones at different stages of infection: progression of disease is associated with a shift from monocytotropic to T-cell-tropic virus population. J Virol 1992; 66:1354–1360.

27. Liu R, Paxton WA, Choe S, Ceradini D, Martin SR, Horuk R, MacDonald ME, Stuhlmann H, Koup RA, Landau NR. Homozygous defect in HIV-1 coreceptor accounts for resistance of some multiply-exposed individuals to HIV-1 infection. Cell 1996; 86:367–377.

28. Samson M, Libert F, Doranz BJ, Rucker J, Liesnard C, Farber CM, Saragosti S, Lapoumeroulie C, Cognaux J, Forceille C, Muyldermans G, Verhofstede C, Burtonboy G, Georges M, Imai T, Rana G, Yi Y, Smyth RJ, Collman RG, Doms RW, Vassart G, Parmentier M. Resistance to HIV-1 infection in caucasian individuals bearing mutant alleles of the CCR-5 chemokine receptor gene [see comments]. Nature 1996; 382: 722–725.

29. Dean M, Carrington M, Winkler C, Huttley GA, Smith MW, Allikmets R, Geodert JJ, Buchbinder SP, Vittinghoff E, Gomperts E, Donfield S, Vlahov D, Kaslow R, Saah A, Rinaldo C, Detels R, O'Brien SJ. Genetic restriction of HIV-1 infection and progression to AIDS by a deletion allele of the CKR5 structural gene. Hemophilia Growth and Development Study, Multicenter AIDS Cohort Study, Multicenter Hemophila Cohort Study, San Francisco City Cohort, ALIVE Study. Science 1996; 273:1856–1862.

30. Trkola A, Dragic T, Arthos J, Binley JM, Olson WC, Allaway GP, Cheng-Mayer C, Robinson J, Maddon PJ, Moore JP. CD4-dependent, antibody-sensitive interactions between HIV-1 and its co-receptor CCR-5. Nature 1996; 384:184–187.

31. Wu L, Gerard NP, Wyatt R, Choe H, Parolin C, Ruffing N, Borsetti A, Cardoso AA, Desjardin E, Newman W, Gerard C, Sodroski J. CD4-induced interaction of primary HIV-1 gp120 glycoproteins with the chemokine receptor CCR-5. Nature 1996; 384: 179–183.

31a. Kwong PD, Wyatt R, Robinson J, Sweet RW, Sodroski J, Hendrickson WA. Structure of an HIV gp120 envelope glycoprotein in complex with the CD4 receptor and a neutralizing human antibody. Nature 1998; 393(6686):648–659.

32. Lapham CK, Ouyang J, Chandrasekhar B, Nguyen N, Dimitrov DS, Golding H. Evidence for cell-surface association between fusin and the CD4-gp120 complex in human cell lines. Science 1996; 274:602–605.

33. Gullough PA, Hughson FM, Skehel JJ, Wiley DC. Structure of influenza haemagglutinin at the pH of membrane fusion. Nature 1994; 371:37–43.

34. Aramori I, Zhang J, Ferguson SS, Bieniasz PD, Cullen BR, Caron M. Molecular mechanism of desensitization of the chemokine receptor CCR-5; receptor signaling and internalization are dissociable from its role as an HIV-1 co-receptor. EMBO J 1997; 16: 4606–4616.

35. Amara A, Gall SL, Schwartz O, Salamero J, Montes M, Loetscher P, Baggiolini M, Virelizier JL, Arenzana SF. HIV coreceptor downregulation as antiviral principle: SDF-1alpha-dependent internalization of the chemokine receptor CXCR4 contributes to inhibition of HIV replication. J Exp Med 1997; 186:139–146.

36. Lu Z, Berson JF, Chen Y, Turner JD, Zhang T, Sharron M, Jenks MH, Wang Z, Kim J, Rucker J, Hoxie JA, Peiper SC, Doms RW. Evolution of HIV-1 coreceptor usage through interactions with distinct CCR5 and CXCR4 domains. Proc Natl Acad Sci USA 1997; 94:6426–6431.

37. Dragic T, Trkola A, Lin SW, Nagashima KA, Kajumo F, Zhao L, Olson WC, Wu L, Mackay CR, Allaway GP, Sakmar TP, Moore JP, Maddon PJ. Amino-terminal substitutions in the CCR5 coreceptor impair gp120 binding and human immunodeficiency virus type 1 entry. J Virol 1998; 72:279–285.

38. Rucker J, Samson M, Doranz BJ, Libert F, Berson JF, Yi Y, Smyth RJ, Collman RG, Broder CC, Vassart G, Doms RW, Parmentier M. Regions in beta-chemokine receptors CCR5 and CCR2b that determine HIV-1 cofactor specificity. Cell 1996; 87:437–446.

39. Farzan M, Choe H, Martin K, Marcon L, Hofmann W, Karlsson G, Sun Y, Barrett P, Marchano N, Sullivan N, Gerard N, Gerard C, Sodroski J. Two orphan seven-transmembrane segment receptors which are expressed in CD4-positive cells support simian immunodeficiency virus infection. J Exp Med 1997; 186:405–411.

40. Wu L, LaRosa G, Kassam N, Gordon CJ, Heath H, Ruffing N, Chen H, Humblias J, Samson M, Parmentier M, Moore JP, Mackay CR. Interaction of chemokine receptor CCR5 with its ligands: multiple domains for HIV-1 gp120 binding and a single domain for chemokine binding. J Exp Med 1997; 186:1373–1381.

41. Picard L, Wilkinson DA, McKnight A, Gray PW, Hoxie JA, Clapham PR, Weiss RA. Role of the amino-terminal extracellular domain of CXCR-4 in human immunodeficiency virus type 1 entry. Virology 1997; 231:105–111.

42. Trkola A, Paxton WA, Monard SP, Hoxie JA, Siani MA, Thompson DA, Wu L, Mackay CR, Horuk R, Moore JP. Genetic subtype-independent inhibition of human immunodeficiency virus type 1 replication by CC and CXC chemokines. J Virol 1998; 72: 396–404.

43. Aiuti A, Webb IJ, Bleul C, Springer T, Gutierrez-Ramos JC. The chemokine SDF-1 is a chemoattractant for human CD34+ hematopoietic progenitor cells and provides a new mechanism to explain the mobilization of CD34+ progenitors to peripheral blood. J Exp Med 1997; 185:111–120.

44. Choe H, Farzan M, Sun Y, Sullivan N, Rollins B, Ponath PD, Wu L, Mackay CR, LaRosa G, Newman W, Gerard N, Gerard C, Sodroski J. The beta-chemokine receptors CCR3 and CCR5 facilitate infection by primary HIV-1 isolates. Cell 1996; 85: 1135–1148.

45. Horuk R, Hesselgesser J, Zhou Y, Faulds D, Halks-Miller M, Harvey S, Taub D, Samson M, Parmentier M, Rucker J, Doranz BJ, Doms RW. The CC chemokine I-309 inhibits CCR8-dependent infection by diverse HIV-1 strains. J Biol Chem 1998; 273: 386–391.

46. Wells TNC, Schwartz TW. Plagiarism of the host immune system lessons about chemokine immunology from viruses. Current Opinion Biotechnology 1997; 8:741–748.

47. Boshoff C, Endo Y, Collins PD, Takeuchi Y, Reeves JD, Schweickart VL, Siani MA, Sasaki T, Williams TJ, Gray PW, Moore PS, Chang Y, Weiss RA. Angiogenic and HIV-inhibitory functions of KSHV-encoded chemokines. Science 1997; 278:290–294.

48. Kledal TN, Rosenkilde MM, Coulin F, Simmons G, Johnsen AH, Alouani S, Power CA, Luttichau HR, Gerstoft J, Clapham PR, Clarklewis I, Wells TNC, Schwartz TW. A broad-spectrum chemokine antagonist encoded by Kaposis sarcoma–associated herpesvirus. Science 1997; 277:1656–1659.

49. Siciliano SJ, Rollins TE, DeMartino J, Konteatis Z, Malkowitz L, van Riper G, Bondy S, Rosen H, Springer MS. Two-site binding of C5a by its receptor: an alternative binding paradigm for G protein-coupled receptors. Proc Natl Acad Sci U S A 1994; 91: 1214–1218.

50. Pakianathan DR, Kuta EG, Artis DR, Skelton NJ, Hebert CA. Distinct but overlapping epitopes for the interaction of a CC chemokine with CCR1, CCR3, and CCR5. Biochemistry 1997; 36:9642–9648.

51. Hebert CA, Vitangcol RV, Baker JB. Scanning mutagenesis of interleukin-8 identifies a cluster of residues required for receptor binding. J Biol Chem 1991; 266:18989–18994.

52. Moser B, Dewald B, Barella L, Schumacher C, Baggiolini M, Clark-Lewis I. Interleukin-8 antagonists generated by N-terminal modification. J Biol Chem 1993; 268: 7125–7128.

53. Baggiolini M, Dewald B, Moser B. Interleukin-8 and related chemotactic cytokines— CXC and CC chemokines. Adv Immunol 1994; 55:97–179.

54. Gong JH, Uguccioni M, Dewald B, Baggiolini M, Clark-Lewis I. RANTES and MCP-3 antagonists bind multiple chemokine receptors. J Biol Chem 1996; 271:10521–10527.

55. Zhang Y, Rollins BJ. A dominant negative inhibitor indicates that monocyte chemo-attractant protein 1 functions as a dimer. Mol Cell Biol 1995; 15:4851–4855.

56. Proudfoot AEI, Power CA, Hoogewerf AJ, Montjovent MO, Borlat F, Offord RE, Wells TNC. Extension of recombinant human RANTES by the retention of the initiating methionine produces a potent antagonist. J Biol Chem 1996; 271:2599–2603.

57. Plater-Zyberk C, Hoogewerf AJ, Proudfoot AEI, Power CA, Wells TNC. Effect of a CC chemokine receptor antagonist on collagen induced arthritis in DBA/1 mice. Immunology Letters 1997; 57:117–120.

58. Lloyd CM, Minto AW, Dorf ME, Proudfoot AEI, Wells TNC, Salant DJ, Gutierrez-Ramos JC. RANTES and monocyte chemoattractant protein-1 (MCP-1) play an important role in the inflammatory phase of crescentic nephritis, but only MCP-1 is involved in crescent formation and interstitial fibrosis. J Exp Med 1997; 185:1371–1380.

58a. Grone HJ, Weber C, Weber KC, Grone EF, Rabelink T, Klier CM, Wells TC, Proudfoot AE, Schlondorff D, Nelson PJ. Met-RANTES reduces vascular and tubular damage during acute renal transplant rejection: blocking monocyte arrest and recruitment. FASEB J 1999; 13:1371–1383.

58b. Gonzalo JA, Lloyd CM, Albar JP, Wen D, Wells TNC, Proudfoot AEI, Martinez-A C, Bjerke T, Coyle AJ, Gutierrez-Ramos JC. The coordinated action of CC chemokines in the lung orchestrates allergic inflammation and airway hyperresponsiveness. J Exp Med 1998; 188:157–167.

59. Simmons G, Clapham PR, Picard L, Offord RE, Rosenkilde MM, Schwartz TW, Buser R, Wells TNC, Proudfoot AEI. Potent inhibition of HIV-1 infectivity in macrophages and lymphocytes by a novel CCR5 antagonist. Science 1997; 276:276–279.

60. Mack M, Luckow B, Nelson PJ, Cihak J, Simmons G, Clapham PR, Signoret N, Marsh M, Stangassinger M, Borlat F, Wells TNC, Schlondorff D, Proudfoot AEI. Aminooxypentane-RANTES induces CCR5 internalization but inhibits recycling: a novel inhibitory mechanism of HIV infectivity. J Exp Med 1998; 187:1215–1224.

61. Arenzana-Seisdedos F, Virelizier JL, Rousset D, Clark-Lewis-I, Loetscher P, Moser B, Baggiolini M. HIV blocked by chemokine antagonist. Nature 1996; 383:400–400.

62. Schmidtmayerova H, Sherry B, Bukrinsky M. Chemokines and HIV replication. Nature 1996; 382:767.

63. Gordon CJ, Muesing MA, Proudfoot AEI, Power CA, Moore JP, Trkola A. Enhancement of human immunodeficiency virus type 1 infection by the CC-chemokine RANTES is independent of the mechanism of virus-cell fusion. J Virol 1999; 73:684–694.

64. Bohm SK, Grady EF, Bunnett NW. Regulatory mechanisms that modulate signalling by g-protein-coupled receptors. Biochem J 1997; 322:1–18.

65. Koenig JA, Edwardson JM. Endocytosis and recycling of g protein-coupled receptors [Review]. Trends Pharmacol Sci 1997; 18:276–287.

66. Solari R, Offord RE, Remy S, Aubry JP, Wells TNC, Whitehorn E, Oung T, Proudfoot AEI. Receptor-mediated endocytosis of CC-chemokines. J Biol Chem 1997; 272: 9617–9620.

67. Signoret N, Oldridge J, Pelchen-Matthews A, Klasse PJ, Tran T, Brass LF, Rosenkilde MM, Schwartz TW, Holmes W, Dalls W, Luther MA, Wells TNC, Hoxie JA, Marsh M. Phorbol esters and SDF-1 induce rapid endocytosis and down modulation of the chemokine receptor CXCR4. J Cell Biol 1997; 139:651–664.

68. Yang AG, Bai XF, Huang XF, Yao CP, Chen SY. Phenotypic knockout of HIV type 1 chemokine coreceptor CCR-5 by intrakines as potential therapeutic approach for HIV-1 infection. Proc Natl Acad Sci U S A 1997; 94:11567–11572.

69. Ponath PD. Chemokine receptor antagonists: novel therapeutics for inflammation and AIDS. Exp Opin Invest Drugs 1998; 7:1–18.

70. Schols D, Struyf S, van Damme J, Este JA, Henson G, De CE. Inhibition of T-tropic HIV strains by selective antagonization of the chemokine receptor CXCR4. J Exp Med 1997; 186:1383–1388.

71. Donzella GA, Schols D, Lin SW, Este JA, Nagashima KA, Maddon PJ, Gallaway GP, Sakmar TP, Henson G, De Clercq E, Moore JP. AMD3100, a small molecule inhibitor of HIV-1 entry via the CXCR4 co-receptor. Nat Med 1998; 4:72–77.

9
Drug Targeting with Colloidal Carriers for Antiretroviral Agents

Hagen von Briesen and Peter Ramge
Georg-Speyer-Haus, Frankfurt am Main, Germany

Jörg Kreuter
Johann Wolfgang Goethe-Universität, Frankfurt am Main, Germany

I. INTRODUCTION

A. General Aspects

One major requirement for the successful use of any drug against retrovirus-related disease is its sufficient bioavailability. However, many promising antiviral agents against human immunodeficiency virus (HIV) are unfortunately compromised by disadvantageous physicochemical properties that lead to poor biodistribution and insufficient cellular uptake. One presupposition for a therapeutical approach is to maintain adequate drug levels at the sites of viral replication over extended periods of time. Moreover, the well-known adverse reactions and side effects of antiviral treatment are often related to the accumulation of the drug at inappropriate sites. Drug carrier systems and dosage forms, such as nanoparticles, liposomes, and others, hold the promise of overcoming these pharmacokinetic obstacles. Following intravenous application, nanoparticles, for example, are known to accumulate in the tissues of the mononuclear phagocyte system (MPS) as a result of a specific enrichment in macrophage-containing organs. Apart from CD4 T lymphocytes, cells of the MPS (i.e., monocytes/macrophages) play a decisive role as a reservoir for HIV. In tissues such as the lung and the brain, HIV is located primarily in macrophage-like cells (i.e., alveolar macrophages and microglia, respectively). In vitro, the incorporation of nanoparticles in primary monocytes/macrophages can be nicely visualized by electron microscopy. In Fig. 1, different steps of phagocytic uptake of nanoparticles made from human serum albumin in

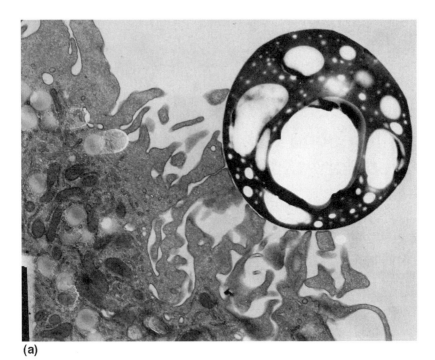

(a)

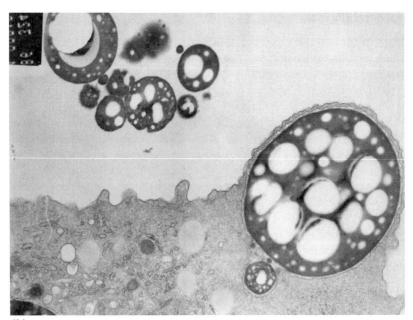

(b)

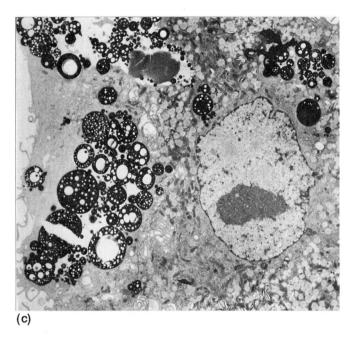

(c)

Figure 1 Phagocytic uptake of nanoparticles. Human serum albumin nanoparticles were phagocytosed by primary macrophages; the transmission electron microscopy shows: (**a**) first contact of pseudopods of a macrophage with a particle ($\times$ 6000); (**b**) total engulfment of the particle into the cytoplasma ($\times$ 8000); (**c**) accumulation of particles within the cytoplasma after 2 hours incubation ($\times$ 1450).

these cells is demonstrated. Therefore, specific drug carrier systems represent interesting vehicles for the transport of antiviral agents to monocytes/macrophages.

B. Colloidal Drug Delivery

Colloidal drug delivery systems differ fundamentally from other pharmaceutical dosage forms. They represent disperse systems in which polymeric (e.g., nanoparticles) or lipid particles (e.g., liposomes or solid lipid nanoparticles [SLN]) are dispersed in a liquid phase. The size of these particles is in the nanometer range. This size range offers the decisive advantage of this class of pharmaceutical dosage forms because it allows the so-called *drug targeting* (see later discussion), which often is not possible with free drug.

Because of their structure, these colloidal particles are recognized and taken up in larger amounts by certain organs (liver, lymphoid tissue) or cell types (macrophages). Drugs bound to the particles thus may be targeted to specific tissues. As a result, the normally occurring nonspecific distribution of the drug throughout the organism is altered. With successful targeting, lower therapeutical dosages may be required to achieve a therapeutical effect. This, in turn, may reduce side effects and yield a better patient compliance.

A large variety of available materials and formulation methods offers the possibility to adjust colloidal drug delivery systems to the needs of the specific applications. In addition to a stabilizing effect on the drug (e.g., protection from degradation by enzymes), the formulations often enable a retardation of the drug liberation, which may positively influence the therapeutical efficacy. By coating the aforementioned systems with surfactants, the biodistribution can be optimized and the targeting properties may be improved and optimized (1). An overview of colloidal drug carriers for therapeutical application is given in a number of reviews (2–6).

C.   Characteristics of Colloidal Drug Carriers

The following chapter gives a short introduction into the physicochemical characteristics of the major classes of colloidal drug carriers. Further in depth information may be found in references 2 through 6.

1.   Nanoparticles

Nanoparticles are solid polymeric colloidal drug carriers ranging in size between 10 and 1000 nm (3,5,6). The polymers employed for their preparation can be of artificial or natural origin. Substances can either be adsorbed onto the surface or be incorporated into these particles. An overview of the different production methods and materials is given by Kreuter (3) and Alleman et al. (4). The coating of these nanoparticles by surfactants plays an important role for the body distribution and for the circulation time of the particles (1). Owing to the wide range of materials and production methods used, nanoparticles can be produced to meet specific requirements for targeting specific sites (3,7).

2.   Liposomes

In contrast to solid nanoparticles, liposomes consist of one or more lipid double layers surrounding a hydrophilic core. The main constituents of the liquid layers are phospholipids and in most cases also cholesterol. Lipophilic drugs can be incorporated into the lipid double layers, and hydrophilic drugs into the aqueous layers between the lipids as well as into the aqueous core. Amphilphilic drugs may be incorporated into both types of layers, but frequently do dissolve the liposomes. Unilamellar and multilamellar systems can be distinguished depending on the number of layers. The size range of liposomes is comparable to that of nanoparticles (7,8). Similarly to nanoparticles, liposomes can be produced to meet different specific application requirements. A large variety of materials allows the formulation of liposomes with the required characteristics. The surface characteristics of liposomes enables the binding of antibodies to the outer shell of the particles, making the targeting to specific receptors possible.

A major disadvantage of liposomes is their relatively lower physical stability. Because of their similarity to biomembranes, some physiological enzyme systems may lead to their destruction. Besides their application for drug targeting, liposomes are widely used in topical dosage forms such as ointments and creams as penetration enhancers or in parenterals for the prevention of incompatibilities in the formulation. For an overview of the different production methods and applications, see a review by Commelin and Schreier (9).

3. Other Small Particulate Drug Carriers

Besides nanoparticles and liposomes, there is a range of other microparticulate systems that can be used as drug carriers. Generally, the prefix "micro" is used for sizes greater than 1 μm and the prefix "nano" for a size range less than 1 μm. Micro- or nanoemulsions are preparations with a liquid inner phase made of droplets in a size range between 30 and 200 nm. Adequate surfactants have to be used in the production process of these emulsions (10). Micro- or nanocapsules are particulate structures in the micro- or nanometer range, respectively, with a solid outer shell and a liquid or solid core containing or representing the drug (11). Solid lipid nanoparticles are manufactured using special O/W (oil in water) emulsions or microemulsions (12). These lipids are solid at room temperature and, because of their physicochemical characteristics, they form a new group of nanoparticles.

4. Drug Targeting

Drug targeting is defined as the delivery of drugs to specific organs or tissues in the body. Besides colloidal drug carriers, other pharmaceutical dosage forms as well as chemically modified drugs (prodrugs) can be used for this purpose. After access of the carrier system or of a prodrug to the targeted site, the release can be controlled by the delivery system (8). A synonym for drug targeting is "site-specific drug delivery" (13). The ability to lower the necessary dosage is the major advantage of targeted delivery, in turn enabling a reduction in side effects. Additionally, the targeting to regions of the body, which so far have been difficult to reach or to reach in insufficient amounts (e.g., tissue macrophages, dendritic cell, or the brain), offers new therapeutic possibilities.

II. DRUG TARGETING WITH ANTIRETROVIRAL AGENTS ENTRAPPED IN COLLOIDAL DRUG CARRIERS

A. Nanoparticles

Because of the particular structure and surface characteristics of nanoparticles, the cells of the reticuloendothelial system (RES), like monocytes/macrophages, are a

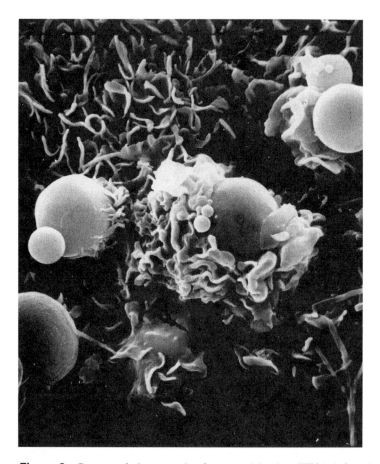

Figure 2   Process of phagocytosis of nanoparticles into HIV-1–infected macrophages. Nanoparticles made from human serum albumin (~ 1.5 μm diameter) attached to the surface of an HIV-1–infected macrophage at day 20 after 30 minutes of incubation with particles. Attachment of nanoparticles is shown to pseudopods (*left*) and engulfment by lamellipods (*right*). Scanning electron microscopy: × 5000.

prime target for them because they are taken up preferentially by these phagocytosing cells. The processes of phagocytosis can be demonstrated by scanning electron microscopy, showing the various states of the uptake of nanoparticles made from human serum albumin (Fig. 2).

In a study of Schäfer et al. (14) phagocytosis of nanoparticles in monocyte-derived macrophages in vitro was investigated with respect to particle material, size, surface properties and other parameters. Phagocytosis is highly dependent on the type of material used for the preparation of particles and on particle size (Table

Table 1 Influence of Particle Size and Material on
Phagocytosis of Nanoparticles by Monocytes/Macrophages

Particle material	Particle size (nm)	Phagocytosed nanoparticles (μg/ml $\pm$ SD)
PHCA	200	3.01 $\pm$ 0.45
PBCA	200	6.56 $\pm$ 0.41
PMMA	130	19.28 $\pm$ 2.82
HSA	200	4.38 $\pm$ 0.29
HSA	1500	15.84 $\pm$ 2.79

Abbreviations: PHCA = polyhexylcyanoacrylate; PBCA = polybutylcyanoacrylate; HSA = human serum albumin; PMMA = poly-
methylmethacrylate.

1). Nanoparticles made from polyhexylcyanoacrylate (PHCA) or human serum albumin with a diameter of 200 nm were found most suitable for targeting antiviral
substances to macrophages. To determine whether HIV-infected macrophages are
compromised concerning phagocytic activity, the influence of HIV-1 infection on
phagocytosis of nanoparticles was examined, either with in vitro HIV-1–infected
macrophages or macrophages derived from HIV-infected patients. For the latter,
no reduction in phagocytic activity was found, especially for cells derived from
symptomatic patients in Centers for Disease Control and Prevention (CDC) stage
IV of the disease. Surprisingly, in vitro infected macrophages showed a 30% increased particle uptake compared to uninfected cells, indicating an activated state
resulting from HIV-1 infection (Fig. 3), which may allow a preferential phagocytosis of drug-loaded nanoparticles, resulting in a targeted delivery of drugs to infected cells. In another study, the process of degradation of nanoparticles was investigated in more detail by Schäfer et al. (15). Therefore, they followed the
intracellular process of biodegradation of human serum albumin (HSA) particles
by transmission electron microscopy. The metabolism started some hours after particle uptake. After 3 days, this process was almost terminated.

Nanoparticles made out of human serum albumin (HSA-NP) and polyhexylcyanoacrylate (PHCA-NP) and loaded with azidothymidine (AZT) and
dideoxycytidine (ddC) were used to examine their potential in inhibition of HIV-
replication in vitro (16). Cultured monocyte/macrophage cells were preincubated
with drug-loaded nanoparticles or with the free drug before infection with HIV-1.
The antiviral effect was monitored by evaluating HIV-production. HSA- and
PHCA-NP either loaded with AZT or ddC were effective against HIV-1 infection.
However, in relation to free drug, they showed no superiority. Because AZT and
ddC can easily diffuse into the cells, these substances do not require drug delivery
by a carrier system. The potential use of these particles for more lipophilic compounds or larger drug molecules with poor bioavailability may profit from this route
of delivery.

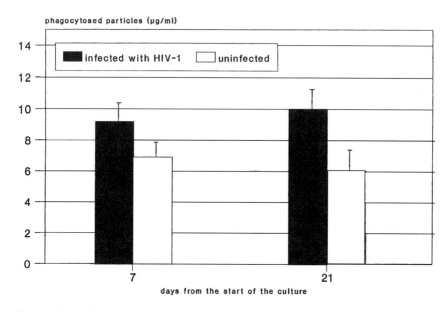

Figure 3 Influence of HIV-1 infection on phagocytosis of nanoparticles by mono-cytes/macrophages (MO/MAC). The MO/MAC were infected in vitro with a monocy-totropic strain of HIV-1 at day 1 after start of culture. At day 7 or 21, nanoparticles made of polybutylcyanoacrylate were added at a final concentration of 0.5 mg/ml and incubated for 6 hours.

This theory was proven by the next investigations of the same authors. The lipophilic HIV protease inhibitor saquinavir was incorporated into PHCA-NP and tested on acutely and chronically HIV-1–infected monocyte/macrophage cells. Also, the prophylactic effect of the preparations was evaluated in comparison to the free drug solution and a simple mixture of nanoparticles and drug solution (17). Efficiency of the preparations was measured by HIV-1 production. In both acutely and chronically infected cells, the nanoparticle preparation showed superior effects to the free solution and the simple mixture. A more than 10-fold increase in an-tiviral activity was shown in acutely infected MO/MAC. The IC_{50} of 0.39 nM was determined for the nanoparticle preparation, whereas the free-drug solution and the simple mixture of free drug and unloaded nanoparticles had an IC_{50} of 4.23 and 5.31 nM, respectively (Fig. 4). These findings indicated that the cellular uptake of protease inhibitors, in contrast to nucleoside analogs, is the limiting factor for their antiviral effectiveness.

In the aforementioned cell culture experiments with human MO/MAC, no difference in the inhibition of the HIV replication between AZT or ddC bound to nanoparticles or in free form was observed. However, in tissue cultures, a homol-

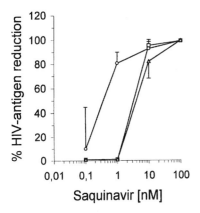

Figure 4 Antiviral activity of saquinavir-loaded hexylcyanoacrylate nanoparticles in acutely HIV-1–infected monocytes/macrophages. Three days after infection, cells were exposed to various concentrations of drug-loaded nanoparticles (○), an aqueous solution of saquinavir (□), or a simple mixture of unloaded nanoparticles and an aqueous drug solution (△). HIV-1 p24 antigen production was measured in cell culture supernatant by enzyme-linked immunosorbent assay. The results are presented as percent reduction of HIV-1 antigen compared with that in infected but untreated control.

ogous cell population exists, which is totally different to the situation in the human or animal body: The body consists of a huge number of different cell types. Macrophages represent only a small percentage of the total number of cells. As a consequence, it was conceivable that AZT or ddC nanoparticles still may achieve a better targeting to these cells despite their inability to show a better antiviral efficacy of these drugs in vitro in the homologous cell cultures. Indeed, that was observable: Löbenberg and Kreuter (18,19) bound [14C]-labeled AZT to nanoparticles using the surfactant bis(2-ethylhexyl) sulphosuccinate sodium (DOSS). After intravenous injection to rats, the liver concentrations of the [14C]-AZT label were about 2.5- to 18-fold higher after binding to nanoparticles than after injection of the solution, with differences increasing with time (Fig. 5). In other organs of the RES, the difference in the uptake rate was not as high as in the liver. Nevertheless, a significant difference between the two preparations occurred in these organs, showing similar trends; in the lungs and in the spleen, about 10-fold differences in favor of the nanoparticles were obtained after 480 minutes. In bone marrow, the difference was about a factor of two after 480 minutes. The total dose of AZT in the organs of the RES after 5 minutes amounted to 23%, whereas the control solutions reached an uptake into the RES of only 9% by the same time. Four hundred and eighty minutes after nanoparticle injection, 60% of the detected AZT label was found in the RES, whereas only 12% of the label was found in the RES after injection of the control solution.

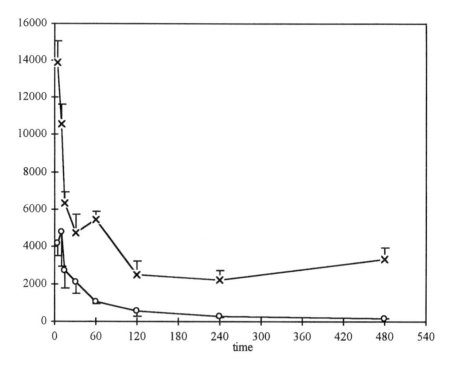

Figure 5   [^{14}C] AZT concentration in the liver after i.v. injection of AZT (3.33 mg/kg) bound to nanoparticles (×) or in form of a solution, identically prepared but without polymer (○). Every time point represents the average concentration of two male and two female rats of a body weight between 180 and 220g.

Autoradiographs after intravenous injection of the solution showed a rather homogeneous, although sparse, distribution of the AZT label in liver and lungs, whereas after intravenous administration of nanoparticles, the radioactive concentrations were much higher (Fig. 6). In this case, not only were the concentrations higher, but they also appeared in clusters. These clusters were ascribed to uptake by macrophages (18,20).

Another study by Löbenberg et al. (18,21) investigated the oral administration of nanoparticles also in rats. Nanoparticles again led to an accumulation of AZT in tissues containing a large number of macrophages. In the liver, the area under the drug concentration versus time curve (AUC) of [^{14}C]-labeled AZT was 30% higher when the drug was bound to nanoparticles. In the brain, the uptake of AZT also was significantly higher when using nanoparticles as the drug-targeting system. Oral absorption of AZT from the solution was very rapid, whereas binding of drug of nanoparticles delayed oral absorption. After administration of nanoparticles, 60 minutes were required to reach the highest concentrations in the RES organs, whereas with a solution, the maximum was reached after 30 minutes.

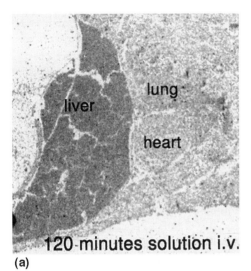 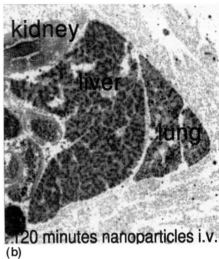

Figure 6 Autoradiographic image of a rat 120 min after i.v. injection of [^{14}C] AZT (3.33 mg/kg), (a) in the form of a solution: AZT was homogeneously distributed in the liver tissue and the lung, up to 94% of AZT was eliminated via kidneys; (b) bound to nanoparticles: AZT was inhomogeneously distributed in the liver tisue and the lung, up to 28% of AZT nanoparticle preparation was eliminated by feces.

The aforementioned spotted appearance of the radioactivity in the organs of the RES is typical for the accumulation in macrophages. In contrast, after administration of the solution, the radioactivity in the aforementioned organs was homogeneously distributed and much lower. These results show that the nanoparticles seemed to have reached their target and that nanoparticles may represent a very promising delivery system for therapy of acquired immunodeficiency syndrome (AIDS).

PH-sensitive nanoparticles produced from the methacrylic acidcopolymers Eudragit L100-55 and S100 were used to increase the bioavailability of the highly lipophilic compound CGP 57813, which is almost not ionizable and nearly insoluble in water, after oral delivery to dogs (22). This compound was shown to be a strong inhibitor of the HIV-protease, which was developed by Ciba-Geigy (Basel, Switzerland), pH-sensitive nanoparticles can be used to specifically control the liberation of incorporated substances in the gastrointestinal tract. Thus, a controlled release can be achieved and higher plasma levels can be obtained resulting from an optimal liberation in the gut. In the study by Leroux et al. (22), no plasma levels were detected after the test substance was given in amorphous form. With nanoparticles, a significant plasma profile was observable, although it was not as high as it was expected from previous results with mice (23). Furthermore, the area under the plasma concentration-time curve (AUC) was highly dependent on the feeding state of the animals. A further optimization of the process seems to be possible because the pH-responsiveness of the nanoparticles may be optimized and adjusted, leading to an increase in AUC.

B. Liposomes

Liposomes are an alternative to nanoparticles and were used in a number of studies to improve the treatment of HIV infections. Besides nanoparticles, the mononuclear phagocyte system was a main target, especially of these drug carriers.

A combined in vitro and in vivo study was performed with two important drugs used for the therapy of HIV infection: AZT and ddC (24). Azidothymidine coupled to a dipalmitoylphosphatidic acid (DPP) and ddC coupled to a dioleoylphosphatidic acid (DOP) were employed in the form of free substances and incorporated into liposomes. As a cell model HT4-6C cells were used, derived from transformed HeLa cells with CD4 gene infected with HIV-1, and the antiviral effect was measured by the plaque reduction assay. Additionally, the human lymphoblastoid cell line CEM-CCRF was infected with HIV-1. In the second case, p24 antigen production was determined to evaluate the efficacy. In the in vivo experiments, the AZT-DPP-liposome formulation was compared to the free drug in Rauscher leukemia virus (RLV)-infected mice. The authors found contradictory results in vitro and in vivo. In the cell systems, the phospholipid liposomal preparations were both active in HIV-infected cells but substantially less effective compared to their free substances. Moreover, they found marked differences in the antiviral activities of AZT and ddC in both cell lines. Both liponucleotides were slightly more active in HT4-6C cells. In contrast, the mouse model gave a clear indication that the liposome formulation was more effective. For liposomal DOP-ddC formulation, they found a 107-fold increased AUC relative to free ddC in the spleen and a 3.8-fold increased AUC in lymph nodes. Although the conjugate as well as the liposome formulation need to be optimized, Hostetler et al. (24) expect that phospholipid prodrugs encapsulated into liposomes may improve HIV therapy by enhancing the efficacies and reducing the toxicities of antiviral agents.

The potential use of liposomes coupled with derivatized human serum albumin (HSA) (cis-aconitic anhydride; Aco-HSA) also could lead to an improved biodistribution and efficacy in HIV therapy (25). The actual mechanism of action of Aco-HSA presently is not clear but it is suspected that it plays a major part in inhibiting the virus–cell binding and the fusion of the virus with the cell membrane. Aco-HSA was shown to have an antiviral effect by itself. PEG was employed to further influence the in vivo distribution of the liposomes. MT-4 cells, a human leukemia cell line, were infected with HIV-1 and used as a cell model. The antiviral assay was measured by the viability of the cells. Although free Aco-HSA showed the best results, the encapsulated formulation also achieved considerable effects in the antiviral assay. In a body distribution study with rats, the liposome formulation showed the most promising results in that most of the injected dose clearly was taken up by liver and spleen. Liver and spleen, as mentioned earlier, are the main organs containing macrophages that represent one of the most important targets for AIDS therapy. The authors speculate that, with Aco-HSA-PEG-liposomes, a dual attack on HIV replication might be accomplished: first on the binding/fusion of the virus with the cell membrane as a result of the coupled Aco-HSA and second, on the reverse transcriptase by including nucleoside analogues such as AZT.

Other researchers incorporated foscarnet into liposomes (26). Foscarnet is effective against cytomegalovirus (CMV) and other forms of the herpes virus family. It also is an inhibitor of the reverse transcriptase of HIV-1 and has a synergistic therapeutic effect with AZT. Dussere et al. (26) investigated the antiviral effect of the liposomal formulation in vitro in HIV-1 infected human promonocytoid U937 cells and additionally the accumulation in murine monocytic RAW 264.7 cells. The in vivo biodistribution of radioactively labeled liposomes was evaluated in rats. The goal was to find a liposomal formulation for the specific macrophage targeting of foscarnet in order to achieve the required high therapeutical concentrations in the organism. Depending on the specific phagocytotic activity, the liposomal formulation was taken up to a much higher extent by both macrophage-related cell lines (RAW cells and U937 cells) than the free compound. The antiviral activity of foscarnet in human U937 cells was slightly increased by the liposomal formulation compared to free foscarnet. In vivo, the liposomal foscarnet showed a distribution pattern that was distinctively different from the free solution. Especially an accumulation in the brain and in the eyes was found that was much higher with the liposomal formulation. Altogether, encapsulation of foscarnet in liposomes improved drug pharmacological parameters, in that plasma half-life was greatly enhanced by suppressing the rapid phase of renal elimination. Higher drug concentrations with the liposomes also were found in the lymph nodes and in the lungs. Both organs are important reservoirs of HIV or CMV, respectively. Liposomal delivery of foscarnet thus seems to increase the efficiency of the therapy of the HIV infection and also that of viral co-infections such as with CMV, because foscarnet also possesses anti-CMV activity.

Two extensive studies on the acute toxicity and body distribution of loaded liposomes containing anti-HIV drugs, including ddC, ddI, foscarnet, and AZT, in mice were presented during the World AIDS Conference 1996 (27,28). The liposome concentration in these studies were 10 and 100 times higher than the dosage suggested for human use. No acute toxicity was found after intravenous injection to the animals. Increased drug concentrations were found in the targeted lymphoid tissue, such as lymph nodes and other organs of the reticuloendothelial system.

New lipophilic alkyl/acyl dinucleoside phosphate derivatives of AZT were incorporated into liposomes by Schwendener et al. (29), and their in vitro and in vivo effects were tested using HIV-1–infected CD4$^+$ HeLa and H9 cells and RLV-infected mice, respectively. Large differences between the two derivatives (N^4-hexadecyldC-AZT and N^4-palmitoyldC-AZT) were observed, and no correlation between the cell and animal models was obtained. The antiviral activity in the cell cultures was evaluated by plaque reduction in the HeLa cells and by the measurement of HIV-1 p24 antigen production in H9 cells. The measurement of spleen size and weight was performed to show the effects of the treatment in vivo. In vitro the lipophilic AZT derivatives inhibited HIV replication in a dose-dependent manner; however, higher concentrations were required to obtain a similar antiviral effect as with free AZT. In contrast to these findings, the results of animal testing were very favorable for the lipophilic derivatives in that they showed a highly improved therapeutic profile. The non-correlation of the effects was attributed to the low phagocytotic activity of the aforementioned cell lines.

A liposome formulation containing the lipophilic muramyl peptide MTP-PE also was shown to have a higher antiviral activity than the free substance (30), although the liposomes showed an antiviral activity of their own. MTP-PE is an immunomodulator with antitumor and antiviral properties in vivo. In vitro, MTP-PE has been characterized as a macrophage-activating agent and is capable of changing several macrophage functions. Freshly isolated human monocytes served as the in vitro model and were infected with the monocytotropic HIV-1 isolate ADA. Measuring reverse transcriptase activity, p24 antigen evaluation, and syncytia formation observation were used for viral detection. The liposomal formulation indeed inhibited HIV replication and had a protective effect on the infection of the cells. If free MTP-PE was used, steady high levels are required to achieve inhibitory effect similar to other antiviral agents like AZT. A liposomal preparation of the drug eliminated this requirement, and a single treatment with relatively low dose was effective in suppressing virus replication.

C. Immunoliposomes

Immunoliposomes enable an even more specific targeting of certain cell types. Monoclonal antibodies directed against cell surface molecules can be attached covalently to the surface of the liposomes. Immunoliposomes enter into lymphoid cells by a receptor-mediated endocytotic pathway. Analogues of 2´, 5´-oligoadenylates (2-5A), cordycepin (3´-deoxyadenosine) core trimer (Co$_3$) and its 5´-monophosphate derivative (pCo$_3$) were shown to inhibit viral replication by nearly 100% if applied with immunoliposomes (31). H9 human T cells were infected with HIV-1 one hour after the application of the liposomes and the reverse transcriptase activity and p24-antigen production was measured. H9 cells were treated before with anti-CD3 antibodies with which protein A coupled to the surface of the liposomes could react. Protein A binds with high affinity to the Fc region of several antibody classes. A similar approach was used also with oligonucleotides (discussed later) (32).

Dideoxyuridine (ddU) is one of the most potent inhibitors of reverse transcriptase of the HIV in vitro. However, ddU itself is a poor substrate for cellular nucleoside kinases; phosphorylated derivatives are not able to cross the cell membrane. For this reason, protein A was coated to drug-loaded liposomes to increase the availability of phosphorylated ddU to cells (33). The HIV-1–infected CCRF-CEM and MT-4 cell cultures were used to examine the effects of the liposome preparations. On CEM cell, antibodies against the CD7 and HLA class I were used; on MT-4 cells, anti-HLA class I as well as II were employed to direct protein A–bearing liposomes to the cells, and RT-activity and p24 antigen expression was measured. The phosphorylated derivatives of ddU encapsulated in these liposomes were able to inhibit replication of HIV in vitro; the efficacy was dependent on the antibody and ddU derivative used. No inhibition was observed with nontargeted liposomes containing phosphorylated ddU, or with empty liposomes, whether targeted or not.

D. Sterically Stabilized Liposomes

An approach to increase the plasma half-life of ddI-loaded liposomes by sterical stabilization with polyethylene glycol (PEG) was described by Harvie et al. (34). This approach is important if tissues outside of the RES are targeted. The PEG hydrophilizes the surface of liposomes and thus inhibits interaction with plasma proteins. These interactions in turn govern the interaction with, for instance, the monocyte/macrophage system. The PEG-stabilized liposomes yielded plasma half-life that were 180 times shorter than that of the free substance. Nevertheless, the PEG-stabilized liposomes prolonged the plasma half-life 3.7-fold compared to conventional liposomes. In this study, the importance of the plasma proteins bound by the liposomes was recognized but was not further evaluated.

E. Red Blood Cells

The possibility of using red blood cells (RBC) to target drugs against HIV and herpes simplex virus (HSV) in in vitro and in vivo systems was demonstrated by several groups. The RBCs are treated by the organism as a physiological part in the biochemical cycle and, therefore, are of large interest as a drug carrier. The RBCs are mostly taken up by macrophages that are a prime target for HIV therapy. Usually, erthrocytes are loaded with drugs by way of hypotonic dialysis, and then resealed and reannealed. The recognition by macrophages can be enhanced by band 3 clustering through treatment with $ZnCl_2$ and BS_3 (bis-sulfosuccinimidyl-suberate) and binding of autologous IgG. Band 3 is the predominant anion transport system in erythrocytes. This system has to be switched off if RBC-encapsulated compounds shall not be pumped out of these cells.

ddC in its 5′-triphosphate form (ddCTP) was encapsulated into autologous RBC to overcome the poor phosphorylation activity or the RES cells. The efficacy of this formulation was tested on HIV-1–infected human monocytes/ macrophages (35). Additionally, the in vivo effects were evaluated in murine leukemia virus infected mice (36). In both models, an increased efficacy of treatment with ddCTP encapsulated in RBC was shown. The p24-antigen production of the HIV-1–infected monocytes/macrophages clearly was reduced. In vivo, the RBC-treated mice exhibited a significant reduction in splenomegaly, lymphoadenopathy, and hypergammaglobulinemy as signs for viral reduction.

In another publication, the same group also was able to show the efficacy of the treatment in a feline model (37). The feline immunodeficiency virus (FIV) causes similar symptoms in cats as HIV in humans. Thus, it is an ideal model to evaluate the treatment with autologous RBCs. In vitro, a cocultivation model of FIV-infected monocyte-derived macrophages with peripheral blood lymphocytes from healthy cats was established. As described earlier, ddCTP-loaded RBCs were used against the infection of FIV. ddCTP-loaded erythrocytes were able to reduce FIV in macrophages infected in vitro or obtained from naturally or experimentally infected cats.

Another drug investigated for its use in anti-HIV therapy incorporated into RBCs (38) was 9-(2-phosphonyl-methoxyethyl)adenine (PMEA). It is a prototype from the family of acyclic nucleoside phosphonates and exhibits strong inhibitory effects on replication of HIV and HSV. The PMEA encapsulated in RBCs was shown to be 500 times more effective than the free substance in inhibiting virus replication in human primary monocyte/macrophage cells, as determined by p24 antigen measurements. Even though empty RBCs showed an effect on their own, the drug-loaded RBCs were the most effective preparation. It can be concluded from these experiments that red blood cells are efficient transporters of drugs into the RES both in vitro and in vivo. The biggest advantage of this carrier is its physiological nature. However, a problem might be the upscaling required for the therapy in humans.

III. ENTRAPMENT OF OLIGONUCLEOTIDES AND THEIR DERIVATIVES IN COLLOIDAL CARRIERS FOR INHIBITION OF HIV EXPRESSION

The use of antisense and sense preparations for the treatment of diseases such as cancer or viral infections is a recent approach. A successful therapy of these diseases in most cases is difficult and often impossible. The strategy of employment of antisense seems to be quite straightforward: by combining sense or antisense oligonucleotides (ON) or oligodeoxynucleotides (ODN) with their respective counterparts in the viral nucleic acids, the translation or transcription is inhibited and, hence, the synthesis of particular viral proteins needed for the assembly of new viruses or for attachment factors will be disturbed. As a result, further infection thus is inhibited and the body might be protected against a further spread of, for example, HIV.

A major disadvantage of these oligonucleotide preparations is their low stability in vitro and their high sensitivity to nuclease digestion. They also show a very low cellular uptake. These problems are combined with the requirement for very high concentrations of the nucleotide preparations at the target site in order to achieve a satisfying therapeutic effect. Because colloidal drug carriers are taken up in significant amounts by a large number of cells, especially macrophages, they thus can act as carriers for the transport of oligonucleotides into these infected cells. In addition, liposomes and nanoparticles were shown to protect oligonucleotides from degradation and nuclease digestion. The latter problem has been addressed by the development of chemically modified forms, including phosphorothioates and methylphosphonates.

In the following discussion, results with different preparations that could effectively bind and protect ON and ODN and derivatives, and show impressive in vitro effects against HIV are summarized.

A. Cationic Lipid Preparation

The lipofection reagent was used by Anazodo et al. (39) to react with specific HIV-1 antisense ODN to enhance uptake into cells. Lipofectin spontaneously forms a cationic lipid complex with DNA, enabling the complete association of the nucleic acid. This complex then may fuse with cell membranes, resulting in an efficient uptake of the encapsulated DNA into the target cell. The antisense construct GPIA2, which was chemically modified at seven different base positions by substitution of nonbridging oxygen atoms of the phosphodiester backbone with sulfur, thus, was directed against a nonregulatory region of the HIV-1 genome. A biologically active provirus was established in a COS-like monkey kidney cell line (B4.14) that transcribes and translates their nucleotide sequences into viral proteins. A sequence as well as dose-dependent inhibition of HIV-1 viral protein synthesis and significant inhibition of the mRNA level could be shown by antisense construct GPI2A. Moreover, encapsulation of the antisense in a cationic lipid preparation significantly enhanced the antiviral effect. The modes of action probably occurred at least partly through a translation arrest associated with RNAse H activation. The ODN preparation described herein will benefit especially in a liposome delivery system, and perhaps eventually as a therapeutic agent.

Newly developed liposomes were used by the group of Puyal (40) to protect unmodified antisense oligonucleotides targeted against the initiation codon region of HIV DNA sequences encoding tat or gag gene. Two kinds of preparations were developed which used different artificial cationic lipids for the encapsulation of the genetic material into liposomes. The basic amino acid L-lysine was covalently coupled to the cationic phospholipid, obtaining more stable liposomes. This cationic formulation achieved a higher entrapment efficiency and protection from extracellular nuclease degradation of the antisense oligonucleotides and better results in delivery toward the tested cells.

To assess the antiviral activity of the different liposomal preparations, they were tested in human peripheral blood mononuclear cells (PBMCs) infected with HIV-1 (40). The reverse transcriptase assay clearly showed significant anti–HIV-1 activity of both free and liposome encapsulated anti-tat. However, the same results were seen with free and encapsulated random oligonucleotides, suggesting that inhibition of viral proliferation was not an specific antisense effect. Nevertheless, they showed that cationic liposomes in principle are able to transport genetic material effectively into mammalian cells.

Sullivan et al. (41) used a slightly different approach. Apart from antisense oligonucleotides, they used sense 20-mer oligodeoxynucleotides (ODN) to the 5´ tat splice acceptor site of HIV-1, which were encapsulated into different liposome preparations containing dipalmitoylphosphatidylcholine (DPPC), distearoylphosphatidylethanolamine acetylthioacetate (DSPE-ATA), or dipalmitoylphosphatidylglycerol (DPPG) and tested for their cellular uptake and antiviral activity against HIV-1. Liposome uptake in lymphocytes and monocytes was evaluated by flow cytometry analysis using fluorescent labeled liposome probes. DSPE-ATA formulated liposomes were taken up at the highest extent by both cell types. These liposomes then were used to examine the inhibitory effect of the sense ODN preparation on viral replication by analysis of the p24 levels. The group was able to show that the sense ODN containing liposomes reduced the number of cells that actively expressed the virus by 71% and reduced the viral protein production by 84%, whereas antisense-ODN loaded liposomes and liposomes containing phosphate buffered saline (PBS) showed no or only minor effects. Also, these authors could not totally explain the effect of the sense ODN-containing liposomes, and, therefore, the mechanism of action remained elusive because, in contrast to other authors, they showed an effect only with the sense ODN preparation.

B. Immunoliposomes

In contrast to "normal" liposomes, immunoliposomes offer the chance to target very specifically certain compounds or regions in the organism, either directly by using coupled antibodies on the surface of the particles or indirectly by coating them with protein A as mentioned earlier. Protein A plays a vital role for targeting because it interacts directly with any antibody (e.g., against the CD3 molecule). Receptor-mediated endocytosis is thus induced, and genetic material, which is entrapped in these immunoliposomes, is transported very efficiently into the cytoplasm.

Protein A–bearing immunoliposomes containing antisense RNA transcripts directed against the HIV-1 *env*- or *pol*-region were used on HIV-1–infected H9 cells to inhibit viral replication (32). The evaluation of the antiviral effect was carried out by measuring reverse transcriptase activity. It was shown that only the protein A–bearing liposomes containing antisense RNA were effective in inhibiting virus replication, whereas the same RNA sequence in sense orientation was not. Before incubation with the liposomes, the human T-cell line H9 was treated with anti-CD3 monoclonal antibodies, which binds to the T cell–specific surface molecule CD3. Only antibody-treated cells showed a clear antiviral effect after incubation with immunoliposomes.

Zelphati et al. (42) found several possible mechanisms for the interaction of immunoliposomes with antisense oligonucleotides leading to the inhibition of HIV-1. Phosphodiester and phosphorothioate derivatives of ON (configuration) against the initiation codon region of the HIV-1 *rev* gene were used on acutely or chronically infected human CEM cells (a T-lymphoblastoid cell line) and co-cultured with the syncytium-forming C-8166 human T-cell line containing a defective genome for the human T-cell leukemia virus type 1 (HTLV-1). Protein A–coupled liposomes containing α and β-phosphorothioate oligonucleotides (anti-rev) were targeted to CEM cells by HLA- specific antibodies (B.1.23.2) against the human major histocompatibility complex (MHC). The antiviral activity was assessed either by a reduction in syncytium formation or by measuring reverse transcriptase activity. The efficiency increased dramatically with the use of protein A–bearing liposomes with ON in β-configuration directed against the HLA-antibody on the surface of the cells compared to the free form.

Similar results were found in the work of Grimaldi et al. (43). It was shown that encapsulated phosphorotioate antisense oligonucleotides directed against HIV-1 gag-encoded region ONs were active against the HIV replication in monocytes/macrophages; 98% virus inhibition was achieved with 0.5 µM.

The 3´-tricholesteryl-modified phosphodiester antisense oligonucleotides incorporated into immunoliposomes were used in a further study of Zelphati et al. (44). The binding of oligonucleotides against the HIV *tat* gene with cholesterol by a reversible disulfide bond (oligodeoxyribonucleotide thiocholesterol conjugates) led to an improvement of binding ratio and association with the immunoliposomes by a factor 10. Additionally, the coupling of the targeting protein with the surface of the liposomes was facilitated. Cholesterol aided interaction with LDL-receptors on cells and may act as a possible trigger for the induced receptor-mediated endocytosis. Again, protein A, as a high-affinity binder for the mouse IgG2a-Fc region of the HLA antibodies, was used to be coupled onto liposomes. The targeted cell surface determinant selected on the CCRF-CEM T-lymphoblastoid cell lines was the HLA class I molecule. No differences were seen between liposomes containing equimolar concentrations of free or cholesterol-coupled oligonucleotides in their capacity to inhibit the replication of HIV-1. Cholesterol-coupled oligonucleotides thus offer increased liposome association without loss of antiviral activity.

It is also possible to bind antibodies directly to the surface of liposomes. This enables the targeting of specific receptors without the use of surface-bound protein A. However, this method is much more complicated and expensive. For this reason, the indirect approach was used.

C. Neoglycoprotein Conjugates

Another approach to increase uptake and intracellular concentration of oligonucleotides and protect them is the conjugation with neoglycoproteins, which also protects them from digestion by nucleases. Neoglycoproteins can be internalized into cells through mediation by sugar-binding receptors (i.e., membrane lectins). The neoglycoproteins still need to carry the relevant sugar to be recognized by the receptor. Membrane lectins can be found and have been characterized on the surface of many normal and malignant cell types, which makes these receptors a prime target as a transport system for drugs into the cell. A cell-specific targeting is possible because different cell types are susceptible for different sugars. For example, a protein such as bovine serum albumin (BSA) bearing mannose-6-phosphate residues (M6P-BSA) could be used as the carrier. This neoglycoprotein then would bind to and would be internalized by cells (i.e., monocytes) expressing M6P- specific membrane lectins.

Bonfils et al. (45) coupled a deoxy-β-ribonucleotide (β-ODN) complementary to a sequence of HIV-1 Bru LTR on their 3′-end thiol function with 6-phosphomannosylated proteins (neoglycoproteins) via a disulfide bridge (45). The 19mer β-ODN, which hybridizes a sequence within the HIV-1 Bru LTR and inhibits the expression of a reporter enzyme in cells transfected with constructs containing LTR, linked to cDNA of that enzyme. The 5′-end was substituted either with a fluorescent probe or with a radioactive label. The neoglycoprotein conjugate was tested on the murine macrophage cell line clone J774E, the human promonocyte cell line U937, and (fibroblast-like) BHK cells that all express the cation independent mannose-6-phosphate specific membrane lectin. The results were evaluated by fluorescence microscopy or scintillation counting and by confocal laser scanning microscopy (CLSM) and flow cytometry. The cells showed different behavior and uptake levels of the conjugate depending on the endocytosis capacity of each cell type. The conjugate also protected the nucleotide against digestion in the medium. Compared to the free oligonucleotide, the ODN bound to the 6-phosphomannoside-bearing neoglycoprotein was internalized to a much higher extent (roughly 20 times). This approach therefore holds promise for the targeting of oligonucleotides to certain cells using the sugar receptors specifically expressed on many different cell types throughout the organism.

D. Fusogenic Peptides

Another approach to transport oligonucleotides into cells is described by Bongartz et al. (46). They used a fusogenic peptide derived from the influenza hemagglutinin envelope protein and conjugated it via thioether linkage or disulfide bond with antisense phosphodiester or phosphorothioate oligonucleotides. Normally, oligonucleotides remain trapped inside endocytic vesicles being degraded in the lysosomes. The fusogenic peptide helps the oligonucleotide to escape the endosomal compartment before the enzymatic degradation becomes prevalent. It could be shown that the peptide alone is capable of disrupting lipid membranes after a conformational change induced by acidification, and subsequently self-assembly of the peptide occurs to form transmembrane channels. The oligonucleotides were directed against the AUG initiation site of the HIV TAT protein (anti TAT-peptide conjugates). The conjugates were tested on HIV-infected CEM-SS lymphocytes in serum-free medium. A stabilization by phospho-groups and an improved delivery by fusogenic peptide to the cytosol were found. BHK 21 fibroblasts were used to observe the distribution of fluorescent-labeled peptide conjugates in the cytosol. An enhanced endosomal efflux of the oligopeptide conjugate was found, resulting in a more diffuse intracellular distribution of the labeled antisense oligonucleotide. However, at the micromolar concentrations used, there was no specific antiviral effect observed. Another problem faced by the authors was the digestion of the oligonucleotides by exonucleases because only the 5′ end was protected by the fusogenic peptide. Experiments to optimize delivery, binding stability, and amount of oligonucleotides have to be performed.

IV. CONJUGATES OF SUBSTANCES

A. LDL-Conjugates

Low density lipoprotein (LDL) particles represent an important part in the metabolization cycle of lipids in the human organism. These particles carry mostly cholesterol to the cells throughout the body. Additionally, they carry apolipoprotein fractions (Apo) on their surface, which are able to dock with different receptors on the cell surfaces. Native LDL is cleared from plasma through a regulated pathway by binding to the apo B/E receptors present on hepatocytes. Chemical modification of apo B, like glucosylation or oxidation, changes the affinity from the apo B receptor toward the scavenger receptor. Scavenger receptors are expressed on the surface of cells of the monocyte/macrophage lineage and on the endothelium. For example, derivatization of the ε-amino group of the apoB-protein abolishes binding to the LDL receptor and initiates the affinity to the scavenger receptor. Thus, coupling antiretroviral substances such as inhibitors of HIV reverse transcriptase to the ε-amino group of the lysine side chain creates a high affinity for monocytes/macrophages. This effect offers the chance to target selectively those cells which are an important reservoir of HIV.

    Radioactively labeled thymidine and AZT were coupled to the ε-amino groups of lysines of LDL-Apo B, and their uptake behavior was studied in human hepatocytes (Hep G2) and murine macrophages (P_{388}) (47). Hep G2 cells do not exhibit a scavenger receptor in contrast to the murine macrophages used in the experiments. Instead, they possess the normal apo B receptor. It was shown that the coupling of the nucleosides induced a shift in affinity to the scavenger receptor of the macrophage cells. By autoradiography, the uptake, lysosomal cleavage from LDL, and triphosphorylation of [³H]-labeled thymidine, LDL in murine macrophages was demonstrated.

In a later work, the antiretroviral effects of these AZT-coupled LDL particles was shown (48). Human macrophage cultures were infected with HIV-1 and subsequently treated with LDL-coupled AZT and with free AZT serving as a control. Additionally, the scavenger-receptor free T-lymphocyte Molt 4/8 cells were infected with HIV-1 and subsequently treated the same way. The results of the treatment were evaluated by measuring the p24 antigen production. It was demonstrated that LDL-coupled AZT was internalized specifically by macrophages via scavenger receptor and had anti-HIV activity comparable to free AZT, whereas the free substance had a better effect on the Molt 4/8 cells. The same results were also found with fluorothymidine, a potent inhibitor of the HIV-1 reverse transcriptase (49). The optimization of the coupling procedures for substances to LDL particles was also described (50). The authors proposed a better efficiency of antiretroviral therapy with the LDL-coupled nucleosides during early stages of infection.

B.   Other Conjugates

A variety of examples can be found in the literature about the synthesis of conjugates consisting of antiviral compounds coupled to lipid derivatives or neoglycoproteins. Steim et al. (51) synthesized monophosphate diglyceride conjugate of AZT containing esterified saturated palmitoyl and unsaturated oleoyl fatty acids (AZTMPDG). Free AZT, the pure conjugate and a formulation as mixed liposomes, was tested in vitro for activity against HIV-1 replication in H9 cells and MOLT-3 cells. Although the conjugates are somewhat less active than free AZT against HIV-1, the authors supposed an advantageous biodistribution of the lipid formulation in vivo. Because, unlike free AZT, glucuronidation of AZTMPDG would not occur and the bound drug would not undergo filtration in the kidneys, a significant increase in plasma lifetime may result.

Van Wijk et al. (52) synthesized nucleoside diphosphate diglyceride that possesses a potential advantage consisting of the release of an antiviral nucleotide monophosphate. They investigated the membrane association and the spontaneous as well as protein-mediated intermembrane transfer of this type of compound, which all showed activity against HIV-1. A different approach is the covalent coupling of the 5´-monophosphate of AZT (AZTMP) to neoglycoproteins. Various mannose-, fucose-, galactose- and glucose-containing neoglycoproteins were created based on phenyl-linkage between sugar and human serum albumin (HSA). T-helper lymphocytes as a primary target for antiviral therapy harbor specific lectins on their surface, recognizing various sugar molecules. The anti-HIV activity of different neoglycoprotein carriers coupled with AZTMP was tested in vitro. Only the derivative having 40 moles mannose per mole protein ($Man_{40}HSA$) showed pronounced anti-HIV-1 activity, itself being more than 30 times as active against HIV-1 compared to HSA-AZTMP. It remains to be investigated whether the marked potency of the $Man_{40}HSA$-AZTMP conjugate can be explained by sugar-specific recognition and subsequent endocytosis of the conjugate into the cells or alternatively by some synergistic action of the glycoprotein and the AZTMP.

REFERENCES

1. Tröster SD, Müller U, Kreuter J. Modification of the body distribution of poly(methylmethacrylate) nanoparticles in rats by coating with surfactants. Int J Pharmacol 1990; 61:85.

2. Courveur P, Vauthier C. Polyalkylcyanoacrylate nanoparticles as drug carrier: present state and perspectives. J Controlled Rel 1991; 17:187–198.

3. Kreuter J. Nanoparticles. In: Kreuter J, ed. Colloidal Drug Delivery Systems. New York: Marcel Dekker, 1994:219–342.

4. Allemann E, Gurny R, Doelker E. Drug-loaded nanoparticles—preparation methods and drug targeting issues. Eur J Pharmacol Biopharmacol 1993; 39:173–191.

5. Kreuter J. Nanoparticles. In: Swarbrick J and Boylan JC, eds. Encyclopedia of Pharmaceutical Technology. New York: Marcel Dekker, 1994:165–190.

6. Kreuter J. Evaluation of nanoparticles as drug-delivery systems. I. Preparation methods. Pharm Acta Helv 1983; 58:196–209.

7. Henry-Michelland S, Alonso MJ, Andremont A, Maincen P, Sauzieres J, Couvreur P. Attachment of antibiotics to nanoparticles: preparation, drug release and antimicrobial activity in vitro. Int J Pharmacol 1987; 35:121–177.

8. Voigt R. Pharmazeutische Technologie für Studium und Beruf. Berlin: Ullstein, Mosby, 1993.

9. Crommelin DJA, Schreier H. Liposomes. In: Kreuter J, ed. Colloidal Drug Delivery Systems. New York: Marcel Dekker, 1994:73–190.

10. Bauer KH, Frömming KH, Führer C. Pharmazeutische Technologie, New York: Thieme, 1991.

11. Birrenbach G, Speiser P. Polymerized micelles and their use as adjuvants in immunology. J Pharmacol Sci 1976; 65:1763.

12. Lucks JS, Müller RH, König B. Solid lipid nanoparticles (SLN)—an alternative parenteral drug delivery system. Eur J Pharmacol Biopharmacol 1992; 38:suppl 33.

13. Speiser PP. Nanopartikel. In: Müller RH, Hildebrand GE, eds. Pharmazeutische Technologie: Moderne Arzneiformen. Stuttgart: WVG, 1998:339–356.

14. Schäfer V, von Briesen H, Andreesen R, et al. Phagocytosis of nanoparticles by human immunodeficiency virus (HIV)-infected macrophages: a possibility for antiviral drug targeting. Pharmacol Res 1992; 9:541–546.

15. Schäfer V, von Briesen H, Rübsamen-Waigmann H, Steffan AM, Royer C, Kreuter J. Phagocytosis and degradation of human serum albumin microsheres and nanoparticles in human macrophages. J Microencapsulation 1994; 11:261–269.

16. Bender A, Schäfer V, Steffan AM, et al. Inhibition of HIV in vitro by antiviral drug-targeting using nanoparticles. Res Virol 1994; 145:215–220.

17. Bender AR, von Briesen H, Kreuter J, Duncan IB, Rübsamen-Waigmann H. Efficiency of nanoparticles as a carrier system for antiviral agents in human immunodeficiency virus-infected human monocytes/macrophages in vitro. Antimicrob Agents Chemother 1996; 40:1467–1471.

18. Löbenberg R, Kreuter J. Macrophage targeting of azidothymidine: a promising strategy for AIDS therapy. AIDS Res Hum Retroviruses 1996; 12:1709–1715.

19. Löbenberg R, Araujo L, Kreuter J. Body distribution of azidothymidine bound to nanoparticles after oral administration. Eur J Pharmacol Biopharmacol 1997; 44:127–132.

20. Löbenberg R, Araujo L, von Briesen H, Rodgers E, Kreuter J. Body distribution of azidothymidine bound to hexyl-cyanoacrylate nanoparticles after i.v. injection into rats. J Controlled Rel 1998; 50:21–30.

21. Löbenberg R, Maas J, Kreuter J. Improved body distribution of ^{14}C-labelled AZT bound to nanoparticles in rats determined by radioluminography. J Drug Target 1998; 5:171–179.

22. Leroux JC, Cozens RM, Roesel JL, Galli B, Doelker E, Gurny R. pH-sensitive nanoparticles: an effective means to improve the oral delivery of HIV-1 protease inhibitors in dogs. Pharmacol Res 1996; 13:485–487.

23. Leroux JC, Cozens R, Roesel JL, et al. Pharmacokinetics of a novel HIV-1 protease inhibitor incorporated into biodegradable or enteric nanoparticles following intravenous and oral administration to mice. J Pharmacol Sci 1995; 84:1387–1391.

24. Hostetler KY, Richman DD, Sridhar CN, et al. Phosphatidylazidothymidine and phosphatidyl-ddC: assessment of uptake in mouse lymphoid tissues and antiviral activities in human immunodeficiency virus-infected cells and in Rauscher leukemia virus-infected mice. Antimicrob Agents Chemother 1994; 38:2792–2797.

25. Kamps JA, Swart PJ, Morselt HW, et al. Preparation and characterization of conjugates of (modified) human serum albumin and liposomes: drug carriers with an intrinsic anti-HIV activity. Biochim Biophys Acta 1996; 1278:183–190.

26. Dusserre N, Lessard C, Paquette N, et al. Encapsulation of foscarnet in liposomes modifies drug intracellular accumulation, in vitro anti-HIV-1 activity, tissue distribution and pharmacokinetics. AIDS 1995; 9:833–841.

27. Gabev EE, Gabev EB, Mitcheva M, Astroug H, Karaivanova M. Acute toxicity study on a new anti HIV liposome combination preparation. Int Conf AIDS 1996; 11:320 (abstract no. Tu.B.2321).

28. Dusserre N, Omar R, Desormeaux A, et al. Entrapment of foscarnet in liposomes: a strategic approach for the treatment of HIV and CMV infections. Int Conf AIDS 1996; 11:63 (abstract no. Mo.A. 1054).

29. Schwendener RA, Gowland P, Horber DH, Zahner R, Schertler A, Schott H. New lipophilic alkyl/acyl dinucleoside phosphates as derivatives of 3′-azido-3′-deoxythymidine: inhibition of HIV-1 replication in vitro and antiviral activity against Rauscher leukemia virus infected mice with delayed treatment regimens. Antiviral Res 1994; 24:79–93.

30. Lazdins JK, Woods-Cook K, Walker M, Alteri E. The lipophilic muramyl peptide MTP-PE is a potent inhibitor of HIV replication in macrophages. AIDS Res Hum Retroviruses 1990; 6:1157–1161.

31. Müller WEG, Weiler BE, Charubala R, et al. Cordycepin analogues of 2´,5´-oligoad-enylate inhibit human immunodeficiency virus infection via inhibition of reverse transcriptase. Biochemistry 1991; 30:2027–2033.

32. Renneisen K, Leserman L, Matthes E, Schroder HC, Muller WE. Inhibition of expression of human immunodeficiency virus-1 in vitro by antibody-targeted liposomes containing antisense RNA to the env region. J Biol Chem 1990; 265:16337–16342.

33. Zelphati O, Degols G, Loughrey H, et al. Inhibition of HIV-1 replication in cultured cells with phosphorylated dideoxyuridine derivatives encapsulated in immunoliposomes. Antiviral Res 1993; 21:181–195.

34. Harvie P, Desormeaux A, Bergeron MC, et al. Comparative pharmacokinetics, distributions in tissue, and interactions with blood proteins of conventional and sterically stabilized liposomes containing 2´,3´-dideoxyinosine. Antimicrob Agents Chemother 1996; 40:225–229.

35. Magnani M, Rossi L, Fraternale A, et al. Targeting antiviral nucleotide analogues to macrophages. J Leuk Biol 1997; 62:133–137.

36. Magnani M, Rossi L, Casabianca A, et al. Red blood cells as advanced drug delivery systems for antiviral nucleoside analogues. In: Magnani M, DeLoach JR, eds. Advances in Experimental Medicine & Biology. New York, 1992:239–245.

37. Magnani M, Rossi L, Fraternale A, et al. Feline immunodeficiency virus infection of macrophages: in vitro and in vivo inhibition by dideoxycytidine-5´-triphosphate-loaded erythrocytes. AIDS Res Hum Retroviruses 1994; 10:1179–1186.

38. Perno CF, Santoro N, Balestra E, et al. Red blood cells mediated delivery of 9-(2-phosphonylmethoxyethyl)adenine to primary macrophages: efficiency metabolism and activity against human immunodeficiency virus or herpes simplex virus. Antiviral Res 1997; 33:153–164.

39. Anazodo MI, Wainberg MA, Friesen AD, Wright JA. Sequence-specific inhibition of gene expression by a novel antisense oligodeoxynucleotide phosphorothioate directed against a nonregulatory region of the human immunodeficiency virus type 1 genome. J Virol 1995; 69:1794–1801.

40. Puyal C, Milhaud P, Bienvenue A, Philippot JR. A new cationic liposome encapsulating genetic material. A potential delivery system for polynucleotides. Eur J Biochem 1995; 228:697–703.

41. Sullivan SM, Gieseler RK, Lenzner S, et al. Inhibition of human immunodeficiency virus-1 proliferation by liposome-encapsulated sense DNA to the 5´ tat splice acceptor site. Antisense Res Dev 1992; 2:187–197.

42. Zelphati O, Imbach JL, Signoret N, Zon G, Rayner B, Leserman L. Antisense oligonucleotides in solution or encapsulated in immunoliposomes inhibit replication of HIV-1 by several different mechanisms. Nucleic Acids Res 1994; 22:4307–4314.

43. Grimaldi S, Lisi A, Pozzi D, Santoro N. Attempts to use liposomes and RBC ghosts as vectors in drug and antisense therapy of virus infection. Res Virol 1997; 148:177–180.

44. Zelphati O, Wagner E, Leserman L. Synthesis and anti-HIV activity of thiocholesteryl-coupled phosphodiester antisense oligonucleotides incorporated into immunoliposomes. Antiviral Res 1994; 25:13–25.

45. Bonfils E, Depierreux C, Midoux P, Thuong NT, Monsigny M, Roche AC. Drug targeting: synthesis and endocytosis of oligonucleotide-neoglycoprotein conjugates. Nucleic Acids Res 1992; 20:4621–4629.

46. Bongartz JP, Aubertin AM, Milhaud PG, Lebleu B. Improved biological activity of antisense oligonucleotides conjugates to a fusogenic peptide. Nucleic Acids Res 1994; 22:4681–4688.

47. von Baeyer H, Neitzel H, Nundel M, Riedel E, Schultis HK. Covalent coupling of nucleosides to low density lipoprotein (LDL) generates macrophage specific (drug)-carriers. Int J Clin Pharmacol Ther Toxicol 1993; 31:382–386.

48. Mankertz J, von Baeyer H, Rokos K, Nundel M, Pauli G, Riedel E. Cell specific uptake of antiretroviral drugs: AZT coupled to LDL inhibits HIV replication in human macrophages. Int J Clin Pharmacol Ther 1995; 33:85–88.

49. Mankertz J, Matthes E, Rokos K, von Baeyer H, Pauli G, Riedel E. Selective endocytosis of fluorothymidine and azidothymidine coupled to LDL into HIV infected mononuclear cells. Biochim Biophys Acta 1996; 1317:233–237.

50. Mankertz J, Nündel M, von Baeyer H, Riedel E. Low density lipoproteins as drug carriers in the therapy of macrophage-associated diseases. Biochem Biophys Res Commun 1997; 240:112–115.

51. Steim JM, Camaioni Neto C, Sarin PS, Sun DK, Sehgal RK, Turcotte JG. Lipid conjugates of antiretroviral agents. I. Azidothymidine-monophosphate-diglyceride: anti-HIV activity, physical properties, and interaction with plasma proteins. Biochem Biophys Res Commun 1990; 171:451–457.

52. van Wijk GMT, Gadella TWJ, Wirtz KWA, Hostetler KY, van den Bosch H. Spontaneous and protein-mediated intermembrane transfer of the antiretroviral liponucleotide 3′-deoxythymidine diphosphate diglyceride. Biochemistry 1992; 31:5912–5917.

10
Nonhuman Primate Models for Testing Anti-HIV Drugs

Koen K. A. Van Rompay and Marta L. Marthas
California Regional Primate Research Center, University of California, Davis, California

I. INTRODUCTION: THE NEED FOR RELEVANT ANIMAL MODELS

During recent years, the development of more potent anti-human immunodeficiency virus (HIV) drugs that inhibit the viral reverse transcriptase (RT) and protease enzymes, and the synergistic effects of combination therapy have led to major improvement in the clinical management of HIV-infected people in the developed countries (1). Despite this success of combination drug therapy in HIV-infected patients, there is still much room for improvement, in that not everyone experiences these "miraculous" effects; in addition, the problems of toxicity, compliance, drug resistance, and costs become very relevant if long-term administration of these drugs is necessary to maintain these benefits. Finally, the majority of HIV-infected people living in the developing countries (2) have not benefited from these recent advances.

Accordingly, the challenge is to find and identify better antiviral drugs. The "ideal" antiviral drug strategy would be one that induces strong and persistent suppression of virus replication, gives prolonged immunological and clinical benefits at the lowest toxicity, can be administered at infrequent dosage intervals, is stable and inexpensive, and can thus benefit the greatest number of HIV-infected people.

For novel compounds, the demonstration of in vitro inhibitory effects on HIV replication are generally the first and prerequisite step for further development. Most compounds that show promising in vitro effects, however, fail when tested in HIV-infected patients, some because of unfavorable pharmacokinetics, others because of toxicity or lack of detectable antiviral effects (3). Hence, there is the need for these promising compounds to be tested in consecutive phase I/II/III clinical trials in HIV-infected patients.

A problem is, however, that, because of the logistics and money- and time-consuming aspects of human clinical trials, only a limited number of drugs can enter these human trials in a given time. In addition, the current availability of quite-effective combinations also impedes progress in the search for better therapeutic strategies: it is becoming increasingly complicated to prove the efficacy of novel antiviral drugs or the superiority of new drug combinations against the existing "gold standard" of combination therapy, because it is unethical to treat "control" groups with anything less than the currently best available treatment (4,5). How can one avoid these dilemmas that threaten to break the stride in finding better treatments against HIV infection? One answer is to use appropriate animal models.

The current turmoil among clinical trial designers (reviewed in Refs. 4 and 5) urges for a reappraisal of the role of animal models in the drug development process. Appropriate animal models that allow rapid evaluation of the efficacy and the toxicity of antiviral compounds would be very useful, because they allow sorting out those drugs that are promising and deserve to enter human clinical trials from those drugs that should probably be discarded. Although this would add an extra step in the already long process of evaluating drugs, in the long run, testing the drug in an appropriate animal model certainly accelerates progress and saves time and money that otherwise would be wasted on testing noneffective or toxic drugs in human trials (Fig. 1).

Several animal models are available for rapid evaluation of antiretroviral compounds (reviewed in Refs. 6–9). Whereas murine and feline models are appropriate for initial screening, further testing can be done in nonhuman primate models that best resemble HIV infection of humans, such as simian immunodeficiency virus (SIV) infection of macaques. During the initial years of the HIV epidemic, the role of nonhuman primate models in the drug development process was limited. In recent years, however, nonhuman primate models for anti-HIV drug testing have improved substantially. This chapter demonstrates the problems that primate investigators were faced with and the solutions that were found. Also discussed are how investigators currently use different study designs (e.g., by manipulating variables such as initiation of drug treatment relative to virus inoculation, the duration of treatment, the age of the animals, the virulence and drug susceptibility of the virus inoculum) to address very specific questions directly relevant to treatment of human HIV infection. In addition to being a test system for preclinical screening of the efficacy of novel drugs, a good animal model can also be used to test hypotheses that are difficult or impossible to study in humans. Examples of this are studies aimed at determining the pre- and post-exposure prophylactic efficacy of antiviral drugs, or studies aimed at determining the in vivo virulence of drug-resistant viral mutants.

As the following discussion will demonstrate, non-human primate models

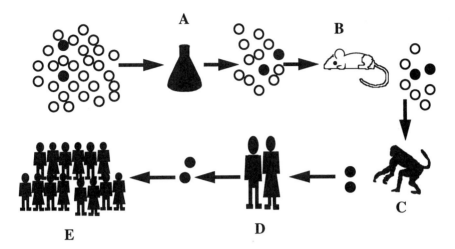

Figure 1 Role of animal models in antiviral drug development. Antiviral drug testing can involve multiple levels of screening; each of these levels includes evaluation of efficacy and toxicity. Ultrarapid test systems with high throughput and relatively low cost, such as in vitro testing (**A**) should be used as an initial level of testing, before proceeding to animal testing. Although murine models (**B**) are useful for initial in vivo screening, nonhuman primate models (**C**) more closely resemble HIV infection of humans and, accordingly, are recommended for a final preclinical evaluation step. Animal models allow rapid screening and can prevent time and resources from being wasted on testing noneffective or highly toxic drugs (*open circles*) in human clinical trials (**D**), and guide effective drugs (*black circles*) more rapidly toward clinical application (**E**).

of HIV infection provide excellent and very adaptable tools to rapidly gather data that can provide a solid scientific basis to guide human clinical trials (Table 1).

II. OVERVIEW OF NONHUMAN PRIMATE MODELS FOR HIV INFECTION

Of all members of the animal kingdom, nonhuman primates are phylogenetically the closest to humans. The higher similarities in physiology (including fetal and infant development, drug metabolism) and immunology allow a more reliable extrapolation of results obtained in nonhuman primate models to clinical applications for the human population. The ideal nonhuman model for AIDS should be permissive to HIV-1/HIV-2 infection and show an identical clinical disease spectrum as that which occurs in human AIDS patients.

Depending on the endpoint used for testing, nonhuman primate models systems can represent models for viremia or models for disease. Models for viremia

Table 1 Value of Nonhuman Primate Models in Anti-HIV Drug Development

---

Toxicity (acute and chronic)
Pharmacokinetics
  Route/dose
  Age-dependency
  Penetration into cerebrospinal fluid; transplacental transfer
Prevention of infection (chemoprophylaxis)
  Occupational exposure (e.g., needlestick)
  Mother-to-infant HIV transmission
Treatment of established infection (chemotherapy)
  Early versus late drug therapy
  Short-term versus prolonged treatment
  Combination versus monotherapy; sequential versus concomitant
  Eradication of viral reservoirs
Drug-resistant viral mutants
  Emergence
  Virulence
  Clinical implications for prophylaxis and therapy

---

are used to study prevention/reduction of acute infection or therapy of chronic viremia. In contrast, animal models that resemble human AIDS (such as SIV infection of macaques) can also be used to evaluate the efficacy of compounds against this type of disease.

A. HIV-1 Infection of Chimpanzees and Pig-Tailed Macaques

HIV-1 can infect chimpanzees. However, except for rare cases, HIV-1 infection does not generally result in the development of clinical disease, even after prolonged follow-up (10–12). Although this model has been used to study chemoprophylaxis or reduction of viremia (13), the lack of availability, the high expense, and their endangered species status make these larger primates unsuitable for general antiviral drug studies.

HIV-1 infection has been demonstrated in pig-tailed macaques (*Macaca nemestrina*) (14,15). However, large inocula were required to result in infection, and even though some aspects of acute HIV-1 infection in humans are replicated in this model, AIDS has not been observed.

B. HIV-2 and SIV Infection of Macaques

Simian immunodeficiency virus (SIV) was originally isolated from rhesus macaques (*Macaca mulatta*) in captivity that showed immunosuppression and lymphomas (16), and was called SIV_{mac}. Since then, SIV strains have also been isolated from other primate hosts. To date, five groups of primate lentiviruses have been identified: (a) SIV_{agm} (African green monkey), (b) SIV_{smm} (sooty mangabey)/ SIV_{mac} (macaque)/SIV_{mne} (nemestrina/SIV_{stm} (stumptail)/HIV-2, (c) SIV_{mnd} (mandrill)/SIV_{lhoest} (l'hoest monkey), (d) SIV_{syk} (sykes monkey), and (e) HIV-1/SIV_{cpz} (chimpanzee) (for review, see Refs. 17–19). The SIV_{smm}/SIV_{mac}/SIV_{mne} group has been used most extensively. These viruses are closely related to HIV-2 and are more distantly related to HIV-1 (80%–90% and 50%–60% amino acid homology in pol, respectively).

The sooty mangabey, African green monkey, mandrill, l'hoest, and chimpanzee isolates have all been derived from African nonhuman primate species, and are found in animals in their natural habitat; none has yet been shown to induce disease in its presumed natural host. Macaques, including rhesus macaques, are Asian Old World primates; evidence suggests that macaques are not naturally infected with SIV but that some captive macaques have acquired their SIV (SIV_{mac}), which is genetically similar to SIV_{smm}, from sooty mangabey monkeys while in captivity at one or more of the Regional Primate Research Centers (for review, see Ref. 20).

The SIV_{mac} and its closely related SIV_{smm} and SIV_{mne}, upon experimental inoculation of a variety of Asian macaque species, induce a disease that resembles human AIDS, including opportunistic infections, tumors, and central nervous system disorders (21). Compared to HIV infection of humans, SIV infection in macaques has an accelerated time course, in that a much greater proportion of infected monkeys die from the infection within a comparatively short period of time (3–30 months compared to 7–10 years for humans) (18). SIV_{smm}PBj14 is a unique case: instead of causing chronic, progressive immunodeficiency, this variant of SIV_{smm} induces an acute clinical disease (characterized by severe diarrhea) in pigtailed macaques within 2 weeks following inoculation (22,23). Evidence suggests that the pathogenesis is due to extensive T lymphocyte activation induced by a particular *nef* allele in the virus (24).

Macaques can be infected with HIV-2. This model, which has the advantage of using a human virus, has been used as a model to test the efficacy of antiviral drugs during acute viremia (25–27), but has some disadvantages for drug testing. In several experiments published, not all inoculated animals became infected; in addition, disease developed rarely, and most animals remained asymptomatic (28,29).

The availability of pathogenic molecular clones as well as attenuated or nonvirulent molecular clones has demonstrated to be an extremely useful tool for studying the determinants of viral virulence, and will continue to be valuable for the development of live-attenuated vaccines (30–34).

In recent years, a pediatric AIDS animal model has been developed using SIV inoculation of newborn macaques; similar to observations in HIV-infected human infants, the disease course in newborn macaques following inoculation with virulent SIV strains is often accelerated (35–37). This model has been proven very useful for antiviral drug testing (see further discussion).

The polymerase region of SIV has about 60% amino acid homology to HIV-1 (18). Not unexpectedly, SIV is susceptible to many of the same inhibitors of reverse transcriptase (RT) (such as zidovudine [AZT], didanosine [ddI], and zalcitabine [ddC]), and protease enzymes at approximately the same in vitro concentrations as HIV-1 (38–42). An exception is the nonnucleoside inhibitors (e.g., the TIBO compounds, and nevirapine), which are specific for HIV-1 and do not inhibit replication of HIV-2 and SIV (43). To overcome this problem, the construction of infectious SIV/HIV-1 chimeric viruses has been proven useful.

C. SIV/HIV-1 Chimeric Viruses

Although SIV infection of macaques is a good animal model for AIDS, the genetic difference between SIV and HIV-1 remains a limitation. In recent years, investigators are overcoming this obstacle by replacing genes (such as envelope) of SIV-mac with their counterparts of HIV-1 and constructing HIV/SIV chimeric viruses (so-called SHIVs), which are infectious and can cause disease following inoculation of macaques (44–54). As mentioned previously, SIV and HIV-2, unlike HIV-1, are not susceptible to inhibition by nonnucleoside RT inhibitors; this excludes the use of SIV-infected macaques for studying drug resistance to this group of antiviral compounds. However, the availability of an infectious RT-SHIV clone, which contains the RT of HIV-1, will enable investigators to use this model in future years to study the efficacy and the emergence of drug resistance for nonnucleoside analogues (54,55).

III. DRUG STUDIES IN NONHUMAN PRIMATE MODELS

A. From Past to Present: Obstacles to Overcome

Because their physiology is very similar to that of humans, the macaque model has been proven very useful for performing toxicity and pharmacokinetic studies of antiviral drugs, including the assessment of drug interactions, the effect of pregnancy, and transplacental drug transfer (56–70). In addition, because SIV infection of macaques closely resembles HIV infection of humans with regard to disease pathogenesis, one would assume that the macaque model would have played a major role in evaluating the efficacy of anti-HIV drugs to inhibit virus replication in vivo. Paradoxically, however, the number of in vivo studies in nonhuman primate models has been limited, and, until recently, testing antiretroviral drugs in clinical trials with HIV-infected patients has largely bypassed preclinical evaluation in nonhuman primate models. Although most anti-HIV drugs inhibit SIV in vitro at similar concentrations as those needed for HIV (38–42,71,72), many initial drug studies in macaques were not highly effective. This was often partially due to the relatively weak potency of the test compounds which were available at that time (although some critics blamed the observed less-than-spectacular efficacy on the so-called inadequacy of the macaque model to recognize "potent" antiviral drugs). In addition, the direct relevance of the results obtained in primate studies to the management of HIV-infected patients was questioned and/or not recognized by clinicians at that time. One of the reasons for this was that most nonhuman primate studies tested the efficacy of short-term drug treatment during the acute viremia stage. At that time, the benefits of early potent antiviral therapy were not recognized for HIV infection, and standard clinical management of HIV infection consisted of initiating therapy late during infection, at the onset of immunodeficiency or $CD4^+$ T-cell reduction. Accordingly, it was unclear whether the results of early drug intervention studies in nonhuman primates could be extrapolated to prolonged drug therapy of chronic HIV infection, especially because short-term studies may not adequately address important issues such as the emergence and clinical implications of drug-resistant viral mutants. However, nonhuman primate models at that time were not practical to reliably evaluate the efficacy of prolonged drug therapy of chronic infection because of a number of problems.

First, most studies used adolescent or adult macaques, and there are several problems associated with this age group for chronic drug studies (Fig. 2). These problems, which are discussed in more detail elsewhere (73), fall into two main categories: the administration of the drug and the detection of antiviral effects.

Because of the problems involved with handling older macaques, difficulties often arise in administering drugs for a prolonged period of time. This is especially problematic for drugs with a short half-life that would need a frequent dosage regimen to maintain adequate blood levels of the drug throughout most of the dosage interval. In addition, the time course of SIV disease progression in older macaques is highly variable, in that the asymptomatic period ranges from months to years and depends on host factors such as the strength of the initial immune response. It is therefore often hard to determine whether a small difference in outcome of infection is due to host factors or to the drug treatment, especially because only small numbers of animals can be used (73). This problem was further compounded when there were no adequate assays to detect antiviral effects of the drug during the asymptomatic stage by monitoring surrogate markers, such as the quantitation of virus levels in blood and tissues (74). Accordingly, testing the efficacy of an antiviral drug was mainly limited to determining its potential to prevent infection or reduce/delay the acute viremia. In recent years, the availability of more sensitive assays to monitor virus replication (such as quantitative viral RNA assays) and the growing evidence that virus levels in HIV-infected patients are the best correlate of disease progression have increased understanding of HIV disease pathogenesis (75–77); the development of similar sensitive assays to quantitate

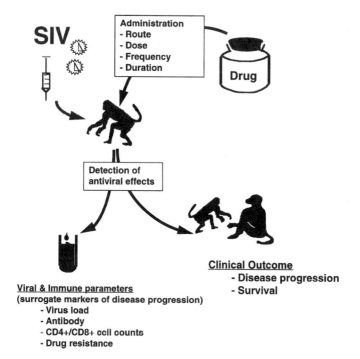

Figure 2   SIV infection of macaques for testing antiretroviral drugs: role of age. The use of adult macaques for prolonged antiviral drug studies is associated with difficulties regarding drug administration as well as detection of antiviral effects. Both groups of problems can be attenuated or solved using newborn or infant macaques. (From Ref. 73.)

virus levels in SIV-infected macaques has spurred the potential of using juvenile/adult macaques with chronic SIV infection for antiviral drug studies (78).

During recent years, SIV infection of newborn and infant macaques has been shown to be a very practical animal model of pediatric HIV infection. In addition, this pediatric animal model has been found to be very attractive for performing antiviral drug studies, because it overcomes many of the difficulties associated with using older macaques. Neonatal macaques can be easily handled and drugs administered more readily for prolonged periods of times by either parenteral or oral routes without the need for sedation and with minimal physical restraint. Animals of this age are also much smaller than adolescent or adult macaques and therefore require less drug, which is important, because many new compounds are very expensive to produce in quantities sufficient for these experiments (73). Although newborn macaques (like human neonates) have a reduced capacity to clear drugs like AZT from the body, resulting in prolonged blood levels following drug administration (57), this is no disadvantage, because once antiviral effects of a drug have been demonstrated in a pediatric population, it will only be a matter of optimizing the dosage regimen in the older population.

An important feature of the newborn model is that the disease course following inoculation with highly virulent SIV isolates is more uniform than in older animals and is characterized by persistently high virus levels, poor antiviral immune response, rapid immunosuppression, and rapid development of clinical disease (in most animals, simian AIDS develops within 2 to 3 months) (36). This disease course resembles that seen in HIV-infected children with rapid disease progression (79–83). Because of the predictably rapid and fulminant disease progression of SIV infection in newborn macaques, effects of drug therapy on disease progression can be evaluated more reliably and quickly than with older animals. Therefore, this animal model of pediatric AIDS is very useful for testing novel intervention strategies, because efficacy can be assessed by monitoring clinical disease progression as well as viral and immune parameters by using a limited number of animals in a relatively short period of time (73,84,85). Information obtained in this pediatric animal model of AIDS applies directly to HIV infection of human infants as well as adults, in that the demonstration of antiviral effects in a "worst-case scenario" is the best indicator of the potency of an antiviral drug strategy (86).

B. Summary of Drug Studies in Nonhuman Primates

1. Prophylaxis: Prevention or Reduction of Acute Viremia

Most studies in nonhuman primates have focused on testing whether drug administration starting around the time of virus inoculation was effective in preventing infection or delaying the appearance of virus or viral antigen in the plasma. Although early studies, which mostly used zidovudine (AZT), were not highly effective in preventing infection, a likely reason for this was the high dose of virus used in these experiments (87–90). More recent studies have shown that antiviral drug administration (AZT, PMEA, FLT) starting before or at the time of virus inoculation can prevent infection when a minimal dose of SIV was used for the inoculation (13,25,91–94). Nevirapine treatment starting before virus inoculation prevented HIV-1 infection of chimpanzees (13). Only a few compounds have prevented infection when treatment was started after virus inoculation: 9-[2-(phosphonomethoxy)prophyl]adenine (PMPA) and 2′,3′-dideoxy-3′-hydroxymethyl cytidine (BEA-005) (26,91,95). Recently, it was found that a two-dose regimen of PMPA was already sufficient to protect newborn macaques against oral SIV infection (92).

The demonstration of AZT chemoprophylaxis in animal models has preceded the demonstration that AZT can prevent infection of humans following exposure to HIV in two clinical settings. The first one is the use of antiviral drugs to prevent infection following needlestick accidents of health care workers. Despite anecdotal reports of the failure of AZT to prevent infection following needlestick accidents (96–98), it has currently been demonstrated that AZT administration following percutaneous HIV exposure reduces the risk of infection by 80% (99–101). A second clinical setting where antiviral drugs are extremely useful is related to vertical transmission of HIV; although vertical transmission can occur in utero or postnatally (through breastfeeding), evidence suggests that a majority of HIV infections occur shortly before or during birth (potentially through contact with maternal blood and fluids). The demonstration that AZT administration to HIV-infected pregnant women beginning at 14 to 34 weeks of gestation, and continuing to their newborns during the first 6 weeks of life, reduces the rate of vertical HIV transmission by two-thirds has been a major advancement in the combat against pediatric HIV infection in developed countries (102). Although recent studies have demonstrated partial efficacy of shorter AZT regimens (103,104), more simple and affordable intervention strategies are urgently needed to curtail vertical HIV transmission in developing countries. The development of antiviral drugs which have even higher chemoprophylactic potential in nonhuman primates (such as PMPA; [91,92,95]), raises the hope that in the future effective and affordable one- or two-dose drug regimens may become available to drastically reduce vertical HIV transmission in developing countries.

Antiviral drug studies in nonhuman primate models demonstrated that even when infection was not prevented, early drug treatment was still able to delay or reduce the peak of rapid virus replication that occurs during the first weeks of infection (87,89,90,93,105–108). Whether this reduction in virus replication during the initial stages of infection also resulted in delayed disease progression was not clear in the initial studies but became apparent in the later studies (27,85,107,109, 110). These studies provided strong evidence that very early events during viral infection determine the ultimate disease course, because short-term suppression of this primary viremia limited the systemic spread of the virus, reduced virus-induced immunosuppression, enhanced antiviral immune responses, and significantly delayed disease progression. This information applies directly to drug treatment of humans during the primary viremia stage. Indeed, in recent years, there is increasing evidence that early drug intervention offers strong benefits for HIV-infected patients in terms of long-term suppression of viral replication, enhanced HIV-specific CD4[+] T-cell proliferative responses, and delayed disease progression (111–113).

2. Chronic Infection

Few nonhuman primate studies have investigated the effects of antiretroviral drug therapy on established, chronic SIV infection (i.e., after the acute viremia stage). Initial studies with AZT were not highly successful to demonstrate therapeutic effects of AZT for macaques once SIV infection was established (74,114). Although this failure to demonstrate therapeutic effects was mainly due to the relative weakness of AZT monotherapy to inhibit virus replication, another confounding problem was the lack of sensitive assays to measure virus replication during the asymp-tomatic stage. The technology to measure viral RNA in plasma was not available at that time. Most juvenile/adult macaques have no detectable p27 antigenemia or infectious virus in plasma during the asymptomatic stage of disease, so the use of these parameters to monitor therapeutic effects is difficult. AZT had little or no im-pact on peripheral blood mononuclear cell (PBMC)-associated infectious virus lev-els once infection was established (114).

During recent years, the discovery of more potent antiviral drugs and the de-velopment of better assays to monitor infection has increased the usefulness of macaques with chronic infection to test the efficacy of novel antiviral drugs. Ad-ministration of PMEA or PMPA to macaques with chronic SIV infection induced strong persistent reduction of infectious PBMC- associated and plasma virus lev-els, and plasma RNA levels (78,84,115,116).

Although the approach of administering antiviral drugs to macaques with chronic SIV infection resembles testing of these compounds in HIV-infected pa-tients in clinical trials, the value of the animal model in the whole process of an-tiviral drug development is multiple. One can rapidly gain preliminary data about the magnitude of antiviral inhibitory effects before starting the first human trials. In addition, and most importantly, animal models can address the duration of viral suppression, and the emergence and clinical implications of drug-resistant mutants.

3. Antiviral Drug Resistance

Introduction: The Value of Animal Models in Studying Drug Resistance. During recent years, the discovery of novel, better antiretroviral drugs and drug combinations, has led to significant advances in the clinical management of HIV-infected patients. Many HIV-1 infected patients, however, do not show the desired strong and persistent suppression of viral replication and eventually show disease progression. Although other factors (such as compliance to the drug dosage regi-men) may contribute to reduced efficacy of antiviral drug therapy, a major limit-ing factor in sustaining durable benefits of antiviral drug therapy appears to be the emergence of viral mutants with reduced in vitro susceptibility to antiviral drugs.

The emergence of these drug-resistant mutants is the inevitable consequence of incomplete suppression of HIV replication, and the high mutation rate and adapt-ability of the virus. With the currently available arsenal of antiviral drugs, the list of drug resistance mutations that can be found in the HIV genome has grown rap-idly and appears limitless (117).

Although the association between the emergence of specific mutations in the viral genome and in vitro reduced susceptibility has been documented well for many antiviral drugs, many questions remain regarding the exact clinical implica-tions of these drug resistant variants in vivo. Because the goal of antiviral therapy is to obtain maximal suppression of virus replication (this would presumably re-sult in maximal delay of disease progression), there is a consensus that the emergence of drug-resistant viral mutants contributes to reduced efficacy of antiviral drug therapy. But, preferably, one should distinguish the situations in which there is no response to treatment (i.e., the disease progresses as if no drugs were present) and those in which the response is less than optimal (in which case it would be wrong to discontinue drug administration unless better alternatives are available) (118–120).

A major question about drug resistance concerns the virulence and replicative fitness of drug-resistant mutants relative to wild-type virus. Because the mutations that cause drug resistance are either undetectable or are present at very low frequency in wild-type virus in the absence of the selection pressure exerted by drug treatment, one would expect that drug resistance mutations reduce the ability of the virus to replicate. But to what degree are drug-resistant mutants attenuated? Are drug-resistant mutants severely attenuated (so that their emergence does not necessarily affect the efficacy of drug treatment as long as replication of wild-type virus is suppressed), or can they be as pathogenic as wild-type virus? Some information regarding the replicative potential and stability of drug-resistant viral mutants can be gathered from anecdotal case reports, such as those documenting primary infection with drug-resistant HIV-1, as well as those monitoring the reversion of drug-resistant virus to wild-type following discontinuation of drug treatment (121–130). In the future, however, it would be more feasible to already have some idea about the virulence and replicative fitness of drug-resistant mutants before the widespread clinical application of a novel antiviral compound.

Many studies have focused on determining the in vitro growth kinetics of drug-resistant viral mutants (131–133). These studies usually involve comparison of molecular clones in which specific drug resistance mutations have been inserted. Although these in vitro studies are scientifically valid for gaining a better understanding of the molecular basis of drug resistance mutations, one should exert caution in extrapolating their conclusions into the clinical practice. Many mutations that emerge during drug therapy in vivo do not directly affect the level of drug resistance, but are compensatory mutations that allow the virus to replicate better in the presence of the mutations that are directly responsible for the drug-resistant phenotype (131,134,135). This observation indicates that the genetic background in which specific mutations emerge is likely to affect the replicative ability of drug-resistant HIV mutants in vivo. Although in vitro studies can incorporate evaluation of compensatory mutations, it is very difficult for in vitro studies to take all these variables appropriately into account. Finally, investigators should not forget that in vitro culture systems can never completely mimic the complex in vivo situation. Studies in the SIV-macaque model have demonstrated repeatedly that the correlation between viral in vitro growth properties/cell tropism and in vivo replicative ability/virulence is often weak, because virus isolates that are able to replicate well in vitro can be severely attenuated following inoculation in macaques (31,34). Also, resistance patterns selected for in vivo can differ from those selected in vitro (135a).

Thus, the extrapolation of results from these in vitro growth kinetic studies to decisions affecting clinical management of HIV-infected patients should be performed with extreme caution.

An animal model allows approaches that are impossible and unethical to do in humans, but that are the most direct way to study the virulence of drug-resistant mutants, namely to inoculate animals with drug-resistant mutants. Although the SIV animal model has been largely underused in this research area, several macaque studies have addressed the emergence or virulence of drug-resistant SIV. Several techniques were used to generate drug-resistant SIV variants, such as site-directed mutagenesis, as well as in vitro and in vivo drug selection procedures.

Site-directed mutagenesis is a useful way to create drug-resistant SIV variants from molecular clones. However, when these drug-resistant variants are found to be attenuated following inoculation in macaques, one can correctly conclude that the introduced mutations interfere with the ability of the specific molecular clone to replicate in vivo, but one cannot exclude that these specific mutations, when present in a different genetic background (with the required compensatory mutations), can give rise to virus with high virulence. Similarly, because of the different requirements for in vitro versus in vivo replication, in vitro selection for drug-resistant virus by passaging virus in the presence of the drug may introduce the correct mutations directly responsible for increased drug resistance, but may not introduce the correct compensatory mutations, but instead, may also induce other mutations which severely attenuate the in vivo replicative potential of the virus. Accordingly, the fact that in vitro generated drug-resistant mutants are not virulent does not guarantee that similar mutations are not compatible with high virulence in vivo. In contrast, in vivo drug selection by administering drugs to SIV-infected macaques involves concomitant selection for drug resistance and in vivo replicative potential. Thus, using in vivo drug selection is the best way to select for highly virulent drug-resistant mutants, which can replicate to high levels in animals and cause fatal disease. This "worst-case scenario" mimics best the situation in HIV-infected patients and is thus a more appropriate way to determine whether certain drug resistance mutations in HIV-1 can be compatible with high in vivo virulence, and whether their emergence in vivo contributes to reduced efficacy of drug therapy and prophylaxis.

Drug Resistance Studies in the SIV Animal Model. In vitro selection of SIV for resistance to 3TC gave rise to the expected mutations M184I and M184V in RT; the role of these mutations in conferring high-level resistance of SIV to 3TC were confirmed by site-directed mutagenesis (136). Using site-directed mutagenesis, the mutations that are most commonly found in AZT- resistant HIV-1 (codons 67, 70, 215, and 219) have been inserted into the molecular clone SIV$_{mac}$239. The resulting SIV$_{mac}$239 mutant was AZT-resistant in vitro; inoculation of macaques with AZT-resistant SIV$_{mac}$239 and short-term treatment with AZT during the primary viremia resulted in reduced efficacy of AZT treatment to delay antibody development in this model (137).

In vivo selection for drug-resistant SIV was performed in several experiments in infant macaques inoculated with wild-type (i.e., drug-sensitive), highly virulent uncloned SIV$_{mac}$251 and treated with antiviral drugs. AZT-resistant SIV$_{mac}$ mutants were isolated from these infant macaques following prolonged (>8 months) AZT therapy (85); these AZT-resistant SIV mutants (with >100-fold level of resistance) had a glutamine-to-methionine substitution at amino acid 151 of RT (Q151M); this mutation is also found in multiple-drug resistant HIV-1, which emerges in patients during sequential or combination therapy with dideoxynucleoside analogues. Inoculation of the Q151M SIV$_{mac}$ mutant into naive newborn macaques demonstrated that this mutation does not significantly reduce viral replication and viral virulence, and that the Q151M mutation is stable, even in the absence of AZT treatment (138). These results suggest that multiple-drug resistant HIV-1 with the Q151M mutation in HIV-infected patients may have high replicative fitness and that its emergence is worrisome and should be avoided. This is confirmed by recent observations demonstrating that multiple-drug resistant HIV-1 with a Q151M mutation can rapidly acquire extra mutations in RT, conferring resistance to additional RT-inhibitors (139,140), which limits the treatment options for these patients (141).

Studies involving PMPA treatment of SIV-infected macaques demonstrated the usefulness of an animal model to study the emergence and decipher the clinical implications of drug resistance for a novel compound before the availability of any such data from human clinical trials. PMPA had only entered human clinical trials recently, so no data were available yet regarding the emergence of PMPA-resistant HIV-1. However, PMPA treatment of SIV-infected infant macaques resulted in the emergence of virus with five-fold decreased susceptibility to PMPA within a few months of PMPA treatment. This was associated with the development of a lysine-to-arginine substitution at amino acid 65 (K65R) or RT and was followed by additional mutations in RT that were likely to be compensatory mutations (84). The K65R mutation has also been found in HIV-1 selected for resistance to PMEA in vitro (142,143); so it is plausible that the K65R mutation will also emerge in HIV-1 infected patients receiving prolonged PMPA treatment. Remarkably, despite this development of low-level resistant SIV$_{mac}$ in PMPA-treated infant macaques, most animals maintained low viremia levels and were still alive and AIDS-free after more than 3 years of PMPA treatment (84,144). Inoculation of the PMPA-resistant SIV$_{mac}$ variants into newborn macaques demonstrated that, in the absence of PMPA treatment, these variants are as virulent as the parental wild-type SIV$_{mac}$, because these animals showed persistently high virus levels, rapid immunosuppression, and rapid development of fatal disease, which is similar to the disease course seen in newborn macaques following inoculation with the parental wild-type uncloned $SIV_{mac}251$ (144). Thus, the RT mutations associated with low-level PMPA resistance do not attenuate the virus significantly. Most importantly, however, PMPA treatment still had very strong therapeutic benefits (in terms of disease-free survival) for infant macaques inoculated with these PMPA-resistant SIV variants (144). These results obtained in infant macaques suggest that PMPA therapy of HIV-infected patients will still offer therapeutic benefits even in the presence of PMPA- resistant virus; in other words, the emergence of PMPA-resistant HIV-1 in patients during prolonged PMPA therapy is, by itself, not a reason to withdraw PMPA therapy unless a better drug regimen, to which the virus is still sensitive, can be initiated. Studies with newborn macaques have also investigated how PMPA resistance affects the efficacy of chemoprophylaxis: A 4-week PMPA treatment regimen partially protected newborn macaques against oral infection with a 100% infectious dose of PMPA-resistant SIV_{mac}. Some animals were protected against infection, whereas other animals became infected despite short-term PMPA treatment, but they survived significantly longer than untreated control animals (145).

IV. CONCLUSIONS

At the start of the HIV pandemic, nonhuman primate models of HIV infection and AIDS had a limited role in the drug development process, and their potential use was largely unexplored. In recent years, however, the optimization of nonhuman primate models for antiviral drug testing, coupled with a better understanding of HIV disease pathogenesis, is leading to a growing recognition of the relevance of results obtained in these animal models to the clinical management of HIV infection in people. It can be expected that, in coming years, the value of these nonhuman primate models will continue to grow as tools to provide a solid scientific basis to guide human clinical trials.

ACKNOWLEDGMENTS

The authors thank N. Aguirre and S. Dillard-Telm for critical proofreading and correcting of the manuscript.

REFERENCES

1. Centers for Disease Control and Prevention. Update: Trends in AIDS incidence-United States, 1996. MMRW 1997; 46:862–867.
2. Mann JM. AIDS—the second decade: a global perspective. J Infect Dis 1992; 165: 245–250.

3. Daar ES, Li XL, Moudgil T, Ho DD. High concentrations of recombinant soluble CD4 are required to neutralize primary human immunodeficiency virus type 1 isolates. Proc Natl Acad Sci U S A 1990; 87:6574–6578.

4. Lange JMA. Current problems and the future of antiretroviral drug trials. Science 1997; 276:548–550.

5. Cohen J. AIDS trials ethics questioned. Science 1997; 276:520–523.

6. Koch JA, Ruprecht RM. Animal models for anti-AIDS therapy. Antiviral Res 1992; 19:81–109.

7. Kindt TJ, Hirsch VM, Johnson PR, Sawasdikisol S. Animal models for acquired immunodeficiency syndrome. Adv Immunol 1992; 52:425–474.

8. Ruprecht R. The use of animal models to evaluate antiretroviral chemotherapy. Int Antiviral News 1994; 2:2–3.

9. Gardner MB, Luciw PA. Animal models of AIDS. FASEB J 1989; 3:2593–2606.

10. Johnson BK, Stone GA, Godec MS, Asher DM, Gajdusek DC, Gibbs CJJ. Long-term observations of human immunodeficiency virus-infected chimpanzees. AIDS Res Hum Retroviruses 1993; 9:375–378.

11. Fultz PN, Siegel RL, Brodie A, Mawle AC, Stricker RB, Swenson RB, Anderson DC. Prolonged CD4+ lymphocytopenia and thrombocytopenia in a chimpanzee persistently infected with human immunodeficiency virus type 1. J Infect Dis 1991; 163:441–447.

12. Novembre FJ, Saucier M, Anderson DC, Klumpp SA, O'Neill SP, Brown CRn, Hart CE, Guenthner PC, Swenson RB, McClure HM. Development of AIDS in a chimpanzee infected with human immunodeficiency virus. J Virol 1997; 71:4086–4091.

13. Grob PM, Cao Y, Muchmore E, Ho DD, Norris S, Pav JW, Shih C-K, Adams J. Prophylaxis against HIV-1 infection in chimpanzees by nevirapine, a nonnucleoside inhibitor of reverse transcriptase. Nat Med 1997; 3:665–670.

14. Frumkin LR, Agy MB, Combs RW, Panther L, Morton WR, Koehler J, Florey MJ, Dragavon J, Schmidt A, Katze MG, Corey L. Acute infection of *Macaca nemestrina* by human immunodeficiency virus type 1. Virology 1993; 195:422–431.

15. Agy MB, Frumkin LR, Corey L, Coombs RW, Wolinsky SM, Koehler J, Morton WR, Katze MG. Infection of *Macaca nemestrina* by human immunodeficiency virus type-1. Science 1992; 257:103–106.

16. Daniel MD, Letvin NL, King NW, Kannagi M, Sehgal PK, Hunt RD, Kanki PJ, Essex M, Desrosiers RC. Isolation of T-cell tropic HTLV-III-like retrovirus from macaques. Science 1985; 228:1201–1204.

17. Hirsch VM, Campbell BJ, Bailes E, Goeken R, Brown C, Elkins WR, Axthelm M, Murphey-Corb M, Sharp PM. Characterization of a novel simian immunodeficiency virus (SIV) from L'Hoest monkeys (*Cercopithecus l'hoesti*): implications for the origins of SIVmnd and other primate lentiviruses. J Virol 1999; 73:1036–1045.

18. Desrosiers RC. The simian immunodeficiency viruses. Ann Rev Immunol 1990; 8:557–578.

19. Hu S-L, Haigwood NL, Morton WR. Non-human primate models for AIDS research. In: Morrow WJW, Haigwood NL, eds. HIV Molecular Organization, Pathogenicity and Treatment. Amsterdam: Elsevier, 1993:294–327.

20. Gardner MB. The history of simian AIDS. J Med Primatol 1996; 25:148–157.

21. Letvin NL, King NW. Immunologic and pathologic manifestations of the infection of rhesus monkeys with simian immunodeficiency virus of macaques. J Acquir Immune Defic Syndr 1990; 3:1023–1040.
22. Fultz PN, McClure HM, Anderson DC, Switzer WM. Identification and biologic characterization of an acutely lethal variant of simian immunodeficiency virus from sooty mangabeys (SIV/SMM). AIDS Res Hum Retroviruses 1989; 5:397–409.
23. Israel ZR, Dean GA, Maul DH, O'Neil SP, Dreitz MJ, Mullins JI, Fultz PN, Hoover EA. Early pathogenesis of disease caused by SIVsmmPBj14 molecular clone 1.9 in macaques. AIDS Res Hum Retroviruses 1993; 9:277–286.
24. Du ZJ, Lang SM, Sasseville VG, Lackner AA, Ilyinskii PO, Daniel MD, Jung JU, Desrosiers RC. Identification of a nef allele that causes lymphocyte activation and acute disease in macaque monkeys. Cell 1995; 82:665–674.
25. Böttiger D, Putkonen P, Öberg B. Prevention of HIV-2 and SIV infections in cynomolgus macaques by prophylactic treatment with 3′-fluorothymidine. AIDS Res Hum Retrovir 1992; 8:1235–1238.
26. Böttiger D, Johansson NG, Samuelsson B, Zhang H, Putkonen P, Vrang L, Öberg B. Prevention of simian immunodeficiency virus, SIVsm, or HIV-2 infection in cynomolgus monkeys by pre- and postexposure administration of BEA-005. AIDS 1997; 11:157–162.
27. Watson A, McClure J, Ranchalis J, Scheibel M, Schmidt A, Kennedy B, Morton WR, Haigwood NL, Hu S-L. Early postinfection antiviral treatment reduces viral load and prevents CD4+ cell decline in HIV type 2-infected macaques. AIDS Res Hum Retroviruses 1997; 13:1375–1381.
28. Dormont D, Livartowski J, Chamaret S, Guetard D, Henin D, Levagueresse R, van de Moortelle PF, Larke B, Gourmelon P, Vazeux R, Metivier H, Flageat J, Court L, Hauw JJ, Montagnier L. HIV-2 in rhesus monkeys: serological, virological and clinical results. Intervirology 1989; 30(suppl 1):59–65.
29. Livartowski J, Dormont D, Boussin F, Chamaret S, Guetard D, Vazeux R, Lebon P, Metivier H, Montagnier L. Clinical and virological aspects of HIV2 infection in rhesus monkeys. Cancer Det Prev 1992; 16:341–345.
30. Kestler H, Kodama T, Ringler D, Marthas M, Pedersen N, Lackner A, Regier D, Sehgal P, Daniel M, King N, Desrosiers R. Induction of AIDS in rhesus monkeys by molecularly cloned simian immunodeficiency virus. Science 1990; 248:1109–1112.
31. Kestler HW III, Ringler DJ, Mori K, Panicalli DL, Sehgal PK, Daniel MD, Desrosiers RC. Importance of the nef gene for maintenance of high virus loads and for development of AIDS. Cell 1991; 65:651–662.
32. Marthas ML, Sutjipto S, Higgins J, Lohman B, Torten J, Luciw PA, Marx PA, Pedersen NC. Immunization with a live, attenuated simian immunodeficiency virus (SIV) prevents early disease but not infection in rhesus macaques challenged with pathogenic SIV. J Virol 1990; 64:3694–3700.
33. Marthas ML, Ramos RA, Lohman BL, Van Rompay KKA, Unger RE, Miller CJ, Banapour B, Pedersen NC, Luciw PA. Viral determinants of simian immunodeficiency virus (SIV) virulence in rhesus macaques assessed by using attenuated and pathogenic molecular clones of SIVmac. J Virol 1993; 67:6047–6055.
34. Lohman BL, McChesney MB, Miller CJ, McGowan E, Joye SM, Van Rompay KKA, Reay E, Antipa L, Pedersen NC, Marthas ML. A partially attenuated simian im-

munodeficiency virus induces host immunity that correlates with resistance to pathogenic virus challenge. J Virol 1994; 68:7021–7029.

35. Bohm RP, Martin LN, Davison-Fairburn B, Baskin GB, Murphey-Corb M. Neonatal disease induced by SIV infection of the rhesus monkey (*Macaca mulatta*). AIDS
Res Hum Retroviruses 1993; 9:1131–1137.

36. Marthas ML, Van Rompay KKA, Otsyula M, Miller CJ, Canfield D, Pedersen NC,
McChesney MB. Viral factors determine progression to AIDS in simian immunodeficiency virus-infected newborn rhesus macaques. J Virol 1995; 69:4198–4205.

37. Otsyula MG, Miller CJ, Marthas ML, Van Rompay KKA, Collins JR, Pedersen NC,
McChesney MB. Virus-induced immunosuppression is linked to rapidly fatal disease
in infant rhesus macaques infected with simian immunodeficiency virus. Pediatr Res
1996; 39:630–635.

38. Ashorn P, McQuade TJ, Thaisrivongs S, Tomasselli AG. An inhibitor of the protease
blocks maturation of human and simian immunodeficiency viruses and spread of infection. Proc Natl Acad Sci U S A 1990; 87:7472–7476.

39. Black PL, Downs MB, Lewis MG, Ussery MA, Dreyer GB, Petteway SRJ, Lambert
DM. Antiretroviral activities of protease inhibitors against murine leukemia virus and
simian immunodeficiency virus in culture. Antimicrob Agents Chemother 1993; 37:
71–77.

40. Grant SK, Deckman IC, Minnich MD, Culp J, Franklin S, Dreyer GB, Tomaszek
TAJ, Debouck C, Meek TD. Purification and biochemical characterization of recombinant simian immunodeficiency virus protease and comparison to human immunodeficiency virus type 1 protease. Biochemistry 1991; 30:8424–8434.

41. Sager PR, Cradock JC, Litterst CL, Martin LN, Soike KF, Murphey-Corb M, Marx
PA, Tsai CC, Fridland A, Bodner A, Resnick L, Schinazi RF. In vitro testing of therapeutics against SIV and HIV. Ann N Y Acad Sci 1990; 616:599–605.

42. Wu JC, Chernow M, Boehme RE, Suttmann RT, McRoberts MJ, Prisbe EJ, Matthews
TR, Marx PA, Chuang RY, Chen MS. Kinetics and inhibition of reverse transcriptase from human and simian immunodeficiency viruses. Antimicrob Agents Chemother 1988; 32:1887–1890.

43. De Clercq E. HIV inhibitors targeted at the reverse transcriptase. AIDS Res Hum
Retroviruses 1992; 8:119–134.

44. Li J, Lord CI, Haseltine W, Letvin NL, Sodroski J. Infection of cynomolgus monkeys with a chimeric HIV-1/SIVmac virus that expresses the HIV-1 envelope glycoproteins. J Acquir Immune Defic Syndr 1992; 5:639–646.

45. Joag SV, Li Z, Foresman L, Stephens EB, Zhao LJ, Adany I, Pinson DM, McClure
HM, Narayan O. Chimeric simian human immunodeficiency virus that causes progressive loss of CD4+ T cells and AIDS in pig-tailed macaques. J Virol 1996; 70:
3189–3197.

46. Igarashi T, Shibata R, Hasebe F, Ami Y, Shinohara K, Komatsu T, Stahl-Hennig C,
Petry H, Hunsmann G, Kuwata T, Jin M, Adachi A, Kurimura T, Okada M, Miura T,
Hayami M. Persistent infection with SIVmac chimeric virus having tat, rev, vpu, env
and nef of HIV type 1 in macaque monkeys. AIDS Res Hum Retroviruses 1994; 10:
1021–1030.

47. Igarashi T, Ami Y, Yamamoto H, Shibata R, Kuwata T, Mukai R, Shinohara K, Komatsu T, Adachi A, Hayami M. Protection of monkeys vaccinated with vpr-and/or

nef-defective simian immunodeficiency virus strain mac/human immunodeficiency virus type 1 chimeric viruses: a potential candidate live-attenuated human AIDS vaccine. J Gen Virol 1997; 78:985–989.

48.   Dunn CS, Beyer C, Kieny MP, Gloeckler L, Schmitt D, Gut JP, Kirn A, Aubertin AM. High viral load and CD4 lymphopenia in rhesus and cynomolgus macaques infected by a chimeric primate lentivirus constructed using the env, rev, tat, and vpu genes from HIV-1 Lai. Virology 1996; 223:351–361.

49.   Kuwata T, Igarashi T, Ido E, Jin MH, Mizuno A, Chen JL, Hayami M. Construction of human immunodeficiency virus1/simian immunodeficiency virus strain mac chimeric viruses having vpr and/or nef of different parental origins and their in vitro and in vivo replication. J Gen Virol 1995; 76:2181–2191.

50.   Kuwata T, Shoida T, Igarashi T, Ido E, Ibuki K, Enose Y, Stahl-Hennig C, Hunsmann G, Miura T, Hayami M. Chimeric viruses between SIVmac and various HIV-1 isolates have biological properties that are similar to those of the parental HIV-1. AIDS 1996; 10:1331–1337.

51.   Quesada-Rolander M, Makitalo B, Thorstensson R, Zhang YJ, Castanos-Yelez E, Biberfeld G, Putkonen P. Protection against mucosal SIVsm challenge in macaques infected with a chimeric SIV that expresses HIV type 1 envelope. AIDS Res Hum Retroviruses 1996; 12:993–999.

52.   Reimann KA, Li JT, Veazey R, Halloran M, Park IW, Karlsson GB, Sodroski J, Letvin NL. A chimeric simian/human immunodeficiency virus expressing a primary patient human immunodeficiency virus type 1 isolate env causes an AIDS-like disease after in vivo passage in rhesus monkeys. J Virol 1996; 70:6922–6928.

53.   Reimann KA, Li JT, Voss G, Lekutis C, Tenner-Racz K, Racz P, Lin WY, Montefiori DC, Lee-Parritz DE, Lu YC, Collman RG, Sodroski J, Letvin NL. An env gene derived from a primary human immunodeficiency virus type 1 isolate confers high in vivo replicative capacity to a chimeric simian human immunodeficiency virus in rhesus monkeys. J Virol 1996; 70:3198–3206.

54.   Überla K, Stahl-Hennig C, Böttiger D, Mätz-Rensing K, Kaup FJ, Li J, Haseltine WA, Fleckenstein B, Hunsmann G, Öberg B, Sodroski J. Animal model for the therapy of acquired immunodeficiency syndrome with reverse transcriptase inhibitors. Proc Natl Acad Sci U S A 1995; 92:8210–8214.

55.   Balzarini J, De Clercq E, Überla K. SIV/HIV-1 hybrid virus expressing the reverse transcriptase gene of HIV-1 remains sensitive to HIV-1-specific reverse transcriptase inhibitors after passage in rhesus macaques. J Acquir Immune Defic Syndr Human Retrovirol 1997; 15:1–4.

56.   Ha JC, Nosbisch C, Conrad SH, Ruppenthal GC, Sackett GP, Abkowitz J, Unadkat JD. Fetal toxicity of zidovudine (azidothymidine) in *Macaca nemestrina*: preliminary observations. J Acquir Immune Defic Syndr 1994; 7:154–157.

57.   Lopez-Anaya A, Unadkat JD, Schumann LA, Smith AL. Pharmacokinetics of zidovudine (azidothymidine). II. Development of metabolic and renal clearance pathways in the neonate. J Acquir Immune Defic Syndr 1990; 3:1052–1058.

58.   Lopez-Anaya A, Unadkat JD, Schumann LA, Smith AL. Pharmacokinetics of zidovudine (azidothymidine). I. Transplacental transfer. J Acquir Immune Defic Syndr 1990; 3:959–964.

59.   Lopez-Anaya A, Unadkat JD, Schumann LA, Smith AL. Pharmacokinetics of zi-

dovudine (azidothymidine). III. Effect of pregnancy. J Acquir Immune Defic Syndr 1991; 4:64–68.

60. Odineces A, Pereira C, Nosbisch C, Unadkat JD. Prenatal and postpartum pharmacokinetics of stavudine (2´,3´-didehydro-3´-deoxythymidine) and didanosine (dideoxyinosine) in pigtailed macaques (*Macaca nemestrina*). Antimicrob Agents Chemother 1996; 40:2423–2425.

61. Odinecs A, Nosbisch C, Unadkat JD. Zidovudine does not affect transplacental transfer of systemic clearance of stavudine (2´,3´-didehydro-deoxythymidine) in the pigtailed macaque (*Macaca nemestrina*). Antimicrob Agents Chemother 1996; 40: 1569–1571.

62. Odinecs A, Nosbisch C, Keller RD, Baughman WL, Unadkat JD. In vivo maternalfetal pharmacokinetics of stavudine (2´,3´-didehydro-3´-deoxythymidine) in pigtailed macaques (*Macaca nemestrina*). Antimicrob Agents Chemother 1996; 40: 196–202.

63. Pereira CM, Nosbisch C, Winter HR, Baughman WL, Unadkat JD. Transplacental pharmacokinetics of dideoxyinosine in pigtailed macaques. Antimicrob Agents Chemother 1994; 38:781–786.

64. Pereira CM, Nosbisch C, Unadkat JD. Pharmacokinetics of dideoxyinosine in neonatal pigtailed macaques. Antimicrob Agents Chemother 1994; 38:787–789.

65. Pereira CM, Nosbisch C, Baughman WL, Unadkat JD. Effect of zidovudine on transplacental pharmacokinetics of ddI in the pigtailed macaque (*Macaca nemestrina*). Antimicrob Agents Chemother 1995; 39:343–345.

66. Qian M, Bui T, Ho RJY, Unadkat JD. Metabolism of 3´-azido-3´-deoxythymidine (AZT) in human placental trophoblasts and Hofbauer cells. Biochem Pharmacol 1994; 48:383–389.

67. Qian M, Chandrasena G, Ho RJH, Unadkat JD. Comparison of rates of intracellular metabolism of zidovudine in human and primate peripheral blood mononuclear cells. Antimicrob Agents Chemother 1994; 38:2398–2403.

68. Ravasco RJ, Unadkat JD, Tsai C-C, Nosbisch C. Pharmacokinetics of dideoxyinosine in pigtailed macaques (*Macaca nemestrina*) after intravenous and subcutaneous administration. J Acquir Immune Defic Syndr 1992; 5:1016–1018.

69. Tuntland T, Nosbisch C, Baughman W, Massarella J, Unadkat J. Mechanism and rate of placental transfer of zalcitabine (2´,3´-dideoxycytidine) in *Macaca nemestrina*. Am J Obstet Gynecol 1996; 174:856–863.

70. Tarantal AF, Spanggord RJ, Hendrickx AG. Pre- and postnatal treatment of the rhesus macaque (*Macaca mulatta*) with azidothymidine: I. Fetal studies. Pediatr AIDS HIV Infect 1994; 5:10–19.

71. Balzarini J, Naesens L, Slachmuylders J, Niphuis H, Rosenberg I, Holy A, Schellekens H, De Clercq E. 9-(2-phosphonylmethoxyethyl)adenine (PMEA) effectively inhibits retrovirus replication in vitro and simian immunodeficiency virus infection in rhesus monkeys. AIDS 1991; 5:21–28.

72. Tsai C-C, Follis KE, Yarnall M, Deaver LE, Benveniste RE, Sager PR. In vitro screening for antiretroviral against simian immunodeficiency virus (SIV). Antiviral Res 1990; 14:87–98.

73. Van Rompay KKA, Otsyula M, Marthas ML, Pedersen NC. Simian immunodeficiency virus infection of newborn and infant rhesus macaques: an animal model for testing antiretroviral drugs. Int Antiviral News 1994; 2:5–6.

74. Böttiger D, Ståhle L, Li S-L, Öberg B. Long-term tolerance and efficacy of 3′-azido-thymidine and 3′-fluorothymidine treatment of asymptomatic monkeys infected with simian immunodeficiency virus. Antimicrob Agents Chemother 1992; 36:1770–1772.

75. Mellors JW, Rinaldo CRJ, Gupta P, White RM, Todd JA, Kingsley LA. Prognosis in HIV-1 infection predicted by the quantity of virus in plasma. Science 1996; 272: 1167–1170.

76. Wei X, Ghosh SK, Taylor ME, Johnson VA, Emini EA, Deutsch P, Lifson JD, Bonhoeffer S, Nowak MA, Hahn BH, Saag MS, Shaw GM. Viral dynamics in human immunodeficiency virus type 1 infection. Nature 1995; 373:117–122.

77. Ho DD, Neumann AU, Perelson AS, Chen W, Leonard JM, Markowitz M. Rapid turnover of plasma virions and CD4 lymphocytes in HIV-1 infection. Nature 1995; 373:123–126.

78. Tsai C-C, Follis KE, Beck TW, Sabo A, Bischofberger N, Dailey PJ. Effects of (R)-9-(2-phosphonylmethoxypropyl)adenine monotherapy on chronic SIV infection. AIDS Res Hum Retroviruses 1997; 13:707–712.

79. European Collaborative Study. Children born to women with HIV-1 infection: natural history and risk of transmission. Lancet 1991; 337:253–260.

80. Blanche S, Rouzioux C, Guihard Moscato M-L, Veber F, Mayaux M-J, Jacomet C, Tricoire J, Deville A, Vial M, Firtion G, de Crepy A, Douard D, Robin M, Courpotin C, Ciraru-Vigneron N, le Deist F, Griscelli C, the HIV Infection in Newborns French Collaborative Study Group. A prospective study of infants born to women seropositive for human immunodeficiency virus type 1. N Engl J Med 1989; 320:1643–1648.

81. Scott GB, Hutto C, Makuch RW, Mastrucci MT, O'Connor T, Mitchell CD, Trapido EJ, Parks WP. Survival in children with perinatally acquired human immunodeficiency virus type 1 infection. N Engl J Med 1989; 321:1791–1796.

82. Epstein LG, Boucher CA, Morrison SH, Connor EM, Oleske JM, Lange JMA, van der Noordaa J, Bakker M, Dekker J, Scherpbier H, van den Berg H, Boer K, Goudsmit J. Persistent human immunodeficiency virus type 1 antigenemia in children correlates with disease progression. Pediatrics 1988; 82:919–924.

83. Pollack H, Zhan MX, Ilmet-Moore T, Ajuang-Simbiri K, Krasinski K, Borkowsky W. Ontogeny of anti-human immunodeficiency virus (HIV) antibody production in HIV-1-infected infants. Proc Natl Acad Sci U S A 1993; 90:2340–2344.

84. Van Rompay KKA, Cherrington JM, Marthas ML, Berardi CJ, Mulato AS, Spinner A, Tarara RP, Canfield DR, Telm S, Bischofberger N, Pedersen NC. 9-[2-(Phosphonomethoxy)propyl]adenine therapy of established simian immunodeficiency virus infection in infant rhesus macaques. Antimicrob Agents Chemother 1996; 40:2586–2591.

85. Van Rompay KKA, Otsyula MG, Marthas ML, Miller CJ, McChesney MB, Pedersen NC. Immediate zidovudine treatment protects simian immunodeficiency virus-infected newborn macaques against rapid onset of AIDS. Antimicrob Agents Chemother 1995; 39:125–131.

86. Ammann AJ. Human immunodeficiency virus infection/AIDS in children: the next decade. Pediatrics 1994; 93:930–935.

87. Wyand MS. The use of SIV-infected rhesus monkeys for the preclinical evaluation of AIDS drugs and vaccines. AIDS Res Hum Retrovir 1992; 8:349–356.

88. Fazely F, Haseltine WA, Rodger RF, Ruprecht RM. Postexposure chemoprophylaxis

with ZDV or ZDV combined with interferon-α: failure after inoculating rhesus monkeys with a high dose of SIV. J Acquir Immune Defic Syndr 1991; 4:1093–1097.

89. Lundgren B, Bottiger D, Ljungdahl-Ståhle E, Norrby E, Ståhle L, Wahren B, Öberg B. Antiviral effects of 3´-fluorothymidine and 3´-azidothymidine in cynomolgus monkeys infected with simian immunodeficiency virus. J Acquir Immune Defic Syndr 1991; 4:489–498.

90. McClure HM, Anderson DC, Ansari AA, Fultz PN, Klumpp SA, Schinazi RF. Nonhuman primate models for evaluation of AIDS therapy. Ann N Y Acad Sci 1990; 616: 287– 298.

91. Van Rompay KKA, Marthas ML, Lifson JD, Berardi CJ, Vasquez GM, Agatep E, Dehqanzada ZA, Cundy KC, Bischofberger N, Pedersen NC. Administration of 9-[2-(phosphonomethoxy)prophyl]adenine (PMPA) for prevention of perinatal simian immunodeficiency virus infection in rhesus macaques. AIDS Res Hum Retroviruses 1998; 14:761–773.

92. Van Rompay KKA, Berardi CJ, Aguirre NL, Bischofberger N, Lietman PS, Pedersen NC, Marthas ML. Two doses of PMPA protect newborn macaques against oral simian immunodeficiency virus infection. AIDS 1998; 12:F79–F83.

93. Böttiger D, Vrang L, Öberg B. Influence of the infectious dose of simian immunodeficiency virus on the acute infection in cynomolgus monkeys and on the effect of treatment with 3´-fluorothymidine. Antivir Chem Chemother 1992; 3:267–271.

94. Tsai C-C, Follis KE, Sabo A, Grant RF, Bartz C, Note RE, Benveniste RE, Bischofberger N. Preexposure prophylaxis with 9-(2-phosphonylmethoxyethyl)adenine against simian immunodeficiency virus infection in macaques. J Infect Dis 1994; 169:260–266.

95. Tsai C-C, Follis KE, Beck TW, Sabo A, Grant RF, Bischofberger N, Benveniste RE. Prevention of simian immunodeficiency virus infection in macaques by 9-(2-phosphonylmethoxypropyl)adenine (PMPA). Science 1995; 270:1197–1199.

96. Lange JMA, Boucher CAB, Hollak CEM, Wiltink EHH, Reiss P, van Royen EA, Roos M, Danner SA, Goudsmit J. Failure of zidovudine prophylaxis after accidental exposure to HIV-1. N Engl J Med 1990; 322:1375–1377.

97. Anonymous. HIV seroconversion after occupational exposure despite early prophylactic zidovudine therapy. Lancet 1993; 341:1077–1078.

98. Durand E, Le Jeunne C, Hugues F. Failure of prophylactic zidovudine after suicidal self-inoculation of HIV- Infected blood. N Engl J Med 1991; 324:1062.

99. Centers for Disease Control and Prevention. Case-control study of HIV seroconversion in health-care workers after percutaneous exposure to HIV-infected blood-France, United Kingdom, and United States, January 1988-August 1994. MMRW 1995; 44:929–933.

100. Centers for Disease Control and Prevention. Update: provisional Public Health Service recommendations for chemoprophylaxis after occupational exposure to HIV. MMRW 1996; 45:468–472.

101. Gerberding JL. Prophylaxis for occupational exposure to HIV. Ann Intern Med 1996; 125:497–501.

102. Connor EM, Sperling RS, Gelber R, Kiselev P, Scott G, O'Sullivan MJ, VanDyke R, Bey M, Shearer W, Jacobson RL, Jiminez E, O'Neill E, Bazin B, Delfraissy J-F, Culnane M, Coombs R, Elkins M, Moye J, Stratton P, Balsley J, for the Pediatric AIDS

Clinical Trials Group Protocol 076 Study Group. Reduction of maternal-infant transmission of human immunodeficiency virus type 1 with zidovudine treatment. N Engl J Med 1994; 331:1173–1180.

103. Centers for Disease Control and Prevention. Administration of zidovudine during late pregnancy and delivery to prevent perinatal HIV transmission-Thailand, 1996–1998. MMWR 1998; 47:151–154.

104. Wade NA, Birkhead GS, Warren BL, Charbonneau TT, French PT, Wang L, Baum JB, Tesoriero JM, Savicki R. Abbreviated regimens of zidovudine prophylaxis and perinatal transmission of the human immunodeficiency virus. N Engl J Med 1998; 12:1409–1414.

105. Martin LN, Murphey-Corb M, Soike KF, Davison-Fairburn B, Baskin GB. Effects of initiation of 3′-azido-3′-deoxythymidine treatment at different times after infection of rhesus monkeys with simian immunodeficiency virus. J Infect Dis 1993; 168: 825–835.

106. Tsai C-C, Follis KE, Grant RF, Nolte RE, Bartz CR, Benveniste RE, Sager PR. Effect of dosing frequency on ZDV prophylaxis in macaques infected with simian immunodeficiency virus. J Acquir Immune Defic Syndr 1993; 6:1086–1092.

107. Joag SV, Li Z, Foresman L, Pinson DM, Stephens EB, Raghavan R, Navé J-F, Casara P, Narayan O. Early treatment with 9-(2-phosphonylmethoxyethyl)adenine reduces virus burdens for a prolonged period in SIV-infected rhesus macaques. AIDS Res Hum Retroviruses 1997; 13:241–246.

108. Le Grand R, Clayette P, Noack O, Vaslin B, Theodoro F, Michel G, Roques P, Dormont D. An animal model for antilentiviral therapy: effect of zidovudine on viral load during acute infection after exposure of macaques to simian immunodeficiency virus. AIDS Res Hum Retroviruses 1994; 10:1279–1287.

109. Van Rompay KKA, Dailey PJ, Tarara RP, Canfield DR, Aguirre NL, Cherrington JM, Lamy PD, Bischofberger N, Pedersen NC, Marthas ML. Early short-term 9-[2-(phosphonomethoxy)prophyl]adenine (PMPA) treatment favorably alters subsequent disease course in simian immunodeficiency virus-infected newborn rhesus macaques. J Virol 1999; 73:2947–2955.

110. Rausch DM, Heyes MP, Murray EA, Eiden LE. Zidovudine treatment prolongs survival and decreases virus load in the central nervous system of rhesus macaques infected perinatally with simian immunodeficiency virus. J Infect Dis 1995; 172:59–69.

111. Rosenberg ES, Billingsley JM, Caliendo AM, Boswell SL, Sax PE, Kalams SA, Walker BD. Vigorous HIV-1-specific CD4+ T cell responses associated with control of viremia. Science 1997; 278:1447–1450.

112. Kinloch-de Loës S, Hirschel BJ, Hoen B, Cooper DA, Tindall B, Carr A, Saurat J-H, Clumeck N, Lazzarin A, Mathiesen L, Raffi F, Antunes F, Von Overbeck J, Lüthy R, Glauser M, Hawkins D, Baumberger C, Yerly S, Perneger TV, Perrin L. A controlled trial of zidovudine in primary human immunodeficiency virus infection. N Engl J Med 1995; 333:408–413.

113. Lafeuillade A, Poggi C, Tamalet C, Profizi N, Tourres C, Costes O. Effects of a combination of zidovudine, didanosine, and lamivudine on primary human immunodeficiency virus type 1 infection. J Infect Dis 1997; 175:1051–1055.

114. Van Rompay KKA, Marthas ML, Ramos RA, Mandell CP, McGowan EK, Joye SM, Pedersen NC. Simian immunodeficiency virus (SIV) infection of infant rhesus

macaques as a model to test antiretroviral drug prophylaxis and therapy: oral 3′-azido-3′-deoxythymidine prevents SIV infection. Antimicrob Agents Chemother 1992; 36:2381–2386.

115. Tsai C-C, Follis KE, Sabo A, Grant R, Bischofberger N. Efficacy of 9-(2-phospho-nylmethoxyethyl)adenine treatment against chronic simian immunodeficiency virus infection in macaques. J Infect Dis 1995; 171:1338–1343.

116. Nowak MA, Lloyd AL, Vasquez GM, Wiltrout TA, Wahl LM, Bischofberger N, Williams J, Kinter A, Fauci AS, Hirsch VM, Lifson JD. Viral dynamics of primary viremia and antiretroviral therapy in simian immunodeficiency virus infection. J Virol 1997; 71:7518–7525.

117. Schinazi RF, Larder BA, Mellors JW. Mutations in retroviral genes associated with drug resistance. Int Antiviral News 1996; 4:95–107.

118. Darby G, Larder BA. The clinical significance of antiviral drug resistance. Res Virol 1992; 143:116–120.

119. Richman DD. The clinical significance of drug-resistant mutants of human immun-odeficiency virus. Res Virol 1992; 143:130–131.

120. Richman DD. Resistance, drug failure, and disease progression. AIDS Res Hum Retroviruses 1994; 10:901–905.

121. Albert J, Wahlberg J, Lundeberg J, Cox S, Sandström E, Wahren B, Uhlen M. Per-sistence of azidothymidine-resistant human immunodeficiency virus type RNA genotypes in posttreatment serum. J Virol 1992; 66:5627–5630.

122. Angarana G, Monno L, Appice A, Giannelli A, Romalli C, Fico C, Pastore G. Trans-mission of zidovudine-resistant HIV-1 through heterosexual contacts. AIDS 1994; 8:1013–1014.

123. Boucher CAB, van Leeuwen R, Kellam P, Schipper P, Tijnagel J, Lange JMA, Larder BA. Effects of discontinuation of zidovudine treatment on zidovudine sensitivity of human immunodeficiency virus type 1 isolates. Antimicrob Agents Chemother 1993; 37:1525–1530.

124. Imrie A, Beveridge A, Genn W, Vizzard J, Cooper DA. Transmission of human im-munodeficiency virus type 1 resistant to nevirapine and zidovudine. J Infect Dis 1997; 175:1502–1506.

125. Imrie A, Carr A, Duncombe C, Finalyson R, Vizzard J, Law M, Kaldor J, Penny R, Cooper D. Primary infection with zidovudine-resistant human immunodeficiency virus type 1 does not adversely affect outcome at 1 year. Sidney Primary HIV In-fection Study Group. J Infect Dis 1996; 174:195–198.

126. Ippolito G, Del Poggio P, Arici C, Gregis GP, Antonelli G, Riva E, Dianzani F. Trans-mission of zidovudine-resistant HIV during a bloody fight. JAMA 1994; 272:433–434.

127. Goudsmit J, De Ronde A, Ho DD, Perelson AS. Human immunodeficiency virus fit-ness in vivo: calculations based on a single zidovudine resistance mutation at codon 215 of reverse transcriptase. J Virol 1996; 70:5662–5664.

128. Masquelier B, Lemoigne E, Pellegrin I, Douard D, Sandler B, Fleury HJA. Primary infection with zidovudine-resistant HIV (letter). N Engl J Med 1993; 329:1123–1124.

129. Sönnerborg A, Johansson B, Ayehunie S, Jolander I. Transmission of zidovudine-re-sistant HIV-1. AIDS 1993; 7:1684–1685.

130. Yerly S, Rakik A, Kinloch S, Hirschel B, Perrin L. Persistence of ZDV resistant mu-tations in patients with primary HIV infection. Fifth International Workshop on HIV

Drug Resistance, Whistler, Canada (July 3–6), 1996:82.

131. Maeda Y, Venzon DJ, Mitsuya H. Altered drug sensitivity, fitness, and evolution of human immunodeficiency virus type 1 with pol gene mutations conferring multi-dideoxynucleoside resistance. J Infect Dis 1998; 177:1207–1213.

132. Caliendo AM, Savara A, An D, DeVore K, Kaplan JC, D'Aquila RT. Effects of zi-dovudine-selected human immunodeficiency virus type 1 reverse transcriptase amino acid substitutions on processive DNA synthesis and viral replication. J Virol 1996; 70:2146–2153.

133. Croteau G, Doyon L, Thibeault D, McKercher G, Pilote L, Lamarre D. Impaired fit-ness of human immunodeficiency virus type 1 variants with high-level resistance to protease inhibitors. J Virol 1997; 71:1089–1096.

134. Iversen AKN, Shafer RW, Wehrly K, Winters MA, Mullins JI, Chesebro B, Merigan TC. Multidrug-resistant human immunodeficiency virus type 1 strains resulting from combination antiretroviral therapy. J Virol 1996; 70:1086–1090.

135. Ho DD, Toyoshima T, Mo H, Kempf DJ, Norbeck D, Chen C-M, Wideburg NE, Burt SK, Erickson JW, Singh MK. Characterization of human immunodeficiency virus type 1 variants with increased resistance to a C2-symmetric protease inhibitor. J Virol 1994; 68:2016–2020.

135a. Rübsamen-Waigmann H, Huguenel E, Shah A, Ruoff H-J, von Briesen H, Immel-mann A, Wainberg MA, Dietrich U. Resistance mutations selected in vivo under ther-apy with anti-HIV drug HBY 097 differ from resistance pattern selected in vitro. An-tiviral Res 1999; 42:15–24.

136. Cherry E, Slater M, Salomon H, Rud E, Wainberg MA. Mutations at codon 184 in simian immunodeficiency virus reverse transcriptase confer resistance to the (-) enan-tiomer of 2´, 3´-dideoxy-thiacytidine. Antimicrob Agents Chemother 1997; 41:2763–2765.

137. Böttiger D, Kemp SD, Larder BA, Zhang H, Vrang L, Öberg B, AZT resistant SIV-mac is refractile to AZT therapy in monkeys. 14th Annual Symposium on Nonhu-man Primate Models for AIDS, October 23–26, Portland, OR, 1996.

138. Van Rompay KKA, Greenier JL, Marthas ML, Otsyula MG, Tarara RP, Miller CJ, Pedersen NC. A zidovudine-resistant simian immunodeficiency virus mutant with a Q151M mutation in reverse transcriptase causes AIDS in newborn macaques. An-timicrob Agents Chemother 1997; 41:278–283.

139. Schmit J-C, Cogniaux J, Hermans P, Van Vaeck C, Sprecher S, Van Remoortel B, Witvrouw M, Balzarini J, Desmyter J, De Clercq E, Vandamme A-M. Multiple drug resistance to nucleoside analogues and non-nucleoside reverse transcriptase in-hibitors in an efficiency replicating HIV-1 patient strain. J Infect Dis 1996; 174:962–968.

140. Shafer RW, Winters MA, Iversen AKN, Merigan TC. Genotypic and phenotypic changes during culture of a multinucleoside-resistant human immunodeficiency virus type 1 strain in the presence and absence of additional reverse transcriptase in-hibitors. Antimicrob Agents Chemother 1996; 40:2887–2890.

141. Schmit JC, Clotet B, Ruiz L, Hermans P, Sprecher S, Arendt V, Leal M, Lissen E, Harrer T, De Clercq E, Witvrouw M, Vandamme A-M. Multiple dideoxynucleoside analogue-resistant HIV-1 in Europe. International Workshop on HIV Drug Resis-tance, Treatment Strategies and Eradication, St. Petersburg, FL, 25–28 June, 1997:38.

142. Foli A, Sogocio KM, Anderson B, Kavlick M, Saville MW, Wainberg MA, Gu X, Cherrington JM, Mitsuya H, Yarchoan R. In vitro selection and molecular characterization of human immunodeficiency virus type 1 with reduced sensitivity to 9-(2-phosphonylmethoxyethyl)adenine. Antiviral Res 1996; 32:91–98.

143. Gu Z, Salomono H, Cherrington JM, Mulato AS, Chen MS, Yarchoan R, Foli A, Sogocio KM, Wainberg MA. K65R mutation of human immunodeficiency virus type 1 reverse transcriptase encodes cross-resistance to 9-(2-phosphonylmethoxyethyl)adenine. Antimicrob Agents Chemother 1995; 39:1888–1891.

144. Van Rompay KKA, Cherrington JM, Marthas ML, Lamy PD, Dailey PJ, Canfield DR, Tarara RP, Bischofberger N, Pedersen NC. 9-[2-(Phosphonomethoxy) propyl]adenine (PMPA) therapy prolongs survival of infant macaques inoculated with simian immunodeficiency virus with reduced susceptibility to PMPA. Antimicrob Agents Chemother 1999; 43:802–812.

145. Van Rompay KKA, Miller MD, Marthas ML, Margot NA, Dailey PJ, Tarara RP, Canfield DR, Cherrington JM, Aguirre NL, Bischofberger N, Pedersen NC. Prophylactic and therapeutic benefits of short-term 9-[2-(phosphonomethoxy)propyl]adenine (PMPA) administration to newborn macaques following oral inoculation with simian immunodeficiency virus with reduced susceptibility to PMPA. J Virol 2000; 74: 1767–1774.

Index